VASCULAR SURGERY

Edited by **Dai Yamanouchi**

Vascular Surgery
Edited by Dai Yamanouchi

Published by InTech
Janeza Trdine 9, 51000 Rijeka, Croatia

Publishing Process Manager Bojan Rafaj

Technical Editor Teodora Smiljanic

Cover Designer InTech Design Team

Additional hard copies can be obtained from orders@intechopen.com

Vascular Surgery, Edited by Dai Yamanouchi
p. cm.
ISBN 978-953-51-0328-8

For EU product safety concerns:
IN TECH d.o.o., Prolaz Marije Krucifikse Kozulić 3, 51000 Rijeka, Croatia,
info@intechopen.com or visit our website at intechopen.com.

Meet the editor

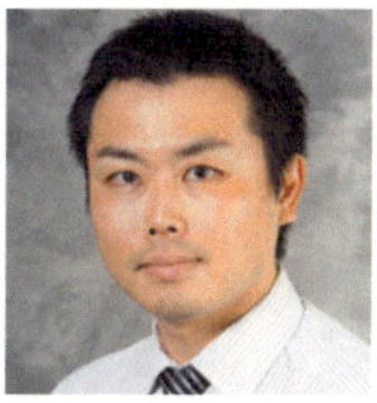

Dr. Yamanouchi is an Assistant Professor of Vascular Surgery at University of Wisconsin School of Medicine and Public health, USA. He finished vascular fellowship both in Japan and also finished advanced endovascular fellowship in the USA. He is board certified by the Japanese Board of Surgery and is a board certified Fellow of the Japanese College of Angiology. His expertise includes treatments for aortic aneurysms, carotid disease, aortic dissection, peripheral arterial disease and other vascular disorders. His research interests include the pathogenesis of abdominal aortic aneurysm and restenosis after angioplasty, including balloon angioplasty and stenting. He is also devoted to the development of novel materials for vascular bypass graft and gene delivery methods to treat patients who suffer from peripheral arterial disease.

Contents

Preface

Vascular surgery is one of the specialties of surgery focusing on the vascular system of the body, i.e. arteries and veins. The unique feature of this specialty is, unlike other surgical specialty, that vascular surgeons routinely perform not only the conventional open surgery but also the diagnostic and interventional endovascular procedures. For that reason, the field of vascular surgery has evolved rapidly since the introduction of the endovascular aneurysms repair (EVAR) as well as the numerous techniques and devices of endovascular procedures for peripheral artery disease and varicose veins.

This book aims to provide a brief overview of conventional open vascular surgery, endovascular surgery and pre- and post-operative management of vascular patients. The first section is focusing on the conventional open vascular surgery with recent consensus and evidence from the literature. The second section addresses the issues of the endovascular surgery. The third section deals with pre- and post-operative management of the vascular patient as well as miscellaneous topics of the vascular surgery.

The collections of contributions from outstanding vascular surgeons and scientists from around the world present detailed and precious information about the important topics of the current vascular surgery practice and research. This book covers a wide variety of issues and topics of the vascular surgery. I would like to acknowledge the authors around the world for their excellent contributions to this book. I also would like to express my special thanks to the managing editor of INTECH for providing me numerous supports and advices.

I hope this book will be used worldwide by young vascular surgeons and medical students enhancing their knowledge and stimulating the advancement of this field.

Dai Yamanouchi, MD, PhD
Assistant Professor of Vascular Surgery,
University of Wisconsin School of Medicine and Public Health,
USA

Part 1

Open Surgery

1

Aortoiliac Occlusive Disease

Tarek Al-Shafie and Paritosh Suman
Harlem Hospital Center,
USA

1. Introduction

Atherosclerotic occlusive (AI) disease of the abdominal aorta and iliac arteries and its clinical manifestation is a common therapeutic challenge encountered by vascular surgeons. It is one subset of peripheral arterial disease which affects 8 to 10 million people in the United States per year. (1)

The aortoiliac occlusive diseases ultimately start at the terminal aorta and the origin of the iliac arteries. The natural history of the disease is slow progression proximally and distally over time to end in complete occlusion of the aorta and iliac arteries. **Fig: 1**

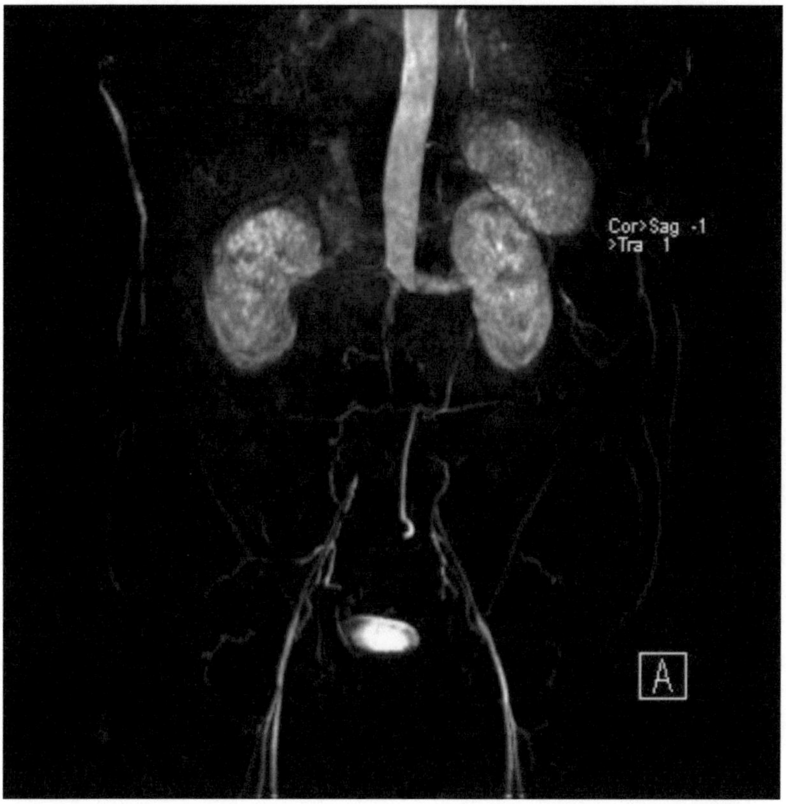

Fig. 1.

Starrett and Stony suggest that the natural history is not always benign and report that in a third of their patients the aortic occlusive disease extends to show thrombosis of the renal arteries over a period of 5 to 10 years. (2)

Others suggest that renal arteries remain open with no incidence of extension of the thrombosis proximally to involve the renal or the mesenteric vessels. (3)

Atherosclerotic occlusive disease is segmental in nature. Stenosis may be in a short or long segment, calcified, ulcerated, concentric or eccentric, single or multiple, unilateral or bilateral and may involve the aorta and iliac arteries alone or together. Approximately 30% of patients with infra inguinal atherosclerotic occlusive disease will have aortoiliac occlusive disease if their circulation is studied carefully.

The majority of patients with atherosclerotic aortoiliac occlusive disease have diffuse disease involving femoro popliteal and infrageniculate vessels. They are commonly older, more likely to be men, have diabetes and hypertension and have concomitant coronary and cerebrovascular diseases. (4)

The aortoiliac occlusive disease can involve isolated segments of the aorta and iliac vessels and usually presents in a younger population, female as male, and have a higher incidence of smoking and hypercholesterolemia as associated risk factors.

Focal infra renal aortic stenosis with no other arteries involved is fairly rare. (5)

Aortoiliac atherosclerotic occlusive disease is characterized by abundant collateralization between abdominal, pelvic and infra inguinal arteries which make the presentation with critical limb ischemia a rare event. A more common presentation is of claudication of varying severity and levels. The two exceptions to this observation are a large thrombus lodged at the narrow aorta causing acute limb ischemia and blue toe syndrome where micro emboli target the small vessels in the toes or the heel.

Being a part of atherosclerotic disease spectrum, aortoiliac occlusive disease has many common risk factors most notably smoking, dyslipidemia, hypertension, diabetes mellitus, male gender, advanced age and high genetic risk.

Isolated aortoiliac occlusive disease primarily occurs in younger patients, more commonly in females and have a higher incidence of smoking and hypercholesterolemia as associated risk factors. They usually have a normal life expectancy. (7) On the other hand, patients with aortoiliac occlusive disease and a more diffuse multilevel pattern of the disease are commonly older, more likely to be male, and more frequently have diabetes and hypertension. They have a higher incidence of concomitant coronary, cerebrovascular, and visceral atherosclerosis. These patients have a significant reduction in their life expectancy when compared with age-matched counterparts. (6) Patients with multi segment diffuse disease present with rest pain, tissue loss and gangrene as opposed to isolated claudication.(8) An aggressive form of the disease was described in a young woman who was a heavy cigarette smoker where a circumscribed calcified occlusive lesion of the middle of the aorta was found. Despite the fact that the upper abdominal aorta is usually spared in the aortoiliac occlusive disease, a minority of such patient has marked involvement of this segment of the aorta with occlusion of the origins of the visceral and renal arteries. (9)

2. Presenting symptoms

Chronic obliterative atherosclerosis of the distal aorta and iliac arteries commonly manifests as symptomatic arterial insufficiency of the lower extremities, producing a range of symptoms from mild claudication to the most severe, critical limb ischemia (CLI).

Claudication, with its characteristic association with ambulation and relief with rest, is the presenting symptom in most of the cases. Severity of claudication and involvement of muscle groups depends on the disease localization.

Intermittent claudication presents with symptoms involving muscles of the thigh, hip and buttock as well as the calf. Because calf claudication is the early manifestation for the infra-inguinal occlusive disease the involvement of more proximal muscle groups may help in identifying the aortoiliac as the diseased level of the circulatory tree. (10)

Unfortunately, sizable numbers of the patient complain of only calf claudication.

Isolated erectile dysfunction is the sole presenting symptom in some men due to significant involvement of hypo gastric arteries. At the other extreme, patients with multilevel disease will suffer from severe rest pain with tissue loss and is usually combined with femoro-popliteal occlusive disease.

Aortoiliac disease can present with classic symptoms of Leriche syndrome- namely bilateral lower extremity claudication, impotence, atrophy of muscles and absence of femoral pulses. (11) The equivalent impact of impaired pelvic perfusion in women remains poorly understood but has recently attracted investigative attention. (12)

3. Diagnosis

3.1 History and physical examination

Evaluation of aortoiliac disease commences with a good history and physical examination. The diagnosis of aortoiliac occlusive disease in patients with vascular risk factors with buttock or high thigh claudication and absent femoral pulses is usually straightforward. Claudication symptoms however must be distinguished from those of nerve root irritation due to spinal stenosis or disk herniation or arthritis. These symptoms are produced by standing as well as by walking and follow sciatic nerve distribution. (13)

The variability of presenting signs and symptoms in patients with AI disease sometimes leads to diagnostic confusion. Although proximal claudication is most common, patients with AI occlusive disease in isolation or those with combined infrainguinal disease may present exclusively with calf claudication.

Acute embolism of the distal extremities and toes could be associated with chronic aortoiliac disease. Rare patients who present with complete acute occlusion of aorta can have symptoms related to intestinal and renal ischemia.

The history will often help in determining the need of any systemic evaluation required including cardiac evaluation.

Physical examination will often reveal an absent or diminished femoral pulse. In a minority of patients, pulses could be palpable but will disappear with ambulatory efforts. An occasional bruit over the lower abdomen or groin can help in unmasking an underlying arterial lesion resulting in a turbulent blood flow. Advanced long-standing aortoiliac disease often has signs of atrophic changes such as cool, shiny, hairless skin with rubor. Patients with chronic multilevel disease can have atrophic leg muscles or in more severe cases gangrene or nonhealing ulcers. (14)

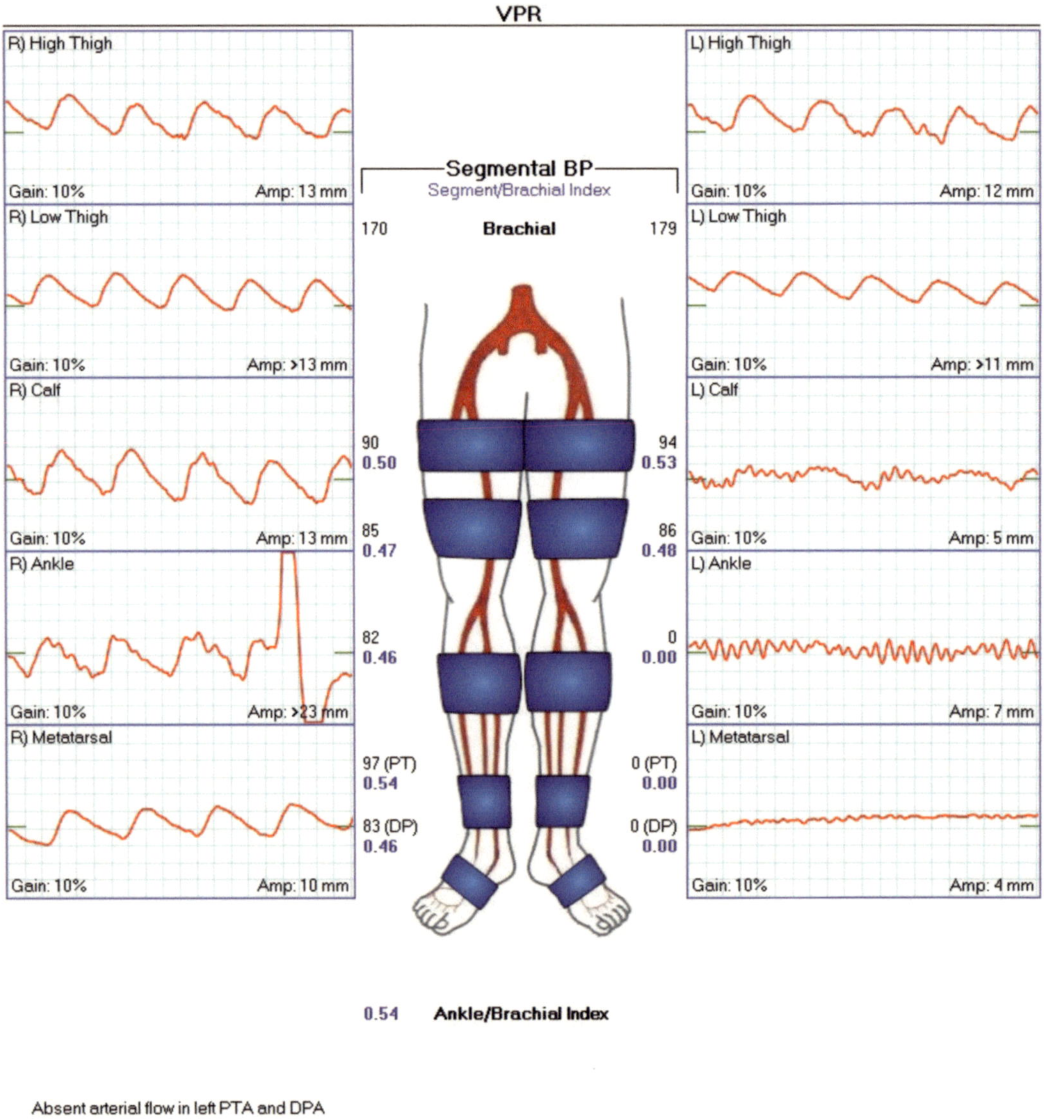

Fig. 2.

3.2 Non invasive arterial studies

Noninvasive laboratory testing serves two major purposes in evaluation of suspected aortoiliac occlusive disease: confirmation of disease when history and physical examination is equivocal; second to establish a baseline for follow up and assessing the therapeutic outcomes.

Ankle-brachial indexes (ABIs), segmental pressure measurement, and pulse volume recordings are the three most common employed modalities. **Fig. 2**

Noninvasive arterial studies show inflow problems and decrease in the thigh brachial index and decrease in the wave amplitude. A difference of at least 20 mm Hg between the brachial pressure and the proximal thigh pressure reflects a significant stenosis in the aorta or iliac arteries, but it may be confused by proximal SFA occlusion. A further reduction in pressure between the thigh and ankle level is consistent with concomitant SFA, popliteal, or tibial outflow disease. (15)

Patients with disabling claudication occasionally demonstrate normal or near normal ankle brachial indices. Repeating the tests after a period of gradual exercise show marked fall in the ankle brachial index if the patients have significant aortoiliac disease. (16)

Noninvasive evaluation is sufficient for diagnosis of aortoiliac occlusive disease in most of the patients. If patient is deemed suitable for operative intervention, further disease localization is determined with Duplex sonography and CT angiography (CTA) or MR angiography (MRA).

4. Imaging

4.1 Duplex ultrasound

By an experienced technician, duplex ultrasound is an excellent noninvasive tool to delineate arterial lesion with further color mapping and stenosis identification. **Fig 3**

Duplex ultrasound is particularly useful in patients with renal insufficiency in whom avoidance of usage of contrast agents is important. Some institutions obtained useful information for preoperative planning. (17).

Duplex assessment of the AI, renal, and visceral arteries is operator dependent, time consuming and needs a dedicated vascular laboratory and trained personnel. The presence of bowel gas, obesity and vessel tortuosity make the precise determination location and the severity of the stenosis difficult. We do not usually use arterial duplex as a sole modality in the management of aortoiliac disease. With the continuous advance in the technology, as operator skill and training improve, and as novel adjunctive duplex imaging agents evolve, this modality will likely play an increasing role in the management of patients with visceral and AI disease. At present, however, it remains inferior to other imaging techniques for preoperative planning. (18)

5. Computerized Tomographic Angiography (CTA)

With the development of the 64-slice multidetector scanner, with shorter acquisition time, high quality, non invasive and three dimensional processing capabilities CTA has become most frequently used imaging modality. The studies are obtained quickly, requiring no more than a few minutes to scan from the proximal abdominal aorta to the feet, which

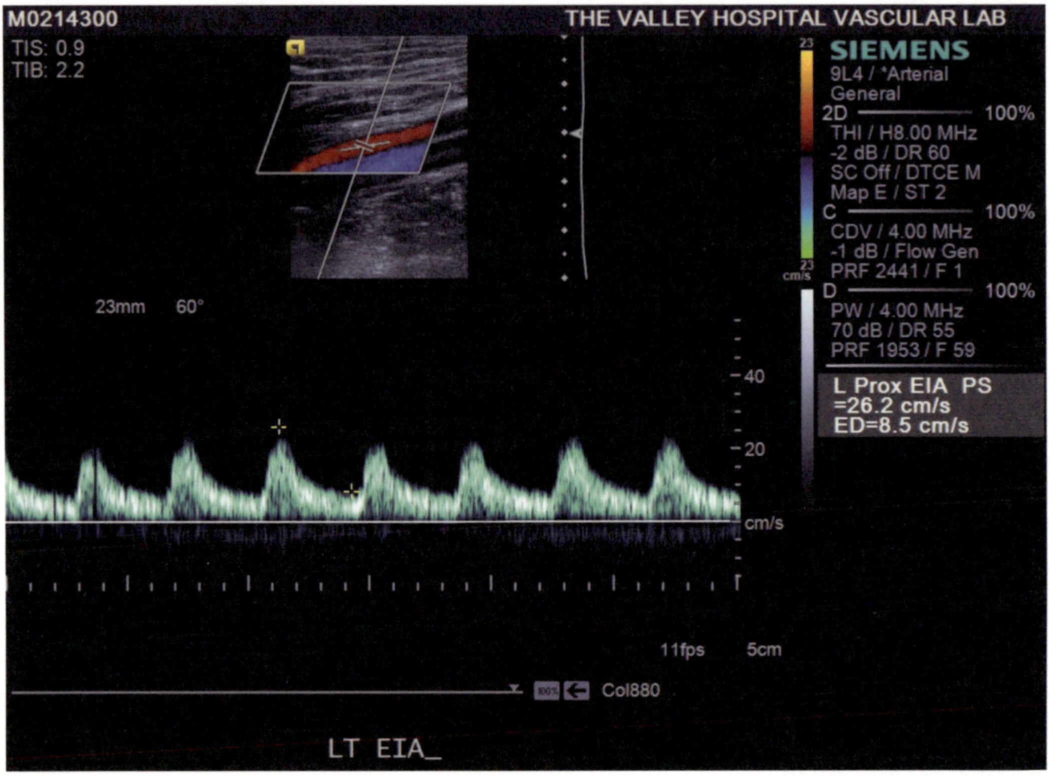

Fig. 3.

minimizes issues related to patient noncompliance. The three-dimensional reconstruction of images provides the physician not only with views of angiographic quality but also with the ability to rotate images along vertical and horizontal axes to obtain a 360-degree assessment of the vessels. A recent meta-analysis of multidetector CTA for the evaluation of the lower extremity arterial tree confirmed the value of this modality. This analysis revealed that CTA has an overall sensitivity and specificity of 96% and 97%, respectively. (19)

Despite these excellent results, there are limitations to the widespread use of CTA. There is concern because of the requirement for an intravenous bolus of iodinated contrast. This high contrast load limits the use of CTA to patients with normal renal function, unless medical necessity dictates otherwise. Also, in the presence of significant amounts of arterial wall calcium, small arteries that are occluded with calcified plaque may be misconstrued as patent. The cross-sectional images must be carefully reviewed and compared with the reconstructed three-dimensional images. Metal artifact may obscure images in patients with metal implants or surgical clips in their legs. (20)

In many centers CT angiography with three dimensional processing capabilities has supplanted contrast angiography and MRA as the initial imaging study of choice for aortoiliac occlusive disease especially for patients who are not candidates for MRA because of the presence of a pacemaker or other metallic implant not suitable for the magnetic field, and those who are unable to lie in the supine position for long periods. (21) **Fig 4**

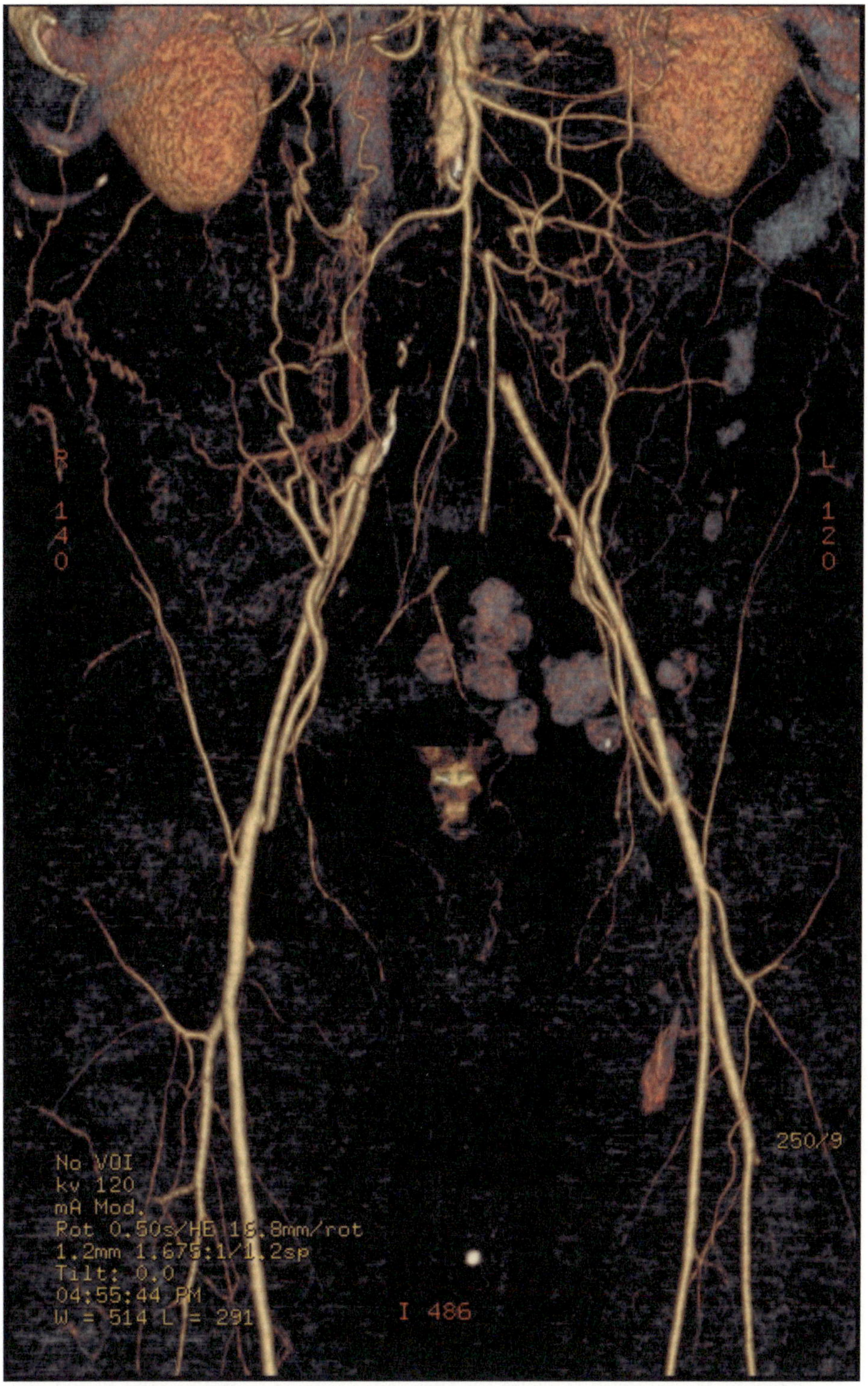
R
140
L
120
No VOI
kv 120
mA Mod.
Rot 0.50s/HE 18.8mm/rot
1.2mm 1.675:1/1.2sp
Tilt: 0.0
04:55:44 PM
W = 514 L = 291
250/9
I 486

Fig. 4.

6. Magnetic Resonance Angiography (MRA)

MRA is used for the evaluation of patients with aortoiliac occlusive disease because it can visualize the entire arterial tree, including pedal vessels, without the use of arterial puncture or standard ionic contrast agents. MRA can reveal a patent pedal vessel suitable for grafting that was not seen on conventional angiography. Exaggeration of the degree of stenosis within a vessel has been noted. Contrast-enhanced MRI had a sensitivity of 92 % and a specificity of 92%. (22)

MRA also has patient-related difficulties. Patients with newly placed metallic implants are frequently not candidates. Others may require sedation because of claustrophobia or difficulty lying flat for a long time. Additionally, although gadolinium is only mildly nephrotoxic, it may adversely affect renal function in patients with preexisting renal insufficiency. (23) More recently, there have been reports of nephrogenic systemic fibrosis related to the administration of gadolinium to patients with a glomerular filtration rate less than 30 mL/min. The incidence may be highest in those with end-stage renal failure who require hemodialysis. Although this complication is infrequent overall, in view of the large number of gadolinium-enhanced magnetic resonance angiograms performed each year, nephrogenic systemic fibrosis is associated with significant disability and mortality. (24) **Fig 1**

7. Arteriography

Digital subtraction angiography (DSA) which is the gold standard for diagnosis of all arterial occlusive diseases, especially if anatomic questions remain, has largely been replaced by computerized tomographic angiography (CTA) and MRA and increasingly been selectively performed for endovascular intervention. **Fig 5**

In many centers magnetic resonance angiography with three dimensional processing capabilities has supplanted contrast angiography as the initial imaging study of choice.

When CTA or MRA show a lesion which is amenable for percutaneous intervention arteriography is then performed for confirming the finding and for treatment. If the anatomic pattern is unfavorable to a percutaneous approach, aortoiliac reconstruction can be planned directly from the information obtained by MRA or CTA. In cases in which the decision has been made to proceed with surgical revascularization, angiography may be undertaken to obtain a final detailed roadmap of the relevant anatomy. (25) Attention should be directed to the inferior mesenteric artery; a large patent inferior mesenteric artery, particularly in the presence of superior mesenteric artery or hypogastric artery occlusive disease, may require preservation during aortic reconstruction to avoid potentially disastrous bowel ischemia. Multiple projections of the iliac and femoral bifurcations are essential to clarify the extent of disease in these regions. Full runoff views of the lower extremities are also needed to assess the presence or absence of femoropopliteal or tibial disease. (26)

Standard retrograde femoral approach is used more frequently despite long-segment near-occlusive or occlusive aortic or bi-iliac disease. Lateral and oblique views of the abdominal aorta are essential to delineate possible concomitant mesenteric or renal artery occlusive disease. Transbrachial approach is sometimes required. (27)

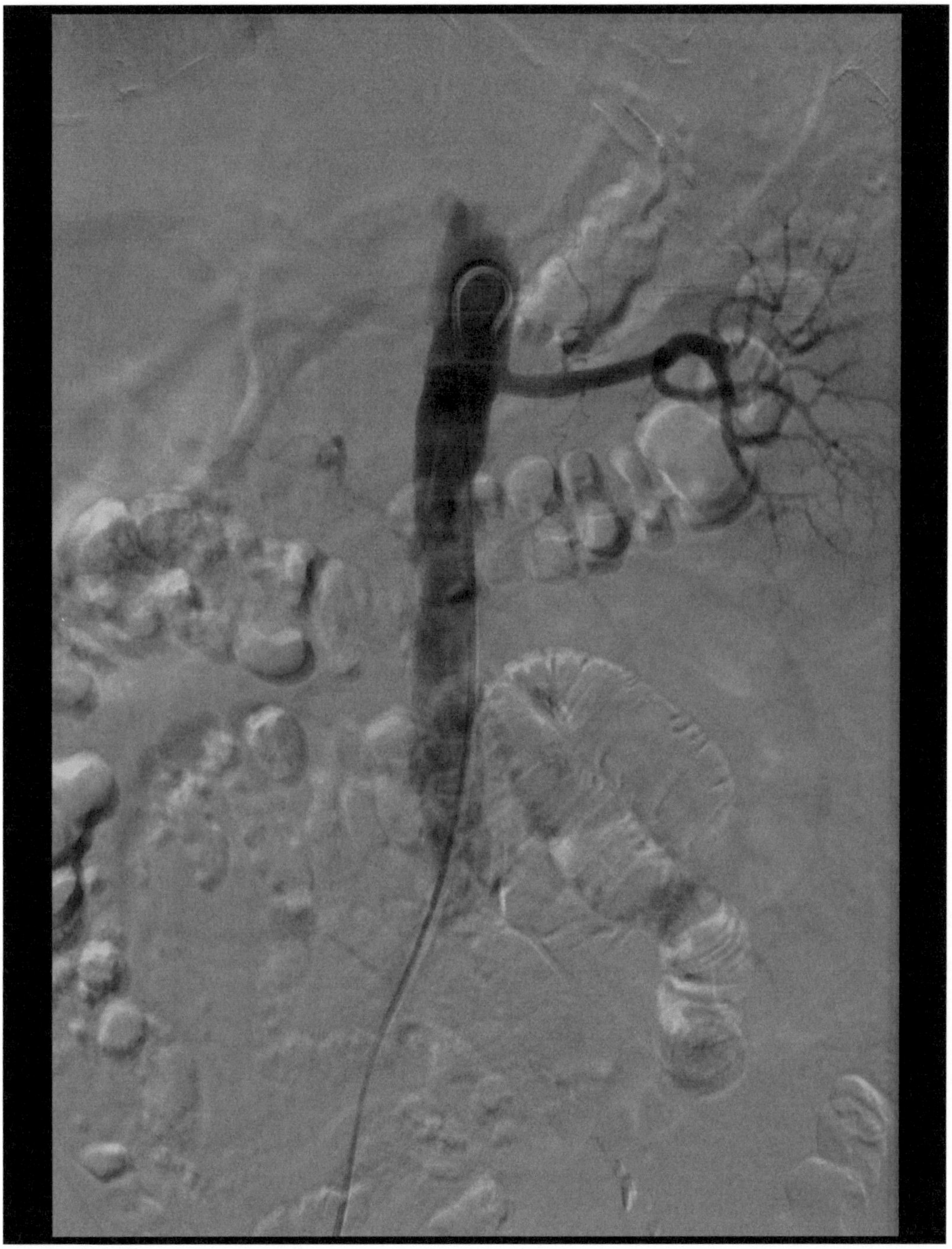

Fig. 5.

At the time of angiogram, obtaining pressure gradient across the iliac artery lesions of doubtful significance is a useful technique to demonstrate whether such lesions are interfering with the blood flow. Measurements should be obtained and if there is no significant difference, it should be repeated after induction of vasodilatation in the arteries of the lower extremities by intra-arterial injection of papaverine. Alternatively, causing reactive hyperemia by applying a tourniquet to the lower extremity. A resting systolic

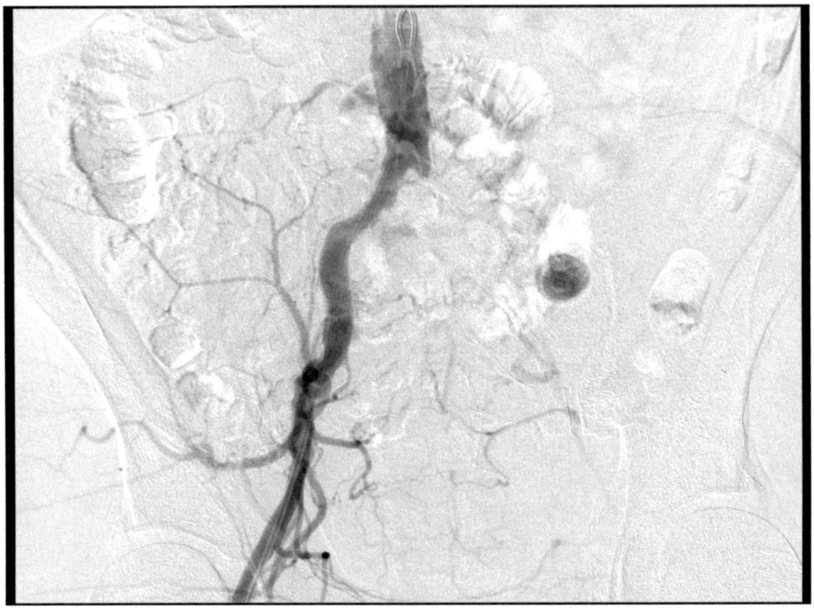

A

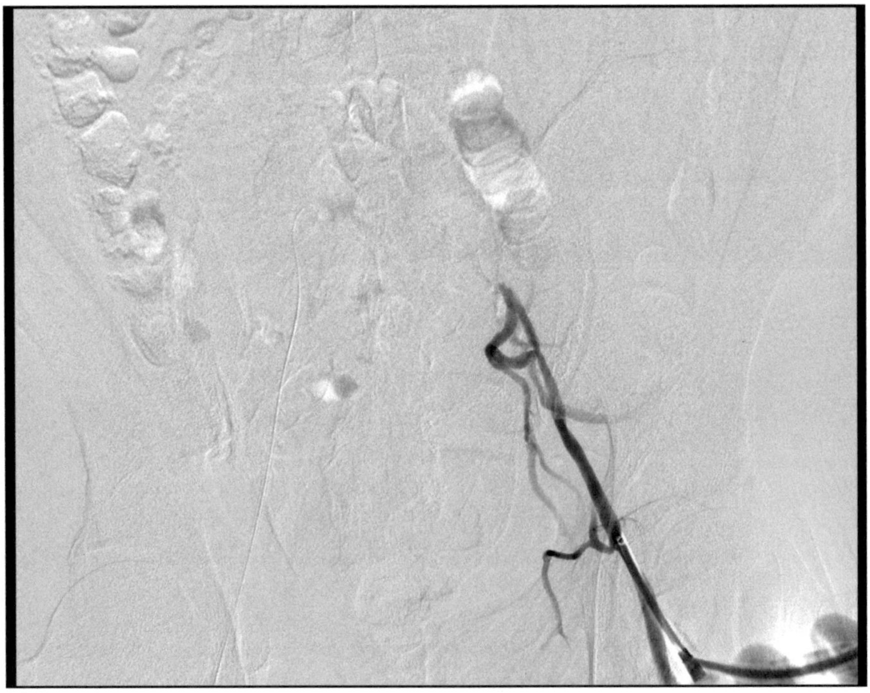

B

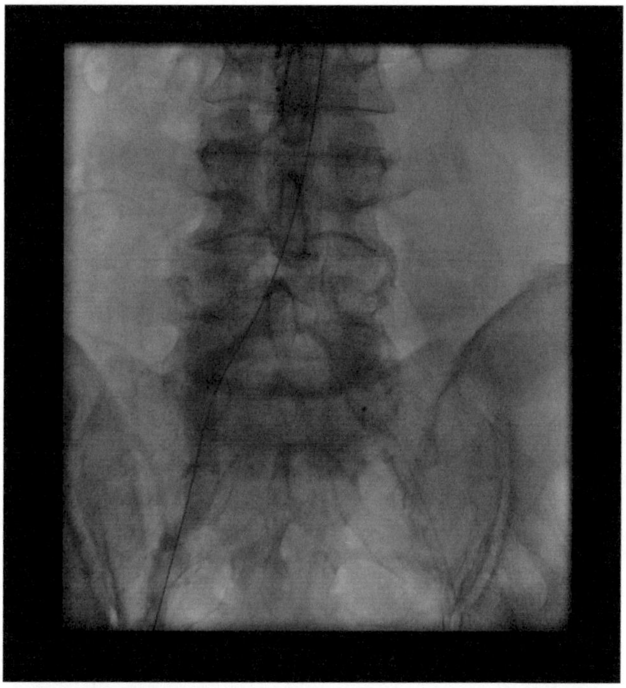

C

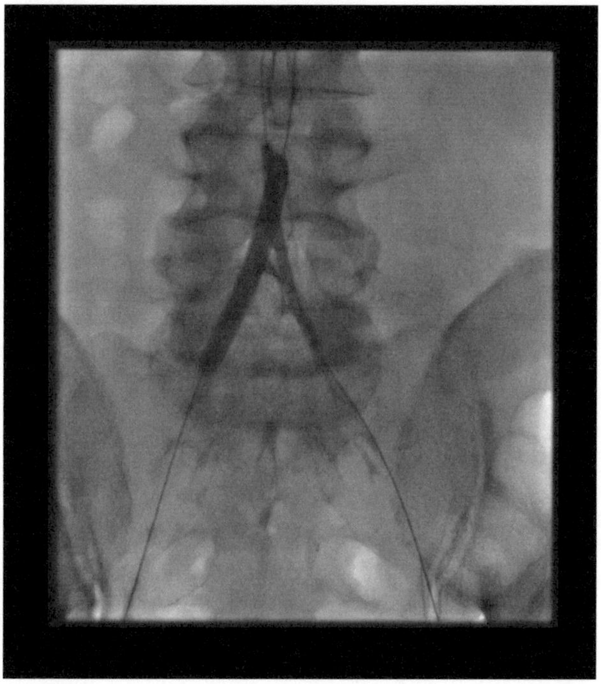

D

Fig. 6.

gradient of approximately 5 to 10 mm Hg or a change in the systolic pressure greater than 15% following pharmacologic vasodilatation is a reliable indicator of disease warranting inflow revascularization. (28) Because there is no image loss induced by arterial wall calcium, angiography is required in patients in whom the distal vasculature cannot be completely evaluated. Angiography is associated with higher morbidity and mortality risks, however, than other imaging modalities. There is an estimated 0.1% risk of a significant reaction to the contrast medium, a 0.16% risk of mortality, and a 0.7% risk of a serious complication adversely affecting planned therapy. (29) Fig 6 (A-D)

Patients with borderline renal function, especially those who are diabetic, present a special challenge. Improvements in image processing have renewed the interest in carbon dioxide angiography, a modality that can clearly delineate both large, high-flow vessels and smaller, distal vessels. The gas infusion is well tolerated and has no adverse effect on renal function, although it may be difficult to clear in patients with severe chronic obstructive pulmonary disease. (30) In patient with renal insufficiency angiography using carbon dioxide as a contrast has been used routinely in our institute.

Whatever the modality used for the diagnosis of aorto iliac occlusive disease, delineation of the infrainguinal arterial tree is essential in the pre intervention planning. **Fig 7**

Adoption of these advanced diagnostic modalities has made the diagnosis of aortoiliac disease very straightforward. Nonetheless, there will always be patients presenting with lower extremity pain when other causes are responsible for the symptoms. Most often neurogenic claudication, arthritis of hip joints and peripheral nerve disease are the culprits. Again a good history and physical examination supplemented with noninvasive evaluations should be sufficient to distinguish these diagnoses. Determination of the contribution of these associated causes in symptomatology prior to any therapeutic intervention will help in avoiding disappointment with the outcome.

8. Treatment of aortoiliac occlusive disease

Management of aortoiliac occlusive disease present a unique challenge due to the complex interplay of factors that must be considered, including the underlying pathology, anatomic defect, presence of distal disease, degree of ischemia, co-morbid conditions, functional status, ambulation potential, and suitability of anatomy for successful revascularization.

In general patients with lower extremity ischemia are typically divided into two groups in regard to their presentation, those with intermittent claudication and those with critical limb ischemia (CLI). (31)

There is an agreement on the treatment of the CLI because the natural history of untreated CLI more frequently leads to limb loss. Patients with CLI often have severe associated cardiovascular co-morbidities and are generally older and in poorer health than those with claudication. In contrast, patients with claudication typically seek treatment for the relief of lifestyle-limiting pain with ambulation. These patients exhibit a more benign natural history with respect to limb viability, with amputation rates of 1% to 7% at 5 years and clinical deterioration of the limb in only 25%.(32)

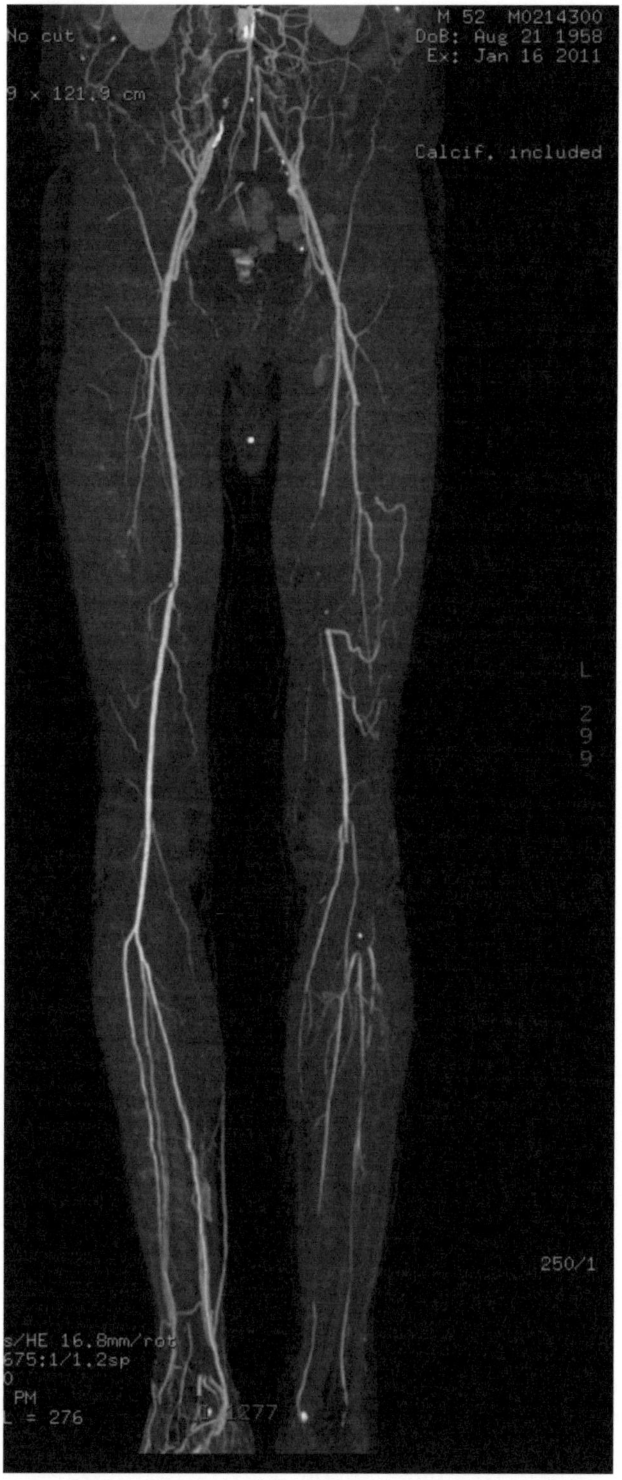
M 52 M0214300
DoB: Aug 21 1958
Ex: Jan 16 2011
Calcif. included
L
2
9
9
250/1
s/HE 16.8mm/rot
675:1/1.2sp
PM
L = 276

Fig. 7.

9. Medical therapy

In patient with CLI, claudication is a marker of significant systemic atherosclerosis, with associated cardiovascular mortality rates at 1, 5, and 10 years as high as 12%, 42%, and 65%, respectively. All patients with PAD require medical management and often benefit from interventional or surgical treatment, as discussed later.(30)

Medical therapy plays an essential part in the management regimen of aortoiliac occlusive disease. It is instituted in all patients with the aims of symptom improvement, prevention of limb loss and reduction of the risk of cardiovascular complications. Risk factor modification is an integral part of medical therapy. Smoking cessation and an optimal control of diabetes mellitus, hypertension and hyperlipidemia has been shown to reduce the proliferation of the atherosclerotic disease process. (32) The primary care physician in collaboration with the vascular surgeon should follow the risk-factor modification guidelines.

Parameter	Target Goal	Therapy
Blood pressure	Systolic <130 to 140 mm Hg Diastolic <80 to 90 mm Hg	β-Blockers, ACE inhibitors
Diabetes mellitus	Hemoglobin A1c <7%	Insulin, ↑ insulin sensitivity
LDL cholesterol	<100 mg/dL	Diet, statins
HDL cholesterol	Men, ≥35 mg/dL Women, ≥45 mg/dL	Diet, fibric acid derivative
Tobacco cessation	Complete abstinence	Nicotine replacement, antidepressants, behavioral therapy
Exercise therapy	All patients	Supervised program three or more times a week
Antiplatelet therapy	All patients	Aspirin (81 or 325 mg/day), clopidogrel (75 mg/day)
Pharmacologic therapy	Trial in all patients with claudication in the absence of heart failure	Cilostazol

Hirsch AT, Haskal ZJ, Hertzer NR, et al: ACC/AHA guidelines for the management of patients with peripheral arterial disease: summary of recommendations,J Vasc Interv Radiol 17(9):1383–1397, 2006.
ACE, Angiotensin-converting enzyme; *LDL,* low-density lipoprotein; *HDL,* high-density lipoprotein.

Table 1. American College of Cardiology/American Heart Association guidelines for the management of patients with peripheral arterial disease

Smoking cessation has been shown to reduce the risk of MI and death in patients with PAD and to delay the progression of lower extremity symptoms from claudication to CLI and limb loss.(34) The importance of smoking cessation extends to patients who have undergone lower extremity revascularization because there is a threefold increased risk of graft failure in smokers compared with nonsmokers. (35)

In association with the risk-factor modification, daily exercise regimen can also significantly alleviate the symptoms and help in regaining some functional capacity. An increased tolerance to demand ischemia has been postulated as a probable mechanism for such observed improvement.

Institution of antiplatelet therapy is often prudent in aortoiliac occlusive disease. Although antiplatelet agents have not been shown to directly improve the outcome of aortoiliac occlusive or peripheral arterial disease, aspirin or clopidigrel do achieve a significant improvement in the treatment of atherosclerotic disease of coronary and cerebral arterial systems. Cilostazol (100 mg two times a day) is effective in increasing overall ambulation distance. This medication is limited to patients with peripheral arterial disease with intermittent claudication and no history of congestive heart failure.

Other pharmacological agents like pentoxifylline can also be used but none of these agents have been shown to gain a significant practical improvement in symptoms.(33)

In claudication there is a convincing data suggesting that the efficacy of medical treatment is comparable to interventional therapy like Edinburgh walking study.

In Critical limb ischemia medical treatment plays a secondary role and revascularization is the essential component for limb salvage.

10. Surgical and endovascular treatment

The indications for surgery and intervention in symptomatic aortoiliac disease are disabling claudication and ischemia at rest manifested by rest pain in the foot, ischemic ulceration or pre gangrenous skin changes. (1)

10.1 Open vs. endovascular

Traditionally aortoiliac occlusive lesions were operated by an open approach. Aortobifemoral bypass is the method of choice. Increasingly endovascular techniques are being adopted for less severe occlusion when there is no extensive involvement of aorta or common iliac arteries. Also for patients with severe comorbidities endovascular methods could be an alternative.

A significant change has occurred in the treatment of atherosclerotic arterial disease. Angioplasty and stenting have become first-line therapy for most patients with aortoiliac occlusive disease. An 850% increase in the use of percutaneous transluminal angioplasty and stenting for AI occlusive disease from 1996 to 2000, along with a simultaneous decrease of 16% in the rate of aortobifemoral grafting. (36)

The Trans-Atlantic Inter-Society Consensus for the Management of Peripheral Arterial Disease (TASC) published a document authored by a working group of representatives from 14 surgical vascular, cardiovascular, and radiologic societies and upgraded document (TASC II) was published in January 2007. These important works interpreted evidence-based data concerning the treatment of lower extremity PAD and offered a series of treatment recommendations based on presentation. (1) **Fig 8**

Whereas percutaneous treatment of the aorta and iliac arteries was previously limited to short-segment, Trans-Atlantic Inter-Society Consensus (TASC) type A or B iliac lesions, wire-based technology has now been successfully applied to even long-segment (TASC type D) occlusions extending for the length of the iliac arteries. (36).

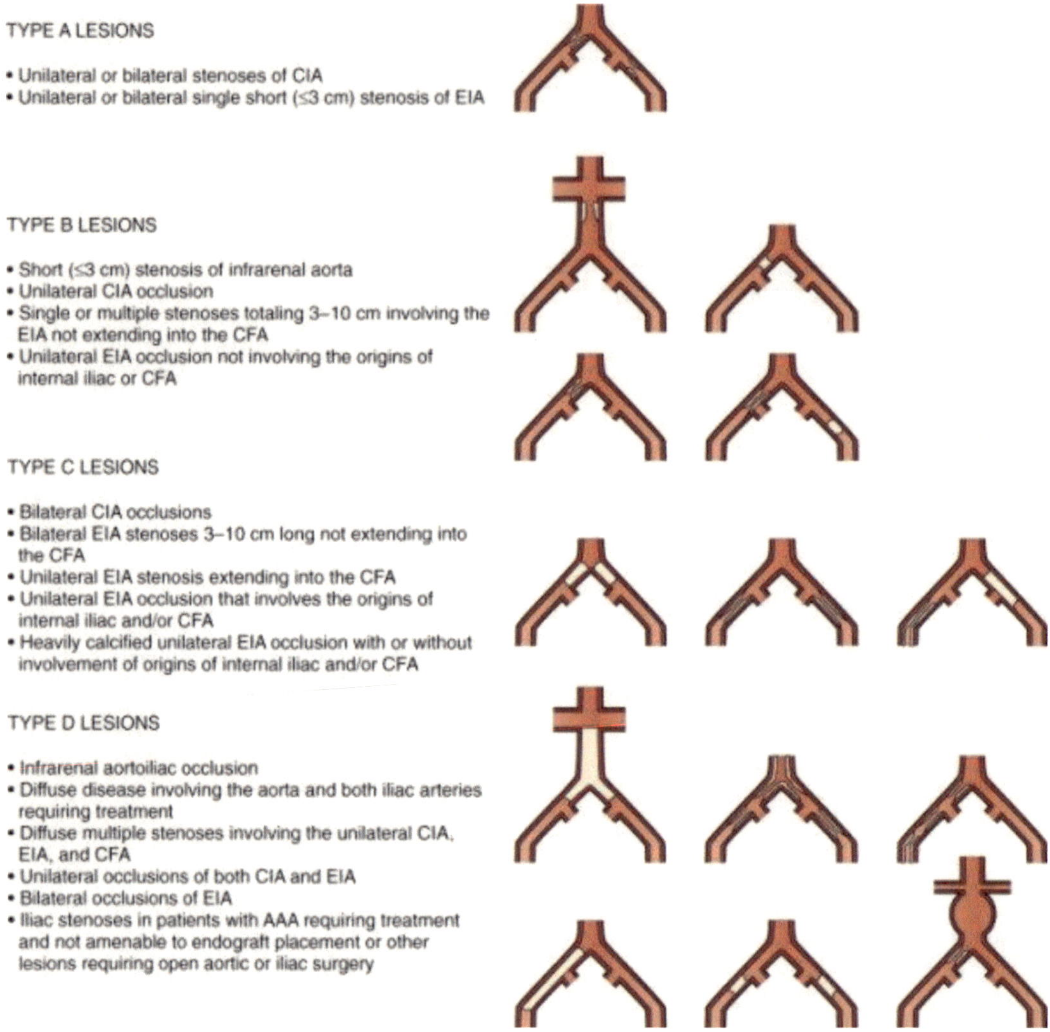

Fig. 8. TASC classification of aortoiliac lesions. AAA, abdominal aortic aneurysm; CFA, common femoral artery; CIA, common iliac artery; EIA, external iliac artery.

Surgical risk assessment is routinely performed preoperatively as coronary artery disease and other comorbidities have frequently been shown to be associated with aortoiliac occlusive disease.

11. Open procedures

Open surgery for aortoiliac disease become a second- or even third-line therapy and is increasingly undertaken in patients in whom endovascular treatment has been technically unsuccessful or in those with such extensive disease that an endovascular approach is deemed inadvisable. Patients with a combination of more proximal aneurysmal disease and common or external iliac occlusive disease continue to be good candidates for open reconstruction. (37) Patients with disease extending to the CFA are can potentially be managed with a hybrid approach, whereby the CFA plaque is treated with a traditional endarterectomy and patch repair and the iliac component is concurrently addressed with endovascular techniques. (38) Patients with significant renal failure in whom endovascular therapy entails a prohibitive risk of triggering dialysis dependence are also considered better suited for operative repair.

Preoperative evaluation of the patients with aortoiliac occlusive disease and assessment of the factors that can increase the intra operative and postoperative complication are essential. About 50% of patients with aortoiliac occlusive disease have evidence of coronary artery disease. Despite the fact that myocardial infarction remains the leading perioperative complication, the reduced perioperative mortality and morbidity after aorto iliac surgery are due to advance in the treatment of concomitant coronary artery diseases. The routine use of perioperative beta blockade is probably the most important practice. The cardioprotective value of continuing aspirin through the time of AI reconstruction has now been clearly documented. Patient with mild or stable coronary artery disease with no recent angina or myocardial infarction can go for surgery without great risk. Patient with unstable angina or recent MI will need more investigation and coronary revascularization first. (39)

Patients with renal insufficiency should be given time for their kidneys to recover from the effect of the contrast and also be hydrated. Pulmonary function should be optimized in patients with restrictive pulmonary disease with bronchodilators and smoking cessation before going for aortoiliac surgery.

Preoperative fluid status optimization, adequate intravenous access, intra-arterial pressure monitoring, Foley catheter placement, and preoperative antibiotics to minimize the risk of prosthetic and wound infection are routine aspects of aortic replacement surgery. (40) Attention should be paid to maintaining normothermia throughout the procedure to reduce the significant organ dysfunction and operative mortality associated with intraoperative hypothermia. An epidural catheter is usually placed for postoperative pain control. (41)

11.1 Aortofemoral bypass graft

As mentioned earlier, aortofemoral bypass graft isthe most preferred surgical method whenever feasible.

In the standard operative technique the femoral vessels are typically exposed first to reduce the time during which the abdomen is open and the viscera exposed. The extent of exposure is dictated by the severity of disease and the level of reconstruction planned at the CFA and its bifurcation. A crossing vein normally present beneath the inguinal ligament must be ligated or carefully avoided to prevent bleeding during the tunneling process.

Infrarenal aortic exposure is often performed through a transperitoneal approach via a longitudinal midline laparotomy; some surgeons prefer a transverse incision. The abdomen is explored for any other pathology. The transverse colon is retracted cephalad, and the small bowel is shifted to the patient's right side. The duodenum is mobilized to the right, allowing access to the infrarenal aorta. The retroperitoneal tissue overlying the aorta is dissected superiorly to the level of the left renal vein, and the larger lymphatic vessels encountered within the retroperitoneal lymphatic network are ligated. Careful dissection should be used below the left renal artery to avoid injury to the lumber vein draining to the left renal and to gonadal vein. Extensive dissection anterior to the aortic bifurcation and proximal left iliac artery should be avoided because the autonomic nerve plexus regulating erection and ejaculation in men sweeps over the aorta in this region.

It is important to extend the reconstruction close to the level of the renal arteries to minimize the risk of failure secondary to disease progression. If end-to-side repair is planned, exposing and controlling all relevant lumbar or accessory renal arteries before performing the aortotomy helps avoid backbleeding.

Creation of the tunnel for the graft is done by finger dissection on the anterior surface of the iliac arteries. On the left side, the tunnel passes beneath the sigmoid mesentery and slightly more laterally in an effort to avoid disruption of the autonomic nerve plexus. Moist umbilical tapes or Penrose drains are passed with a smooth aortic clamp to mark the tunnels. With vessel exposure and tunnel creation complete, but before vascular occlusion, heparin for anticoagulation is given as an intravenous bolus and repeated doses may be necessary, depending on the length of the clamp placement.

The aorta is clamped first proximally at the site of least disease to avoid dislodgement and potential distal embolization of plaque. If an end-to-end anastomosis is planned, the aorta is transected below the proximal clamp, and the distal aorta is oversewn in two layers with running monofilament suture.

Although some surgeons prefer polytetrafluoroethylene (PTFE) grafts, knitted polyester (Dacron) grafts are more commonly used.

There is still considerable debate involves the type of proximal anastomosis, both end-to-end and end-to-side techniques are acceptable and effective and each may be preferred in certain circumstances.

Surgeons favoring an end-to-end anastomosis claim that it has less turbulence, lower rates of proximal suture line pseudoaneurysm and better long-term patency rates reported in some series. (42) The graft lies flatter in the retroperitoneum, this enhances the ability to close the retroperitoneum over the graft, resulting in a lower rate of late graft infection and aortoenteric fistulae.

There are certain circumstances when an end-to-side proximal anastomosis is advantageous. The most common indication is in patients with occluded or severely diseased external iliac arteries but patent common and internal iliac arteries. Without the retrograde flow through the external iliac arteries normally present in an end-to-end configuration, pelvic ischemia, ranging from mild hip claudication to severe buttock rest pain or ulceration, may result. (43) Additional ischemic complications, such as erectile dysfunction in males and rarely seen paraplegia. (44)

Large inferior mesenteric artery with little back flow and important accessory renal artery can be re-implanted to the graft.

The graft limbs are then passed through the retroperitoneal tunnels, taking care to prevent twisting and to eliminate excess redundancy. Care is taken to match graft size to femoral artery diameter. Arteriotomy limited to the distal CFA sometimes is sufficient. More commonly, extension of the arteriotomy across the profunda femoris artery origin and profundaplasty will prove necessary. The distal anastomoses are completed in an end-to-side fashion using flushing maneuvers before completing the anastomoses. It is very important to alert the anesthetic team before releaseing the clamp, to be prepared to avoid blood pressure drop with reperfusion.

Once hemostasis is sufficient, the abdomen is irrigated and the retroperitoneum is closed. If adequate retroperitoneal coverage is not possible, particularly with an end-to-side proximal anastomosis, a sleeve of omentum should be fashioned to cover any exposed segment of the anastomosis and to separate the graft from the adjacent bowel. The groin wounds are copiously irrigated with antibiotic solution, and the deeper tissue is closed in several layers using absorbable Vicryl sutures.

Confirm adequate distal perfusion and ensure that no distal embolization has occurred.

Although aortobifemoral bypass is easier and has better long term patency compared to aortobiiliac bypass, in certain circumstances performing an aortobiiliac bypass remains advantageous. In patients with hostile groin creases from prior surgery or radiation therapy, or are obese, diabetic patients with an intertriginous rash at the inguinal crease and patent external iliac arteries, the impact of synchronous SFA disease on the results of AI revascularization remains undefined. Although up to 80% of patients with claudication and both inflow and outflow disease manifest symptomatic improvement following aortofemoral bypass grafting alone. (45) If significant tissue loss is present, concurrent inflow and outflow procedures are likely warranted if limb salvage is to be achieved. (46)

The graft patency rates continues to improve and the accumulated experience to date has shown that 5-year primary patency rates between 85% and 90% and 10-year rates between 75% and 85% can be expected with aortobifemoral grafting

Similarly the perioperative mortality rate continues to decline and less than 2% mortality is a standard now. (47, 48) Age has proved to be a significant predictor of outcome; in one report, primary patency rates at 5 years were greater than 95% for patients older than 60 years but only 66% for those younger than 50 years. (49)

11.2 Complications

Reported overall morbidity rates range from 17% to 32% following aortic surgery for occlusive disease include cardiac complications which are the most common cause of mortality and result from the hemodynamic stress associated with major vascular surgery and the obligatory fluid shifts during the early postoperative period. Pulmonary complications are most likely to occur in the elderly or those with chronic obstructive pulmonary disease. Acute renal failure following aortic reconstruction for occlusive disease is relatively uncommon in patients with normal preoperative renal function.

Adequate hydration and avoiding repetitive aortic cross-clamping and perioperative hypotension are valuable prophylactic maneuvers; the adjunctive use of mannitol and furosemide (Lasix) prior to aortic cross-clamping is less documented despite its wide use. Intraoperative injury to the ureters during dissection, graft tunneling, intraoperative injury to the small and large bowel can usually be avoided with careful surgical technique. For patients undergoing aortobifemoral grafting, postoperative hemorrhage is a relatively rare event, occurring in 1% to 2% of cases. (37, 47)

Careful postoperative monitoring of the abdominal girth, hematocrit, bladder pressure, coagulation parameters, and hemodynamic status is paramount to identify ongoing bleeding significant enough to require urgent reoperation.

Intestinal ischemia following aortic reconstruction has been reported in 2% of cases.

If compromised bowel perfusion is recognized intraoperatively inferior mesenteric artery re-implantation is indicated. Maintaining a high index of suspicion and having a low threshold for performing sigmoidoscopy during the early postoperative period are critical (50)

Spinal cord ischemia is a devastating complication of aortic surgery and the main component of prophylaxis is careful preservation of hypogastric perfusion. Fortunately, this complication is uncommon, occurring in only 0.3% of AI reconstructions for occlusive disease in one series. (51)

Late complications following aortobifemoral grafting include graft limb thrombosis, graft infection, aortoenteric fistula, and anastomotic pseudoaneurysm

Graft thrombosis is the most frequently encountered late complication. It occurs in as many as 30% of cases in some series in which the grafts were observed for 10 years or longer. (52) Inflow can frequently be restored with aggressive efforts using special thrombectomy catheters. If successfully restored, revising the distal anastomotic site with a profundaplasty or extension of the graft may prove necessary. If restoring the flow through the graft is unsuccessful a femorofemoral or axillofemoral graft usually suffices as a secondary source of inflow.

Prosthetic graft infection is a particularly feared complication of aortic reconstruction, given its high associated morbidity and mortality. Diagnosis can be established with CT if there is clinical suspicion. Once infection is diagnosed, graft excision is usually indicated and inflow established with extra anatomical bypass. (53)

Aortoenteric fistula is another rare but potentially devastating late complication associated with aortobifemoral. The most common pathophysiologic process is erosion of the proximal aortic suture line through the third or fourth portion of the duodenum, although fistulae between the iliac anastomoses into the small bowel or colon are also well described. Commonly presented with a small, self-limited bleed then become large or massive bleeding. Treatment is usually similar to that for graft infection; extra-anatomic bypass and graft removal are usually required, covering the aortic stump with adequate tissue coverage and repair of the involved gastrointestinal tract. (54)

Pseudoaneurysm of the anastomotic line are far less but they continue to be seen as a late complication in 1% to 5% of patient after aortobifemoral bypass. They arise secondary to a weakening in the suture line as a result of structural fatigue or fabric degeneration. Undue tension, poor suturing technique, and focal weakening of the recipient arterial wall have been implicated as causative factors. Infection undoubtedly plays a role in many cases, despite the frequent absence of any obvious clinical signs; Staphylococcus species are the predominant organisms identified in culture. Femoral anastomotic false aneurysms are most common and typically present as a slowly enlarging, asymptomatic groin bulge. Given the potential complications of thrombosis, embolization, or rupture, repair is generally recommended for femoral false aneurysms larger than 2 cm or aortic false aneurysms greater than 50% of the graft diameter. Proximal anastomotic false aneurysms are often discovered incidentally or noted when they rupture. Treatment usually consists of débridement of the degenerated tissue and placement of a short interposition graft. (55)

11.3 Aortoiliac endarterectomy

During the 1950s and 1960s, endarterectomy was the standard therapy for severe AI occlusive disease. Enthusiasm for the procedure dimmed, however, with the introduction of prosthetic graft. An obvious benefit of endarterectomy is the elimination of the need for a prosthetic graft, making it an appealing alternative in the setting of infection. Advocates have likewise pointed to the advantages of endarterectomy for younger patients or those with small vessels who are less than ideal candidates for endovascular therapy or aortobifemoral grafting.

In patients with localized aortoiliac disease, aortoiliac endarterectomy may be suitable options and have excellent long-term patency rates, compare with aortic bypass grafting, have been reported. (56) In contrast, results in cases of long-segment disease involving the entire infrarenal aorta and extending into the external iliac arteries have been disappointing. (57) In our practice, aortiliac endarterectomy is rarely done. The increasing popularity of endovascular therapy is further decrease the small proportion of patients considered suitable for this reconstructive approach.

11.4 Crossover bypass

A few patients with only one iliac artery involvement with good aortic and contralateral iliac artery can be offered the choice of supra pubic ilioiliac and femorofemoral bypass graft. Hemodynamic studies confirm that one iliac artery can support both legs, at least at rest, in the absence of flow-limiting lesions in the planned donor iliac arterial system. (58, 59) Even a diseased donor iliac arterial system may be improved with endovascular techniques to allow a less invasive yet effective femorofemoral bypass when a more invasive procedure would otherwise be required. The majority of the studies published have found that iliofemoral bypass yields somewhat better patency than femorofemoral bypass, assuming the presence of an appropriate common iliac artery for inflow to the graft. (60-62) Ipsilateral iliofemoral bypass is a good procedure when anatomically feasible. Kretschmer and colleagues found no difference between femorofemoral bypass and unilateral iliofemoral bypass with respect to patency. (63) Van der Vliet and associates, in a truly remarkable study, compared the results of 184 unilateral iliac reconstructions (62% based on iliac artery inflow) to 350 contemporaneous patients undergoing aorta-to-bilateral iliac or femoral reconstruction over a 10-year period and found no difference in patency between the groups, implying that iliofemoral bypass yields results comparable to the "benchmark" aortofemoral bypass. (64) The abdomen is prepped along with the groins and anterior thighs to allow access to the abdomen in case of unexpected findings during surgery. Longitudinal incisions and less frequent oblique incisions are generally used to expose and control the femoral arteries on both sides. The graft is tunneled from one groin incision to the other within the abdominal wall superior to the pubis. The tunnel is created bluntly with fingers, a large clamp, or a tubular tunneler. The graft tunneled in the prefascial subcutaneous plane or in the preperitoneal position if unfavorable conditions exist in the abdominal wall, such as prior surgery, radiation-damaged skin or other skin changes, an unusually thin subcutaneous fat layer, or obesity. (65) If the inflow provided in by a contralateral iliac artery, these iliac origin crossover grafts are usually most conveniently placed in the preperitoneal position. (66) Anastomoses are end-to-side anastomoses in nearly all cases. Kinking of the graft should be avoid by taking the graft lower on the common femoral to the origin of the profunda parallel to the artery. A prosthetic graft is now used in nearly all cases.

Exposure for the iliac site of the anastomosis usually done through suprainguinal curved incision which is simple also in the obese patient avoid the groin and the graft is more deepley placed and more cushioned than in the femoro femoral bypass.

It is not surprising that endovascular procedures to improve suboptimal donor iliac arteries might be considered prior to or concomitant with femorofemoral bypass. the results of these studies generally support the view that donor iliac artery balloon angioplasty with stenting in selected cases is associated with a satisfactory hemodynamic outcome and patency rate. (67)

The perioperative mortality associated with femorofemoral bypass is highly dependent on patient selection but should be well under 5% in elective operations. Estimated 3-year survival rates of 71% for patients undergoing femorofemoral bypass, versus 35% for those having axillofemoral bypass. (67, 68) The primary and secondary patency rates for femorofemoral bypass at 3 to 5 years should be about 60% and 70%, respectively. (67, 69) There is a trend toward better patency in claudicants, consistent with observations in virtually every other arterial intervention. (70)

11.5 Axillofemoral bypass

In high risk patient with a combination of aortic and proximal iliac occlusive disease, those with other co-morbidities such as multiple prior abdominal operations, abdominal stomas, or prior radiation therapy, axillofemoral bypass is a valuable alternative for distal revascularization. Axillofemoral bypass is an essential tool for the treatment of many patients with infected aortic or prosthetic arterial grafts or aortoenteric fistulae (53,54)

Axillofemoral bypass is nearly always performed with general anesthesia. Supine position. Either axillary artery can be chosen as a donor unless there is disease in the subclavian or axillary artery. The axillary artery on the side with the higher blood pressure is chosen if there is a 10 mm Hg or greater systolic pressure discrepancy between the arms. (71) A transverse infraclavicular incision is carried through the clavipectoral fascia, exposing the pectoralis major muscle. The pectoralis major muscle fibers are pushed superiorly and inferiorly, exposing the deep fascia and, beneath that, the fat containing the axillary vein, artery, and brachial plexus elements. The axillary artery is exposed from the clavicle medially to the pectoralis minor muscle laterally, often requiring the ligation of crossing veins or small arterial branches. Conventional longitudinal or oblique groin incisions are used for femoral artery exposure. It is very important to place the axillary graft anastomosis as medially as possible to avoid tension on the axillary anastomosis when the arm is abducted. (72) The axillofemoral graft must be tunneled in the midaxillary line to prevent kinking of the graft. The anastomosis of the proximal end of the graft to the side of the axillary artery is generally performed first. The distal anastomosis is conventionally performed end to side to an appropriate artery in the groin. It is important to ensure adequate outflow. (72) It is very important to confirm distal flow using continuous-wave Doppler after the anastomoses are completed and all clamps are removed. It is also essential to ensure adequate blood flow in the donor arm beyond the axillary anastomosis. Patency rates with axillofemoral bypass varies widely between 30% to as high as 85%. (73) The reasons for this variability is due to in part to patient selection, indication and status of the outflow arteries. Patient with claudication do better than limb salvage patients because of the inherent outflow restriction in the latter group. Patients with a previous distal bypass have better results. 25% of declotted grafts go on to long term patency. (74) Due to co morbidities estimated survival of only 43% at 28 months after axillofemoral bypass. (75) Devolfe and coworkers observed an approximately 35% 3-year survival. (76) Patients whose initial presentation was CLI 3-year limb salvage estimates ranging from 69% to slightly more than 80%. (77)

11.6 Axillopopliteal bypass

Occasionally axillofemoral bypass has been extended to the popliteal artery, primarily for cases in which there is groin sepsis and the superficial femoral artery is an unacceptable distal target vessel. Patency was inferior to that expected with more conventional reconstructions. Nevertheless, this technique is occasionally the only reasonable approach to patients with groin sepsis. (78)

11.7 Obturator bypass

Obturator bypass used to avoid frankly contaminated fields during reconstruction after the removal of infected grafts in the groin, but obturator bypass can also be used for reconstruction in patients after the removal of infected ePTFE dialysis access grafts based on the femoral arteries; in patients with infected femoral pseudoaneurysms after diagnostic or therapeutic femoral arterial access or recreational drug use; in those with groin neoplasms requiring en bloc removal of tumor and artery, with a residual soft tissue defect that would expose an in situ reconstruction and in patients who have undergone therapeutic radiation in the groin. (79, 80)

11.8 Thoraco-femoral and supraceliac to iliofemoral bypass

These procedures have most often been applied to patients with failure or infection of previous infrarenal aortic reconstructions, previous abdominal surgery for other than aortic pathology, prior radiation treatment, or other reasons that would make a conventional transperitoneal or retroperitoneal approach to infrarenal aortic surgery difficult or impossible and who are not candidates for endovascular intervention. Passman and colleagues reported a 5-year primary patency rate of 79% in 50 patients. (81)

11.9 Laparoscopic aortic surgery

Laproscopic general surgery shows tremendous advance s, new applications in different fields. However, its role in vascular surgery has yet to be defined. Several authors report aorto iliac surgical reconstruction performed laparoscopic ally or hand assisted. (82) As the technology evolves and intracorporeal anastomotic techniques are refined the rule of aortofemoral bypass will expand and become clear.

11.10 Endovascular treatment

The advent of endovascular surgery has resulted in a dramatic shift in the treatment of patients with aortoiliac occlusive disease. It is likely that even patients with more advanced aortoiliac occlusive disease will be candidates for endovascular therapy by means of stent-grafts and hybrid open-endovascular approaches. The indication for therapy is similar to the indication of open surgery. Patients with disabling claudication constitute the largest group of patients who undergo aortoiliac endovascular revascularization. Patients with critical limb ischemia (CLI) manifesting as either rest pain or tissue loss frequently have multilevel occlusive disease. In patients with a significant CFA disease burden, combined femoral artery endarterectomy and patch angioplasty with simultaneous aortoiliac stenting or stent-grafting often provides adequate perfusion to treat CLI. Juxta renal aortic occlusion, circumferential heavy calcification, hypo plastic aortic syndrome, and adjacent aneurysmal disease. Renal insufficiency is also a relative contraindication owing to potential contrast-induced nephropathy, although preventive regimens and minimal contrast techniques have reduced the impact of this complication. (1, 83)

Endovascular therapy is the recommended first-line therapy for TASC A and B lesions and increasingly for TASC C lesions as endovascular techniques improve. Good-risk patients with TASC type C disease can also be treated with open surgery, depending on patient preference. Surgery is usually recommended for TASC D lesions, but advanced endovascular approaches are now being applied in these lesions as well, with good results. (1)

High-risk patients with TASC C and D disease, CLI may be treated with endovascular therapy, acknowledging that this approach will be less durable than open surgical options. (84) Once a decision has been made that intervention is indicated, information must be gathered to determine the location and extent of the atherosclerotic occlusive disease. Evaluation of the femoral artery as an access for intervention is crucial. Patients with greater than 50% CFA stenosis on duplex arterial mapping, MRA, or CTA are usually treated with a hybrid approach that entails open femoral endarterectomy, patch angioplasty, and simultaneous stent or stent-graft placement. In patients with less severe CFA disease, a percutaneous approach can be under taken and ipsilateral retrograde, contralateral, bilateral femoral, or brachial approach can be planned. (85)

Aortic lesions are frequently calcified, exophytoc and have a higher risk of rupture and embolization and stent graft may warranted.

Different techniques are used for the endovascular treatment of aortoiliac occlusive diseases. Common iliac artery (CIA) disease is generally treated through an ipsilateral, retrograde approach. A complete diagnostic angiogram can be performed through a catheter in the contralateral femoral artery before any intervention; this also provides access to protect the contralateral CIA from injury during ipsilateral CIA intervention.

In general, the contralateral oblique projection shows the iliac artery bifurcations, whereas the ipsilateral oblique projection best displays the profunda origins at the femoral artery bifurcations. The infrainguinal runoff is visualized before inflow intervention. If the obstruction is distal in the external iliac artery it may be better to approach from the contralateral because it permits more extensive treatment of the external iliac artery (EIA) into the proximal portion of the CFA if needed

An arterial sheath to facilitate catheter exchanges. The lesion is crossed with a floppy-tipped glide wire is used to cross the lesion supported by soft low profile catheter. After advancing the catheter across the lesion, the wire is removed, and free aspiration of blood ensures that the catheter tip is intraluminal. Injection of contrast follows to confirm the position. Pressure measurements across the lesion should be obtained as mentioned in the angiogram technique earlier.

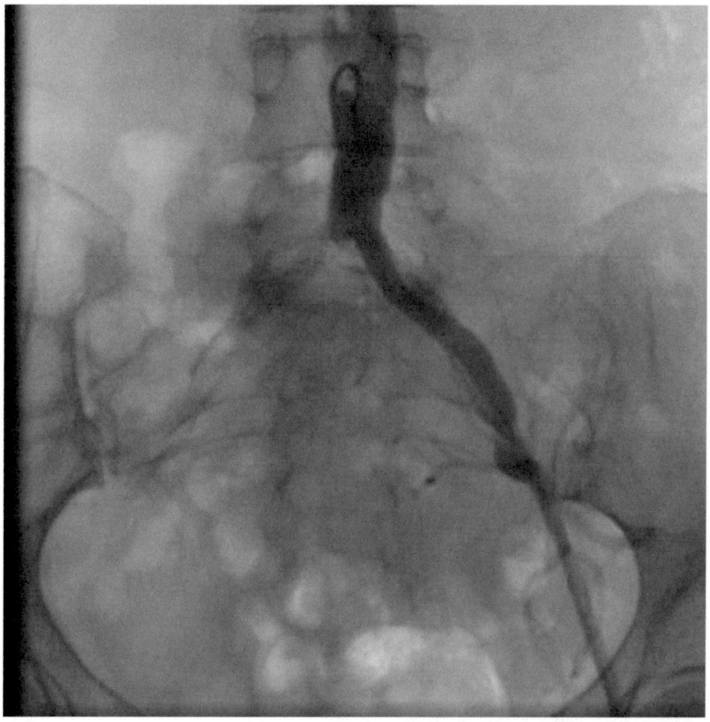

A

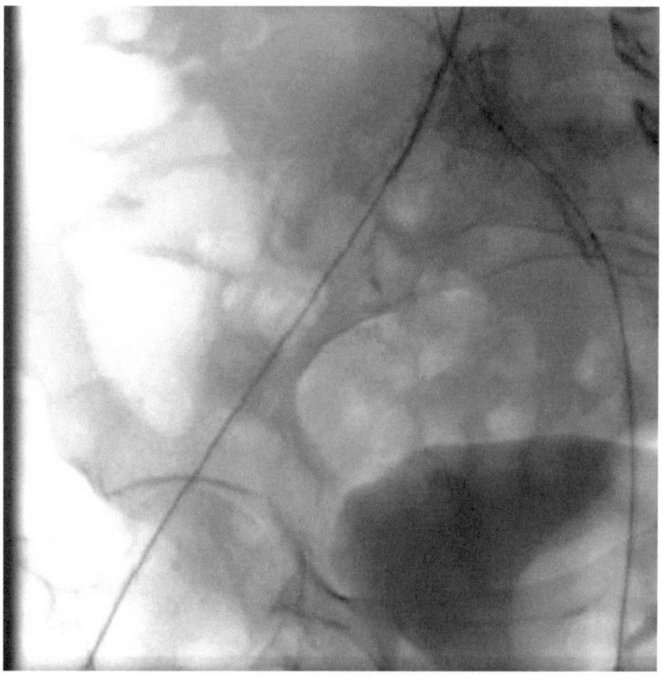

B

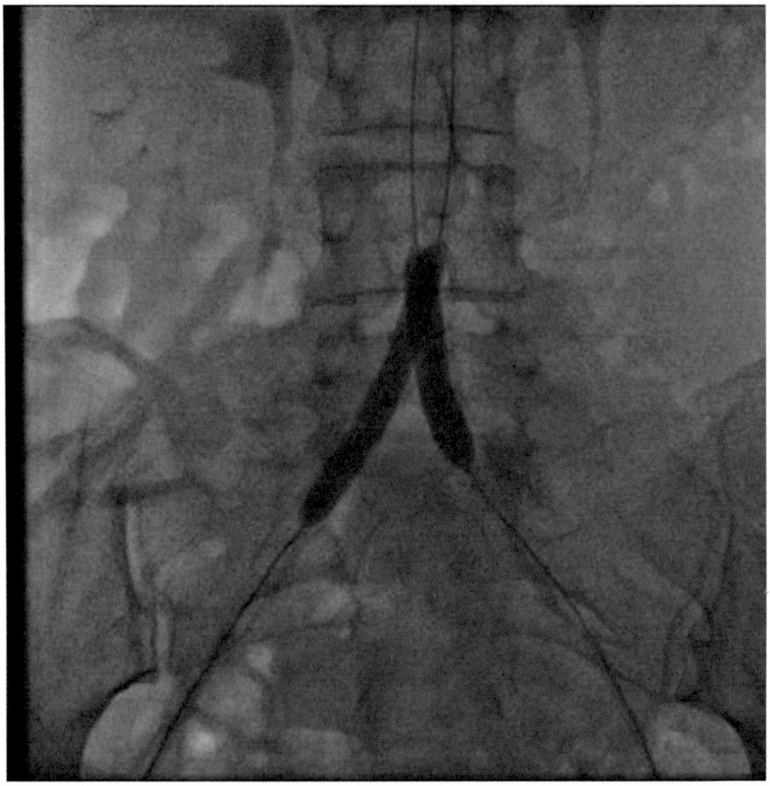

C

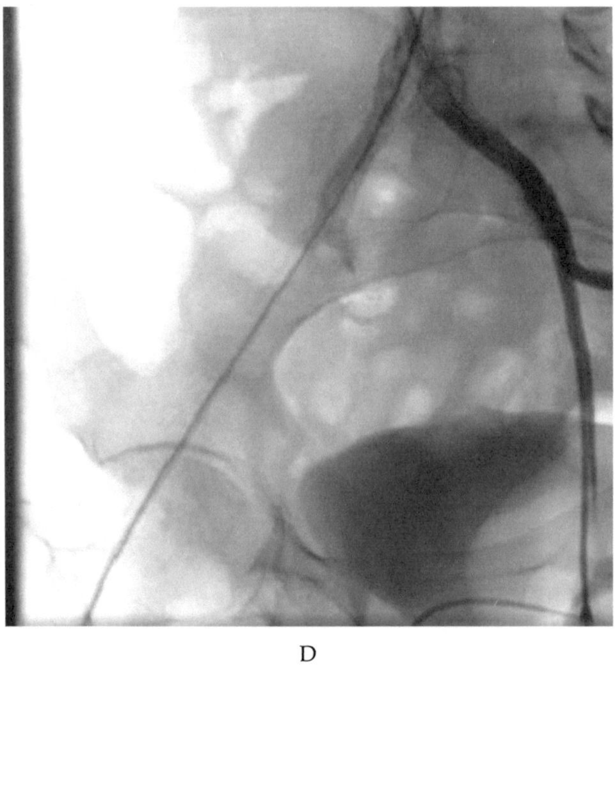

D

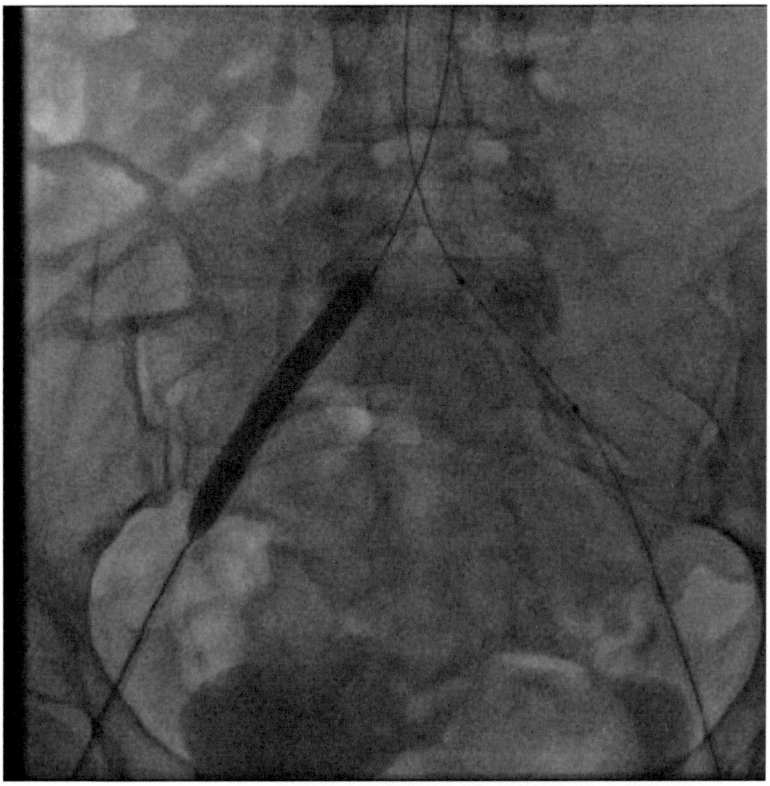

E

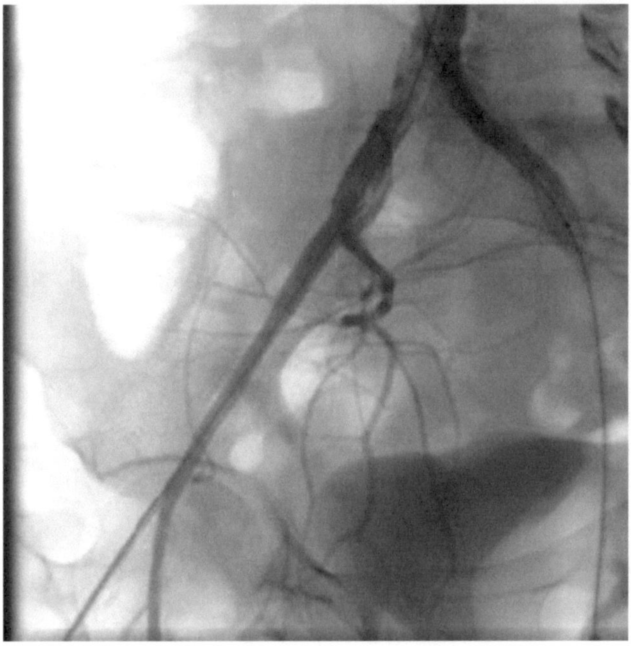

F

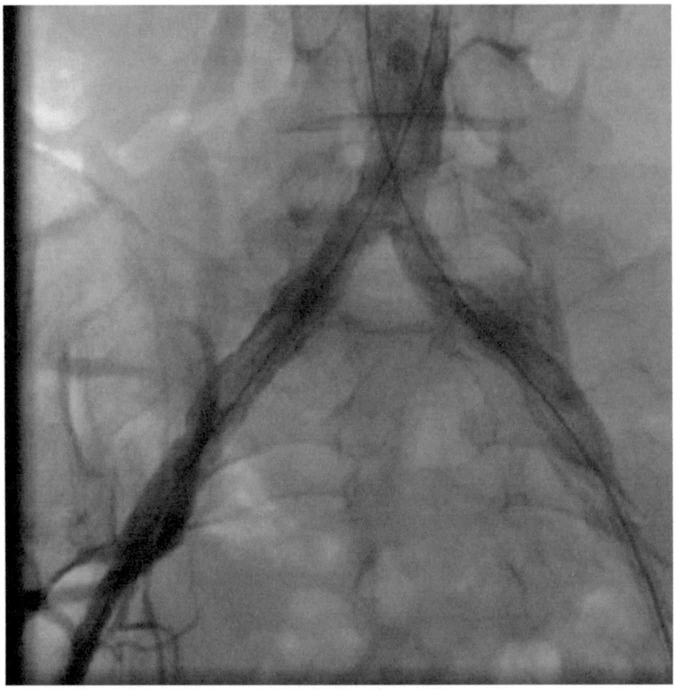

G

Fig. 9.

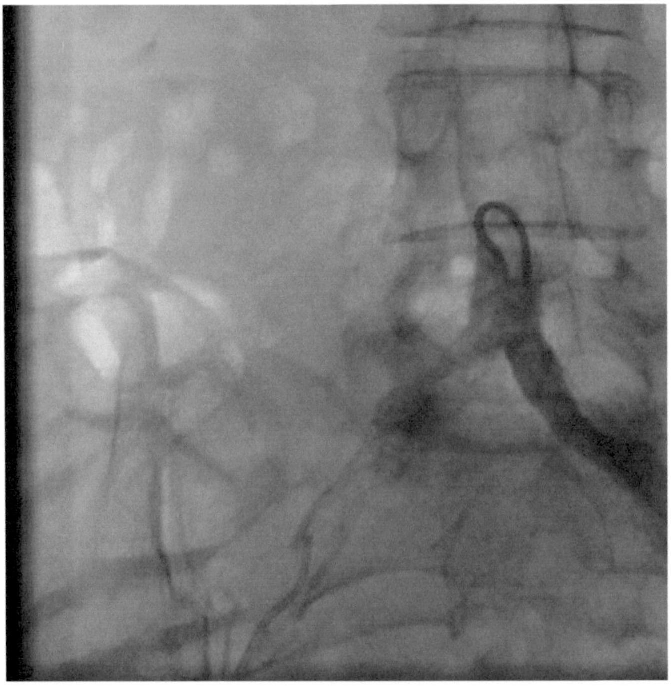

Fig. 10.

During the attempt to recanalize an occluded iliac artery in a retrograde fashion, the guide wire frequently follows a subintimal path. Once this has occurred, it may be difficult to redirect the guide wire into the lumen. Fig 9 (A-G)

An antegrade approach from the contralateral CFA is frequently successful. As soon as the guide wire has crossed the obstructive lesion and lies within the ipsilateral EIA lumen, it is snared from the ipsilateral CFA. The hydrophilic guide wire is then removed, and a working guide wire is inserted to facilitate the intervention. Fig 10

If the CIA occlusion is flush with aorta a contralateral femoral approach to cross the lesion is generally unsuccessful; transbrachial or ipsilateral femoral approaches are more likely to achieve success.

The recent development of reentry catheters has greatly increased the technical success of crossing complete arterial occlusions.

On angioplasty of the common iliac arteries a 'Kissing Balloon' technique which involves simultaneous balloon dilatation at the origins of both CIAs is advocated, even in the presence of a unilateral lesion, to protect the contralateral CIA from dissection, plaque dislodgement, or subsequent embolization.

If significant CFA disease, a' hybrid technique', open femoral approach with combined endovascular iliac therapy and femoral endarterectomy should be strongly considered

Selection of the appropriate balloon or stent diameter is of utmost importance for a successful intervention. Slight oversizing of 5% to 10% is recommended, except in the case of heavily calcified lesions that may rupture. A calibrated catheter inserted into the vessel allows measurement of the artery. The length of the balloon or stent should cover the diseased area without damaging the normal vessel. The lesion cause a waist on the balloon and the waist disappears after successful dilatation. Mild pain during dilatation is acceptable excessive or persistent pain may indicate arterial rupture. Less than 20% residual stenosis and less than 10 mm Hg pressure gradient consider a technical success. (86) Contrast-induced nephropathy oncidenec can be decreased by preprocedural volume loading and the use of low-osmolar or iso-osmolar contrast agents. (87)

The reported 4-year success rates for iliac angioplasty are approximately 44% to 65%. (88) In another study kissing iliac stents showed good results in aortic bifurcation disease with primary and secondary patency rates of 78% and 98%, respectively, at 3 years. (89)

Comparing stenting with stand-alone PTA, he Dutch Iliac Stent Trial Study Group performed a randomized comparison of primary balloon-expandable stent placement with primary angioplasty followed by selective stent placement in patients with iliac artery occlusive disease. Iliac patency ranged from 97% at 3 months to 83% at 5 years in the patients with primary stent placement; it ranged from 94% to 74% in the patients treated with PTA and selective stent placement. This difference was not significant. (90)

Other randomized trials have shown primary stenting to be superior to selective stent placement The 4-year primary patency rate for claudication, with technical failures excluded, was 68% (range, 65% to 74%) after PTA, compared with 77% (range, 72% to 81%) after stenting. The 4-year primary patency rate for critical ischemia, with technical failures excluded, was 55% (range, 48% to 63%) after PTA, versus 67% (range, 55% to 79%) after stenting. The authors concluded that stent placement reduced the risk of long-term failure by 39% compared with PTA alone. (91)

Meta-analysis of primary iliac artery stent placement in a total of 2058 limbs shows the technical success rate was 97%, the complication rate was 6%, and the 5-year primary and secondary patency rates were 73% and 85%, respectively.(92)

Outcomes of iliac intervention depend on TASC lesion classification. Galaria and associates examined reported 10-year patency results for patients with TASC types A and B lesions. Sixty-two percent of the lesions were TASC type A, and the remainder were type B. Of the 394 primary interventions, 51% included the placement of stents. Technical success (defined as <30% residual stenosis) was achieved in 98% of treated vessels. The procedure-related mortality rate was 1.8% at 30 days and 4.7% at 90 days; the procedure-related complication rate was 7%. A rise in the ABI >0.15) was achieved in 82%.. Within 3 months, 84% of patients demonstrated clinical improvement. The cumulative assisted patency rate was 71% ± 7 at 10 years. (93)

Although iliac angioplasty and stenting of TASC types A and B common iliac lesions achieve a patency similar to that of open surgical reconstruction, patients with diffuse aortoiliac occlusive disease (TASC types C and D lesions) have markedly inferior patency with stenting when compared with aortobifemoral bypass.

Recently, several authors have documented more promising results in the treatment of more complex TASC types C and D iliac lesions with 2-year primary patency ranges from 69% to 76%, with secondary patency rates of 85% to 95%. (94, 95)

In a series of 212 patients with chronic iliac occlusions, successful recanalization was accomplished in nearly 90% of patients, with marked clinical improvement in the vast majority. The primary patency at 4 years was 75.7%. (96)

The primary patency at 4 years was 75.7%. Leville and coworkers recently reported late results of the treatment of complex iliac occlusive disease. Three-year primary patency, secondary patency, and limb salvage rates were 76%, 90%, and 97%, respectively. (97)

Extension of disease into the EIA increases procedural complexity and decreases the durability of the intervention. (93)

Rzucidlo and colleagues the use of stent-grafts, (85% TASC types C and D lesions) increased the primary and primary assisted patency at 1 year to 70% and 88%, respectively, compared with patients treated with stents alone, and led to 100% early hemodynamic and clinical success. (98)

12. References

[1] Norgren L. Hiatt WR, Dormandy JA. El at. Inter-Society Consensus for the Management of the Peripheral Arterial Disease (TASC II). J Vasc Surg 2007, 45(SupplS) S5-S67.
[2] Starrett RW, Stoney RJ: Juxtarenal Aortic occlusion. Surgery 76:890, 1974.
[3] Reilly LM, Sauer I, L, Weinstein ES, et al; Infra renal aortic occlusion. Does it threaten renal perfusion or function? J Vasc Surg 11:216, 1990.

[4] Debakey ME, Lawrie GM, Glaeser DH: Patterns of atherosclerosis and their surgecial significance. Ann Surg 201:1115-131, 1985.
[5] Brewster DC. Clinical and anatomical consideration for surgery in aortoiliac disease and result of surgical treatment. Circulation 83, (2 suppl) I42-I52, 1991.
[6] Darling RC, Brewster DC, Hallett Jr JW, et al: Aortoiliac reconstruction. *Surg Clin North Am* 1979; 59:565.
[7] Malone JM, Moore WS, Goldstone J: Life expectancy following aortofemoral arterial grafting. *Surgery* 1977; 81:551.
[8] Brewster DC, Perler BA, Robison JG, et al: Aortofemoral graft for multilevel occlusive disease: predictors of success and need for distal bypass. *Arch Surg* 1982; 117:1593.
[9] Krug RT, Calligaro KD, Dougherty MJ: Claudication in the young patient. *Perspect Vasc Surg* 2000; 13:27.
[10] Flanigan DP, Schuler JJ, Keifer T, et al: Elimination of iatrogenic impotence and improvement of sexual dysfunction after aortoiliac revascularization. *Arch Surg* 1982; 117:544.
[11] Leriche R, Morel A: The syndrome of thrombotic obliteration of the aortic bifurcation. *Ann Surg* 1948; 127:193.
[12] Berman JR, Berman LA, Goldstein I: Female sexual dysfunction: incidence, pathophysiology, evaluation and treatment options. *Urology* 1999; 54:385.
[13] Hirsch AT, Haskal ZJ, Hertzer NR, et al: ACC/AHA 2005 Practice Guidelines for the management of patients with peripheral arterial disease. *J Am Coll Cardiol* 2006; 47:1239.
[14] Cournot M, Boccalon H, Cambou JP, et al: Accuracy of the screening physical examination to identify subclinical atherosclerosis and peripheral arterial disease in asymptomatic subjects. *J Vasc Surg* 2007; 46:1215-1221.
[15] Gahtan V: The noninvasive laboratory. *Surg Clin North Am* 1998; 78:507-518.
[16] Eva*luation of claudication. Vascular Diagnosis*, Philadelphia: Elsevier, Inc.; 2004.
[17] Platt JF: Doppler ultrasound of the kidney. *Semin Ultrasound CT MR* 1997; 18:22.
[18] Soares GM, Murphy TP, Singha MS, et al: Renal artery duplex ultrasonography as a screening and surveillance tool to detect renal artery stenosis: a comparison with current reference standard imaging. *J Ultrasound Med* 2006; 25:293.
[19] Heijenbrok-Kal MH, Kock MC, Hunink MG: Lower extremity arterial disease: multidetector CT angiography—meta-analysis. *Radiology* 2007; 245:433-439.
[20] Ota H, Takase K, Igarashi K, et al: MDCT compared with digital subtraction angiography for assessment of lower extremity arterial occlusive disease: importance of reviewing cross-sectional images. *Am J Roentgenol* 2004; 182:201-209.
[21] Ouwendijk R, Kock MC, van Dijk LC, et al: Vessel wall calcifications at multi-dectector row CT angiography in patients with peripheral arterial disease: effect on clinical utility and clinical predictors. *Radiology* 2006; 241:603-608.
[22] Kreitner KF, Kalden P, Neufang A, et al: Diabetes and peripheral arterial occlusive disease: prospective comparison of contrast-enhanced three-dimensional MR angiography with conventional digital subtraction angiography. *Am J Radiol* 2000; 174:171-179.
[23] Sam AD, Morasch MD, Collins J, et al: Safety of gadolinium contrast angiography in patients with chronic renal insufficiency. *J Vasc Surg* 2003; 38:313-318.

[24] Othersen JB, Maize JC, Woolson RF, Budisavlievic MN: Nephrogenic systemic fibrosis after exposure to gadolinium in patients with renal failure. *Nephrol Dial Transplant* 2007; 22:3179-3185.
[25] Bostrom AA, Karacagil S, Hellberg A, et al: Surgical reconstruction without preoperative angiography in patients with aortoiliac occlusive disease. *Ann Vasc Surg* 2002; 16:273.
[26] Bettmann MA, Heeren T, Greenfield A, et al: SCVIR contrast agent registry report. *Radiology* 1997; 203:611-620.
[27] Armstrong P, Han D, Baxter J, et al: Complication rates of percutaneous brachial artery access in peripheral vascular angiography. *Ann Vasc Surg* 2003; 17:107.
[28] Udoff EJ, Barth KH, Harrington DP, et al: Hemodynamic significance of iliac artery stenosis: pressure measurements during angiography. *Radiology* 1979; 132:289.
[29] Waugh JR, Sacharias N: Arteriographic complications in the DSA era. *Radiology* 1992; 182:243-246.
[30] Back MR, Caridi JG, Hawkins IF, Seeger JM: Angiography with carbon dioxide (CO2). *Surg Clin North Am* 1998; 78:575-591
[31] O'Riordan DS, O'Donnell JA: Realistic expectations for the patient with intermittent claudication. *Br J Surg* 1991; 78:861-863.
[32] Muluk SC, Muluk VS, Kelley ME, et al: Outcome events in patients with claudication: a 15 year study in 2777 patients. *J Vasc Surg* 2001; 33:251-257.
[33] Hirsch AT, Haskal ZJ, Hertzer NR, et al: ACC/AHA guidelines for the management of patients with peripheral arterial disease: summary of recommendations, sc Interv Radiol 17(9):1383–1397, 2006.
[34] Creager MA, Jones DW, Easton JD: Atherosclerotic Vascular Disease Conference: Writing Group V: Medical decision making and therapy. *Circulation* 2004; 109:2634-2642.
[35] Tonstad S, Farsang C, Klaene G, et al: Bupropion SR for smoking cessation in smokers with cardiovascular disease: a multicentre, randomised study. *Eur Heart J* 2003; 24:946-955.
[36] Upchurch GR, Dimick JB, Wainess RM, et al: Diffusion of new technology in health care: the case of aorto-iliac occlusive disease. *Surgery* 2004; 136:812.
[37] Hertzer NR, Bena JF, Karafa MT: A personal experience with direct reconstruction and extra-anatomic bypass for aortobifemoral occlusive disease. *J Vasc Surg* 2007; 45:527.
[38] Chang RW, Goodney PP, Baek JH, et al: Long-term results of combined common femoral endarterectomy and iliac stenting/stent grafting for occlusive disease. *J Vasc Surg* 2008.Jun:epub
[39] Stevens RD, Burri H, Tramer MR: Pharmacologic myocardial protection in patients undergoing noncardiac surgery: a quantitative systematic review. *Anesth Analg* 2003; 97:623.
[40] Hoeks SE, Scholte Op Reimer WJ, van Urk H, et al: Increase of 1-year mortality after perioperative beta-blocker withdrawal in endovascular and vascular surgery patients. *Eur J Vasc Endovasc Surg* 2007; 33:13.
[41] Bush Jr HL, Hydo LJ, Fischer E, et al: Hypothermia during elective abdominal aortic aneurysm repair: the high price of avoidable morbidity. J Vasc Surg 1995; 21:392.

[42] Juleff RS, Brown OW, McKain MM, et al: The influence of competitive flow on graft patency. J Cardiovasc Surg 1992; 33:415.
[43] Pierce GE, Turrentine M, Stringfield S, et al: Evaluation of end-to-side v end-to-end proximal anastomosis in aortobifemoral bypass. Arch Surg 1982; 117:1580.
[44] Gloviczki P, Cross SA, Stanson AW, et al: Ischemic injury to the spinal cord or lumbosacral plexus after aorto-iliac reconstruction. Am J Surg 1991; 162:131.
[45] Brewster DC, Perler BA, Robison JG, et al: Aortofemoral graft for multilevel occlusive disease: predictors of success and need for distal bypass. Arch Surg 1982; 117:1593.
[46] Martinez BD, Hertzer NR, Beven EG: Influence of distal arterial occlusive disease on prognosis following aortobifemoral bypass. Surgery 1980; 88:795.
[47] Ballard JL, Bergan JJ, Singh P, et al: Aortoiliac stent deployment versus surgical reconstruction: analysis of outcome and cost. J Vasc Surg 1998; 28:94.
[48] Faries PL, LoGerfo FW, Hook SC, et al: The impact of diabetes on arterial reconstructions for multilevel arterial occlusive disease. Am J Surg 2001; 181:251.
[49] Reed AB, Conte MS, Donaldson MC, et al: The impact of patient age and aortic size on the results of aortobifemoral bypass grafting. J Vasc Surg 2003; 37:1219.
[50] Steele SR: Ischemic colitis complicating major vascular surgery. Surg Clin North Am 2007; 87:1099.
[51] Gloviczki P, Cross SA, Stanson AW, et al: Ischemic injury to the spinal cord or lumbosacral plexus after aorto-iliac reconstruction. Am J Surg 1991; 162:131.
[52] Nevelsteen A, Suy R: Graft occlusion following aortofemoral Dacron bypass. Ann Vasc Surg 1991; 5:32.
[53] O'Connor S, Andrew P, Batt M, Becquemin JP: A systematic review and meta-analysis of treatments for aortic graft infection. J Vasc Surg 2006; 44:38-45.
[54] Armstrong PA, Back MR, Wilson JS, et al: Improved outcomes in the recent management of secondary aortoenteric fistula. J Vasc Surg 2005; 42:660.
[55] Hagino RT, Taylor SM, Fuitani RM, et al: Proximal anastomotic failure following infrarenal aortic reconstruction: late development of true aneurysms, pseudoaneurysms, and occlusive disease. Ann Vasc Surg 1993; 7:8.
[56] Connolly JE, Price T: Aortoiliac endarterectomy: a lost art?. Ann Vasc Surg 2006; 20:56.
[57] Van der Akker PJ, van Schilfaarde R: Long-term results of prosthetic and non-prosthetic reconstruction for obstructive aorto-iliac disease. Eur J Vasc Surg 1992; 6:53.
[58] Sumner DS, Strandness Jr DE: The hemodynamics of the femorofemoral shunt. Surg Gynecol Obstet 1972; 134:629-636.
[59] Nicholson ML, Beard JD, Horrocks M: Intra-operative inflow resistance measurement: a predictor of steal syndromes following femoro-femoral bypass grafting. Br J Surg 1988; 75:1064-1066.
[60] Couch NP, Clowes AW, Whittemore AD, et al: The iliac-origin arterial graft: a useful alternative for iliac occlusive disease. Surgery 1985; 97:83-87.
[61] Sidawy AN, Menzoian JO, Cantelmo NL, LoGerfo FW: Retroperitoneal inflow procedures for iliac occlusive vascular disease. Arch Surg 1985; 120:794-796.

[62] Ricco J-B, Probst H: Long-term results of a multicenter randomized study on direct versus crossover bypass for unilateral iliac artery occlusive disease. J Vasc Surg 2008; 47:45-54.
[63] Kretschmer G, Niederle B, Schemper M, Polterauer P: Extra-anatomic femoro-femoral crossover bypass (FF) vs. unilateral orthotopic ilio-femoral bypass (IF): an attempt to compare results based on data matching. Eur J Vasc Surg 1991; 5:75-82.
[64] Van der Vliet JA, Scharn DM, de Waard J-WD, et al: Unilateral vascular reconstruction for iliac obstructive disease. J Vasc Surg 1994; 19:610-614.
[65] Tyson RR, Reichle FA: Retropubic femorofemoral bypass: a new route through the space of Retzius. Surgery 1972; 72:401-403.
[66] Mosley JG, Marston A: Long term results of 66 femoral-to-femoral by-pass grafts: a 9-year follow-up. Br J Surg 1983; 70:631-634.
[67] Schneider JR, Besso SR, Walsh DB, et al: Femorofemoral versus aortobifemoral bypass: outcome and hemodynamic results. J Vasc Surg 1994; 19:43-57.
[68] Schneider JR, McDaniel MD, Walsh DB, et al: Axillofemoral bypass: outcome and hemodynamic results in high-risk patients. J Vasc Surg 1992; 15:952-963.
[69] Brener BJ, Brief DK, Alpert J, et al: Femorofemoral bypass: a twenty-five year experience. In: Yao JST, Pearce WH, ed. Long-term Results in Vascular Surgery, East Norwalk: Appleton & Lange; 1993:385-393.
[70] Pursell R, Sideso E, Magee TR, Galland RB: Critical appraisal of femorofemoral crossover grafts. Br J Surg 2005; 92:565-569.
[71] Calligaro KD, Ascer E, Veith FJ, et al: Unsuspected inflow disease in candidates for axillofemoral bypass operations: a prospective study. J Vasc Surg 1990; 11:832-837.
[72] Sullivan LP, Davidson PG, D'Anna Jr JA, Sithian N: Disruption of the proximal anastomosis of axillobifemoral grafts: two case reports. J Vasc Surg 1989; 10:190-192.
[73] LoGerfo FW, Johnson WC, Corson JD, et al: A comparison of the late patency rates of axillobilateral femoral and axillounilateral femoral grafts. Surgery 1977; 81:33-40.
[74] Harris Jr EJ, Taylor Jr LM, McConnell DB, et al: Clinical results of axillobifemoral bypass using externally supported polytetrafluoroethylene. J Vasc Surg 1990; 12:416-421.
[75] Bliss BP, Barrett GS: Axillo-femoral and axillo-profunda bypass grafts. Their use for limb salvage in the bad-risk patient with occlusion or infection of the abdominal aorta and iliac arteries. Ann R Coll Surg Engl 1972; 50:268-273.
[76] Devolfe C, Adeleine P, Violet F, Descotes J: La revascularisation des membres inférieurs à partir de l'artère axillaire est-elle fiable? Analyse informatique de 98 pontages. Lyon Chir 1981; 77:88-93.
[77] Naylor AR, Ah-See AK, Engeset J: Axillofemoral bypass as a limb salvage procedure in high risk patients with aortoiliac disease. Br J Surg 1990; 77:659-661.
[78] Keller MP, Hoch JR, Harding AD, et al: Axillopopliteal bypass for limb salvage. J Vasc Surg 1992; 15:817-822.
[79] Tilson MD, Sweeney T, Gusberg RJ, Stansel HC: Obturator canal bypass grafts for septic lesions of the femoral artery. Arch Surg 1979; 114:1031-1033.

[80] Mentha C, Launois B, Delaere J: Les pontages artériels ilio-fémoraux par le trou obturateur [Ilio-femoral arterial bridging by the obturator foramen]. J Chir (Paris) 1965; 90:131-140.
[81] Passman MA, Farber MA, Criado E, et al: Descending thoracic aorta to iliofemoral artery bypass grafting: a role for primary revascularization for aortoiliac occlusive disease?. J Vasc Surg 1999; 29:249-258.
[82] Said S, Mall J, Peter F, et al: Laparoscopic aorto-femoral bypass grafting: human cadaveric and initial clinical experiences. J Vasc Surg 1999; 29:639-648.
[83] Briguori C, Airoldi F, D'Andrea D, et al: Renal Insufficiency Following Contrast Media Administration Trial (REMEDIAL): a randomized comparison of 3 preventive strategies. Circulation 2007; 115:1211-1217.
[84] Leville CD, Kashyap VS, Clair DG, et al: Endovascular management of iliac artery occlusions: extending treatment to TransAtlantic Inter-Society Consensus class C and D patients. J Vasc Surg 2006; 43:32-39.
[85] Rzucidlo EM, Powell RJ, Zwolak RM, et al: Early results of stent-grafting to treat diffuse aortoiliac occlusive disease. J Vasc Surg 2003; 37:1175-1180.
[86] Haulon S, Mounier-Vehier C, Gaxotte V, et al: Percutaneous reconstruction of the aortoiliac bifurcation with the "kissing stents" technique: long-term follow-up in 106 patients. J Endovasc Ther 2002; 9:363-368.
[87] Aspelin P, Aubry P, Fransson SG, et al: Nephrotoxic effects in high-risk patients undergoing angiography. N Engl J Med 2003; 348:491-499
[88] Parsons RE, Suggs WD, Lee JJ, et al: Percutaneous transluminal angioplasty for the treatment of limb threatening ischemia: do the results justify an attempt before bypassgrafting?. J Vasc Surg 1998; 28:1066-1071.
[89] Haulon S, Mounier-Vehier C, Gaxotte V, et al: Percutaneous reconstruction of the aortoiliac bifurcation with the "kissing stents" technique: long-term follow-up in 106 patients. J Endovasc Ther 2002; 9:363-368.
[90] Tetteroo E, van der Graaf Y, Bosch JL, et al: Randomised comparison of primary stent placement versus primary angioplasty followed by selective stent placement in patients with iliac-artery occlusive disease. Dutch Iliac Stent Trial Study Group. Lancet 1998; 351:1153-1159.
[91] Bosch JL, Hunink MG: Meta-analysis of the results of percutaneous transluminal angioplasty and stent placement for aortoiliac occlusive disease. Radiology 1997; 204:87-96.
[92] Murphy TP: The role of stents in aorto-iliac occlusive disease. New York, Thieme, 1998.
[93] Galaria II, Davies MG: Percutaneous transluminal revascularization for iliac occlusive disease: long-term outcomes in TransAtlantic Inter-Society Consensus A and B lesions. Ann Vasc Surg 2005; 19:352-360.
[94] Carnevale FC, De Blas M, Merino S, et al: Percutaneous endovascular treatment of chronic iliac artery occlusion. Cardiovasc Intervent Radiol 2004; 27:447-452.
[95] Uher P, Nyman U, Lindh M, et al: Long-term results of stenting for chronic iliac artery occlusion. J Endovasc Ther 2002; 9:67-75.
[96] Scheinert D, Schroder M, Ludwig J, et al: Stent-supported recanalization of chronic iliac artery occlusions. Am J Med 2001; 110:708-715.

[97] Leville CD, Kashyap VS, Clair DG, et al: Endovascular management of iliac artery occlusions: extending treatment to TransAtlantic Inter-Society Consensus class C and D patients. J Vasc Surg 2006; 43:32-39.

[98] Rzucidlo EM, Powell RJ, Zwolak RM, et al: Early results of stent-grafting to treat diffuse aortoiliac occlusive disease. J Vasc Surg 2003; 37:1175-1180.

2

Vascular Trauma: New Directions in Screening, Diagnosis and Management

Leslie Kobayashi and Raul Coimbra
University of California San Diego, USA

1. Introduction

Major vascular injury following trauma is uncommon, however, it can result in extremely high mortality and morbidity, particularly if diagnosis or treatment are delayed. Physical examination has historically been the mainstay of diagnosis, and open repair the mainstay of treatment for these injuries. However, as advanced imaging technologies and endovascular treatment modalities become more common, and validated in the literature the diagnosis and treatment of traumatic vascular injuries has evolved. While patients with classic "hard signs" of vascular injury such as arterial bleeding, expanding hematoma, lack of pulses, bruit, thrill, or shock should still be taken immediately to the operating theater for open exploration with, or without on table angiography if necessary; patients with soft signs of injury or concerning mechanisms now have a myriad of screening options available. Additionally, in vascular injuries that are difficult to diagnose, expose and definitively treat, such as thoracic aortic and subclavian artery injury, minimally invasive diagnostic and treatment options have significantly altered the course of care of these trauma patients. One of the most important advancements in the diagnosis of vascular injury has been the development of computed tomography (CT), specifically CT angiography (CTA). CT scanning is widely available in most hospitals in the United States, is rapid, immediately and easily performed, and does not require the presence of specially trained radiologists and technologists as in traditional angiography. CT angiography has now become the screening tool of choice for traumatic aortic injury, and is becoming more commonly utilized in the diagnosis of upper and lower extremity vascular injury. In the therapeutic realm, minimally invasive endovascular techniques such as stent graft deployment and embolization with coils, glue or gelfoam are increasingly utilized in the treatment of vascular injury. This review will discuss the use of modern imaging techniques such as CT angiography and magnetic resonance imaging (MRI) in the screening and diagnosis of thoracic aortic and upper and lower extremity vascular injuries. We will also discuss the indications for, efficacy and complications of, and outcomes in endovascular therapies for traumatic vascular injuries.

2. Diagnosis

2.1 Peripheral vascular injury

Peripheral vascular injuries, defined as injuries of, or distal to, the axillobrachial and femoropopliteal vessels, while uncommon overall, account for the majority of civilian vascular trauma (Mattox, et al., 1989). Lower extremity injuries are more common than upper, and the majority of injuries are due to penetrating trauma, which accounts for 75-80% of cases (Dente, et al., 2008). In contrast to injuries of the thoracoabdominal vessels where injury can result in significant occult hemorrhage into the thorax, abdomen, or retroperitoneum; peripheral vascular injury generally results in bleeding or hematoma formation that is clearly visible on clinical exam. Additionally, peripheral injuries can be easily controlled in the field by direct pressure or tourniquet application. These factors combine to improve the chances of patients with peripheral vascular injury presenting to the hospital alive, and in stable condition.

Because of the peripheral and more superficial location of these vessels clinical exam is very sensitive for detection of arterial injury (Gonzalez & Falimirski, 1999; Hood, et al., 1998; Modrall, et al., 1998). The classical hard signs of vascular injury include arterial bleeding, expanding or pulsatile hematoma, lack of distal pulse, bruit, thrill, and shock without other explanation. Patients with any hard signs of injury should be taken to surgery immediately. The one exception would be in blunt trauma patients or patients with multi-level penetrating trauma such as shotgun wounds where angiography or CTA can be a helpful roadmap for surgical planning and exploration.

In stable patients lacking hard signs of vascular injury physical examination should include visual inspection, palpation for edema, compartment tension and tenderness, as well as range of motion across all joints to assess for associated fracture or dislocation. Complete neurologic examination of the affected extremity should also be performed in cooperative patients, as there is a high rate of nerve injury associated with vascular trauma, and neurologic defect should be considered a soft sign of vascular injury. Other soft signs include non-expanding non-pulsatile hematomas and history of profuse or pulsatile bleeding. A complete assessment of all peripheral pulses should be performed. If any asymmetry is noted, and in cases of obvious fracture or deformity, an ankle-brachial index (ABI) or brachial-brachial index (BBI) should be performed to rule out occult vascular injury. The blood pressure should be taken below the level of injury in the affected extremity. If the ABI/BBI is less than 0.9, or any soft signs of injury are present further imaging is mandatory as up to 35% of these patients will have a surgically significant injury (Gonzalez & Falimirski, 1999). ABI as a screening tool for diagnosis of arterial injury has a very good sensitivity ranging from 95-100% and a negative predictive value of 98% (Levy, et al., 2005; Sadjadi, et al., 2009). Unfortunately, a normal ABI may occasionally miss injuries that do not inhibit distal flow such as pseudoaneurysm, arterio-venous fistula, and intimal flap. However, the majority, 87-95%, of these lesions heal spontaneously and in follow up only 1-4% of these patients with missed injuries require intervention at 1 year, and 9% at 5-10 years (Dennis, et al., 1998; Frykberg, et al., 1991).

Patients with no hard or soft signs of injury, and with normal ABI/BBI's may be discharged if there is no other indication for admission (Figure 1). Advanced imaging or surgical exploration solely for proximity of injury is neither cost effective nor advocated in the absence of concerning ABI or physical exam findings as the likelihood of finding a surgically significant injury is very low (Hood, et al., 1998; Modrall, et al,. 1998; Weaver, et al., 1990).

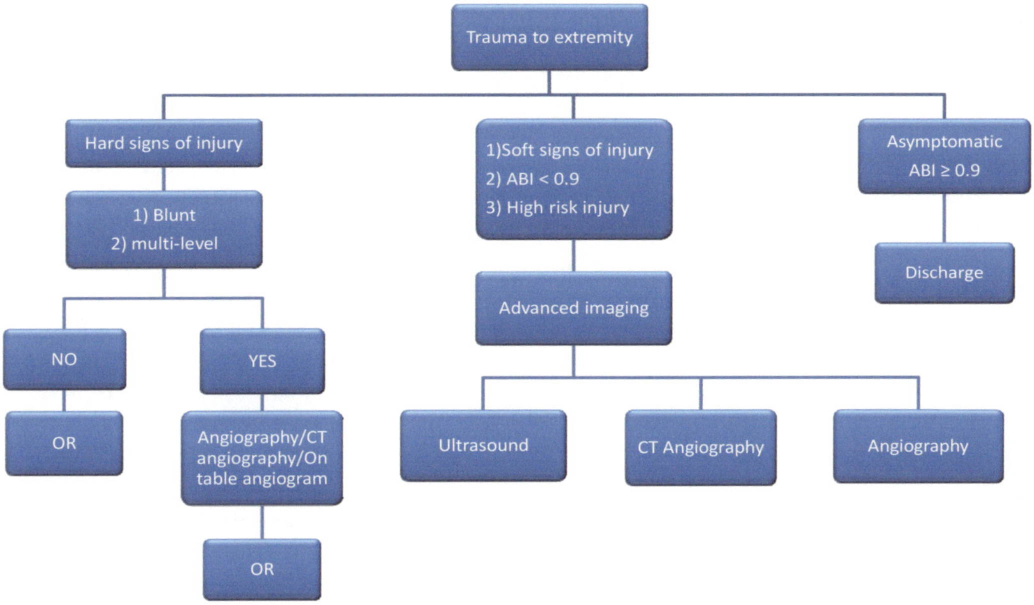

Fig. 1. Diagnostic and treatment algorithm for extremity trauma

Imaging options include MRI and MR angiography (MRA), ultrasound, angiography, and CTA. Studies of MRA in non-traumatic vascular lesions produce very accurate images of the vasculature. Among patients undergoing MRA for peripheral arterial disease sensitivity and specificity range from 92-99.5% and 64-99% respectively (Collins, et al., 2007). A single study of MRA in 12 cases of penetrating trauma revealed satisfactory studies in all patients, and successfully identified 3 injuries confirmed by angiography (Yaquinto, et al., 1992). However, MRA is not commonly utilized for diagnosis of peripheral arterial injury as it can be a lengthy and difficult to obtain exam, and may not be advisable in victims of shotgun, gunshot, or blast injuries as metallic fragments present in the patient may not be compatible with the machine. Additionally, because of the longer image acquisition time, MRA is more susceptible to motion artifact than ultrasound or CTA.

Ultrasound is an excellent option in the lower extremity below the inguinal ligament and in the upper extremity below the shoulder, however the examination can be quite limited in the presence of soft tissue injury, and is less useful for imaging proximal vessels. Ultrasound has the benefit of being portable, and imaging can be obtained quite rapidly in the emergency room, trauma bay, and operating room. It is non-invasive and does not require contrast administration or ionizing radiation. However, reported sensitivities range quite broadly from 50-100% and are highly operator dependent (Feliciano, et al., 2011). When injuries are detected specificity and accuracy are quite high ranging from 95-99% (Doody, et al., 2008; Feliciano, et al., 2011). The largest drawback for ultrasound is availability as a vascular technologist or experienced vascular surgeon with ultrasound training, are required to perform the exam.

Traditional angiography as a screening tool has a reported sensitivity and specificity of 95-100%, and 90-98% respectively (Levy, et al., 2005). Surgeon performed angiography is also quite sensitive and specific with a low complication rate of 1-4% (Itani, et al., 1992;

O'Gorman, et al., 1984). However, both methods are invasive, require administration of iodinated contrast, and in the case of traditional angiography may be quite lengthy and require transportation to the interventional radiology suite.

Because both ultrasound and angiography require mobilization of advanced imaging teams with specialized training and are unlikely to be immediately available in most centers after hours or on holidays/weekends, CTA has become an attractive alternative screening method. It has the benefit of speed, ease and a low rate of complications, can be performed without arterial puncture, does not require an interventional radiology team, and can be performed with significantly less contrast and radiation exposure than traditional angiography (Willmann & Wildermuth. 2005). CTA also has the benefit of giving additional information on non-vascular structures such as the bone, joint, and soft tissue. It may be of particular benefit in children as traditional angiography has an increased risk of complications among pediatric patients (Feliciano, et al., 2011). Because of these benefits CTA has now become the dominant mode of screening for peripheral vascular injury in many centers (Anderson, et al., 2008; Fleiter&Mervis. 2007; Peng, et al., 2008). Injury can present as focal narrowing, occlusion, thrombosis, pseudoaneurysm, extravasation, arteriovenous fistula, dissection, and intimal flap (Figure 2a, 2b). There is some evidence that arterial spasm may result in false positives on CTA (Figure 3), while conversely small intimal flaps may not be detected and result in false negatives (Rieger, et al., 2006; Soto, et al., 2001). Confirmatory angiography may be useful in cases of suspected spasm, vs. repeat imaging following resuscitation, while in the case of intimal flaps, the need for endovascular or open intervention is rare even in series with long term follow up (Dennis, et al., 1998). Overall CT angiography has excellent sensitivity (90-100%) and specificity (87-100%) for detecting both upper and lower extremity vascular injuries (Doody, et al., 2008; Fleiter & Mervis. 2007; Inaba, et al., 2006; Peng, et al., 2008; Rieger, et al., 2006; Seamon, et al., 2009). Accuracy appears to be particularly good when using multi-detector 16 and 64 slice scanners, and reformatting such as maximum intensity projections (MIP) and 2 and 3-dimensional reconstruction (Figure 4). Initial studies validated CTA as an excellent screening tool for proximal extremity injuries, but more recent studies have also shown good sensitivity, specificity and image quality for distal portions of extremities (Rieger, et al., 2006). One prospective study revealed a sensitivity and specificity of 100%, as compared to surgery and angiography as the gold standard, including injuries as distal as the posterior tibial trunk and radial artery. This study also found a significant cost savings with CTA over traditional angiography if it had been used as the sole screening modality (Seamon, et al., 2009). Lastly, CT is reported as being the least uncomfortable vascular exam in many series comparing it to MRA, ultrasound and traditional angiography (Collins, et al., 2007).

Limitations of CTA include the need to transport the patient to the radiology suite and exposure to contrast and ionizing radiation. Additionally, in victims of gunshot and shotgun wounds images may be compromised by metallic fragments, which occurs in 3.6-19% of cases (Anderson, et al., 2008; Soto, et al., 2001). However, metallic artifact when present did not appear to significantly limit the utility of CTA in two recent series (Anderson, et al., 2008; White, et al., 2010). Complications of CT are rare and include anaphylaxis (0.004-0.22%) and contrast infiltration (0.2-2.2%). Contrast induced nephropathy can occur in 1.2-2.6% of patients, however this can increase to 11-33% in high risk groups (Bellin, et al., 2002; Haveman, et al., 2006; Lencioni, et al., 2010; Morcos. 2005; Nguyen, et al., 2009; Pucelikova, et al., 2008; Rashid, et al., 2009; Wang, et al., 2007).

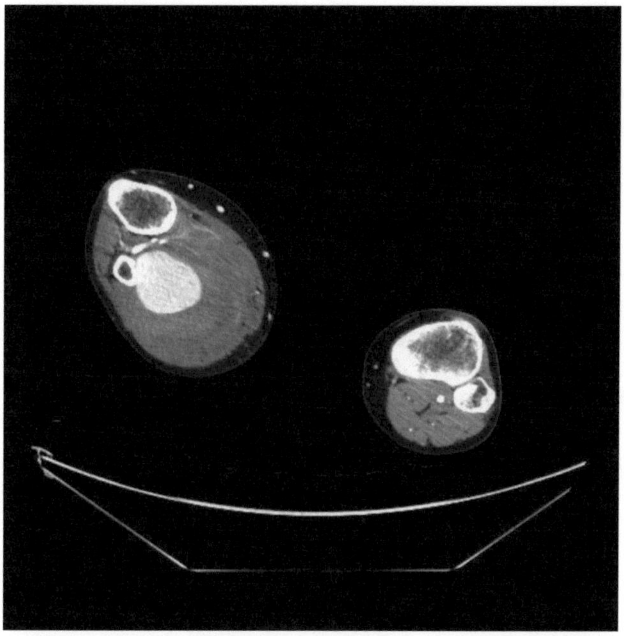

(a)

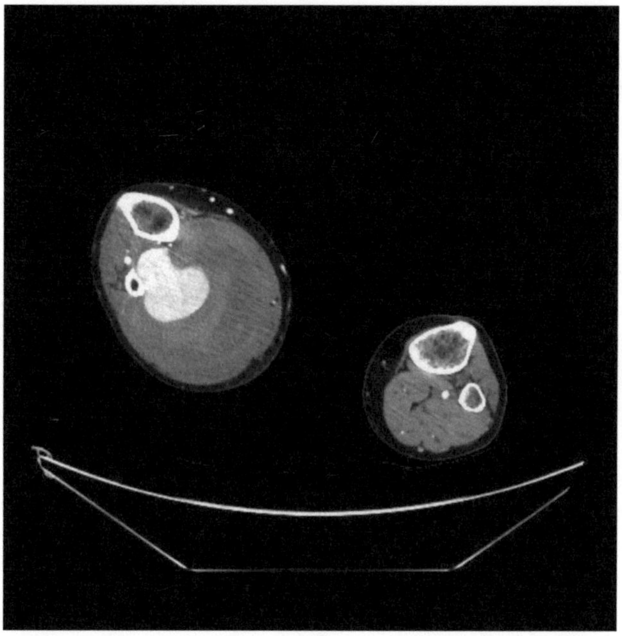

(b)

Fig. 2. a) Lower extremity pseudoaneurysm, b) pseudoaneurysm with its feeding vessel, the posterior tibial artery

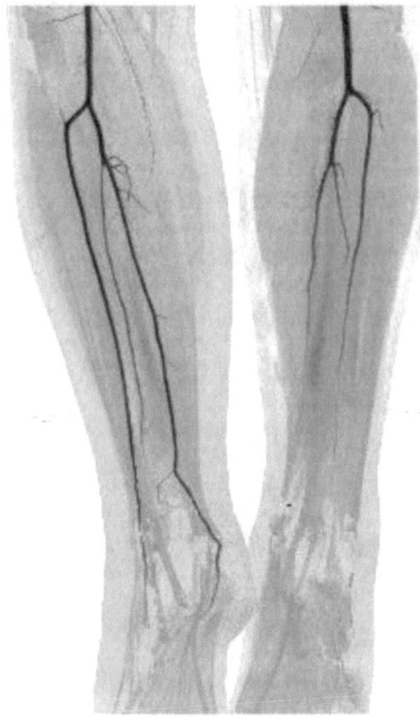

Fig. 3. Lower extremity demonstrating multivessels vasospasm of the anterior tibial, peroneal and posterior tibial arteries.

2.2 Thoraco-abdominal vascular injury

Thoraco-abdominal vascular trauma is a rare entity accounting for 0.01-2% of all trauma admissions (Asensio, et al., 2000; Asensio, et al., 2002; Dente, et al., 2008; Hoyt, et al., 2001). Penetrating mechanisms are responsible for the vast majority of injuries accounting for 70-95% of patients (Asensio, et al., 2000; Asensio, et al., 2002; Hoyt, et al., 2001; Mattox, et al., 1989). Of blunt causes motor vehicle crashes are the most common followed by falls from height and pedestrians struck by vehicles (Asensio, et al., 2001b; Bertrand, et al., 2008; Mirvis & Shanmuganathan. 2007; Neschis, et al., 2008; Wintermark, et al., 2002). Unlike extremity vascular injury where bleeding, hematomas, pulsations, thrills, bruits, and in some cases the vessels themselves are easily examined clinically, outside of hypotension, there are few clinical signs of truncal vascular injury. Because of this radiographic adjuncts are of great importance in the diagnosis of truncal vascular injury. Increasingly CT scanning is being utilized for diagnosis of thoraco-abdominal vascular injury. Intravascular interventions such as covered stents have been increasingly utilized for treatment of thoracic, subclavian and iliac arterial injuries, structures which have classically been difficult to expose and treat surgically (Asensio, et al., 2001a; Boufi, et al., 2011; Carrick, et al., 2010; Castelli, et al., 2005; Cestero, et al., 2009; Demetriades, et al., 2008a; Demetriades, et al., 2008b; Starnes & Arthurs. 2006).

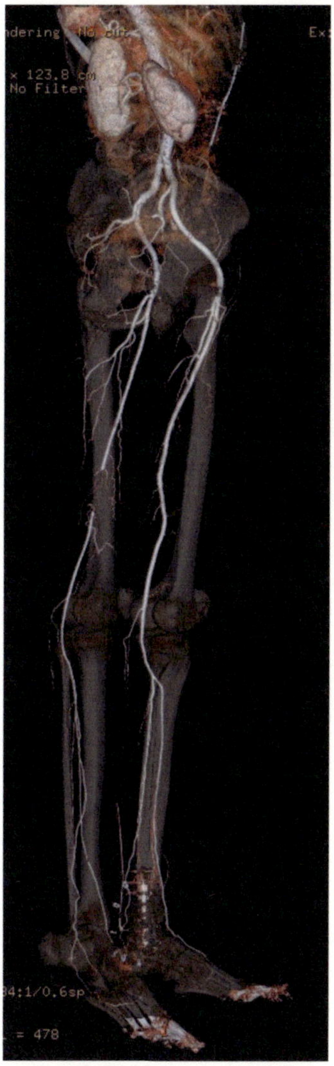

Fig. 4. 3-Dimensional reconstruction of SFA injury with occlusion and reconstitution of flow distal to the injury.

2.2.1 Thoracic aorta

Blunt thoracic aortic injury (TAI) is a rare but potentially lethal result of thoracic trauma. The result of acceleration-deceleration injuries, the most common mechanisms are falls and motor-vehicle crashes. Unfortunately the majority of patients with TAI do not reach the hospital alive, 80-90% die prior to hospital arrival, and TAI accounts for between 16-29% of motor-vehicle fatalities (Bertrand, et al., 2008; Mirvis, et al., 1987; Neschis, et al., 2008; O'Conor. 2004). Of patients surviving to evaluation TAI is present in approximately 0.3-2.8% of patients (Arthurs, et al., 2009; Bertrand, et al., 2008; Fitzharris, et al., 2004; Ungar, et al., 2006; Wintermark, et al., 2002). Detection of these few patients has long been a subject of debate. Chest x-ray is the primary screening exam, however, it can be normal in up to 44%

of patients with TAI, and positive findings are nonspecific (Demetriades, et al., 1998; Neschis, et al., 2008; Raptopoulos, et al., 1992; Woodring. 1990). Abnormalities associated with TAI include widened mediastinum, apical capping, left pleural effusion, loss of aorto-pulmonary window, depression of the left mainstem bronchus, deviation of the trachea or nasogastric tube to the right, and widening of the right paratracheal stripe (Woodring & Dillon. 1984). All patients with abnormalities on chest x-ray should rapidly undergo further imaging. Additionally, when the is a very high index of suspicion for TAI advanced imaging can be considered even with a normal chest x-ray. Risk factors include fall from height, high speed motor-vehicle crash particularly with a side impact, which carries a 2-fold higher risk of TAI compared to head on collision, patients with associated injuries such as traumatic brain injury, pelvic and multiple rib fractures (Bertrand, et al., 2008; Fitzharris, et al., 2004; O'Conor. 2004). Several studies also suggest a lower threshold for imaging patients ≥ 65-70 years, and in one study for patients as young as 30 years (Bertrand, et al., 2008; Fitzharris, et al., 2004; Kaiser, et al., 2011; Smith, et al., 1995).

Imaging options include traditional angiography, CTA, echocardiography, and MRI/MRA. Each of these techniques has its own set of advantages and limitations, and the choice of imaging technique will be determined not solely by sensitivity and specificity, but also by the patient's clinical condition, concomitant injuries, and institutional availability.

The historical gold standard, angiography/aortography is decreasing in popularity. While older studies of aortography, reported sensitivity nearing 100%, others utilizing modern technologies have revealed sensitivities of 38-92% (Azizzadeh, et al., 2011; Fabian, et al., 1998). The majority of missed injuries appear to be intimal tears and small intramural hematomas which are more likely to be diagnosed by echocardiography or CTA (Azizzadeh, et al., 2011; Fabian, et al., 1998; Smith, et al., 1995). Aortography has excellent specificity, ranging from 98-100% in most series and provides detailed information on the location and morphology of the aortic injury which can be used for operative planning (Fabian, et al., 1998; Mirvis, et al., 1987; O'Conor. 2004). Complications of angiography include access site thrombosis or hemorrhage with significant bleeding occurring in 3-17% of cases; compartment syndrome in 0.004% of patients; and injury to the access vessel including dissection occurring in ~0.5% of patients, pseudoaneurysm, and arteriovenous fistula complicating 0.1% of cases (Bellin, et al., 2002; Fruhwirth, et al., 1996; Meyerson, et al., 2002; Tizon-Marcos & Barbeau. 2008). Systemic complications include anaphylaxis which is rare, and contrast induced nephropathy which occurs in 3.3-14.5% of cases overall, but can increase to 15-62% in high risk populations (Haveman, et al., 2006; Morcos. 2005; Pucelikova, et al., 2008). Additionally, angiography requires specialized equipment and personnel with advanced training which may not be present in all centers, and requires the patient be transported to an angiography suite and remain there for a prolonged period of time. Because of these limitations, aortography to screen for TAI is primarily utilized in patients with other indications for angiography, such as pelvic or solid organ injury requiring angioembolization.

In contrast to angiography CT is widely available, can be performed at any time, is fast, requires a lower contrast load, and avoids arterial puncture. Because of these benefits CT is increasing in popularity. A comparison of trauma practices from the time periods 1994-1996 and 2005-2007 revealed an increase in the use of CT scan for diagnosis of TAI from 34.8% to

93.3%. In that same time period the authors also noted a decrease in use of aortography from 87% to 8.3% (Demetriades, et al., 2008b). Indications of TAI include mediastinal or intramural hematoma, pseudoaneurysm, contrast extravasation, variation in aortic contour, and intimal flap (Figure 5, 6a, 6b). More subtle changes may include aortic dilation around and narrowing distal to the injury. While early trials of CT scan were met with skepticism due to highly variable sensitivity and low specificity. Multi-detector helical scanners now have the ability to acquire more data in less time (20-35 seconds), with improved definition, and MIP and 3-dimensional reconstruction has allowed even greater anatomical accuracy. Modern series reliably report sensitivity between 95-100% (Bruckner, et al., 2006; Dyer, et al., 2000; Exadaktylos, et al., 2005; Fisher, et al., 1994; Raptopoulos, et al., 1992; Wintermark, et al., 2002). Specificity, initially a drawback ranging from 83-86% (Fabian, et al., 1998; Raptopoulos, et al., 1992), has improved with modern technology as well and now ranges between 94-99.8% (Mirvis & Shanmuganathan. 2007; Wintermark, et al., 2002; Wong, et al., 2004). These advances have come at the price of higher radiation doses due to the greater number of detectors. However, there have been a number of protocol changes that have been able to significantly reduce the amount of radiation required for scans without apparently diminishing the image quality. Particularly in multi-trauma patients who require CT imaging of multiple body parts, the use of single pass whole body protocols result in significantly decreased radiation dose, contrast dose, and scan time, as well as total time in the CT suite (Fanucci, et al., 2007; Flamm. 2007; Loupatatzis, et al., 2008; Nguyen, et al., 2009; Ptak, et al., 2003).

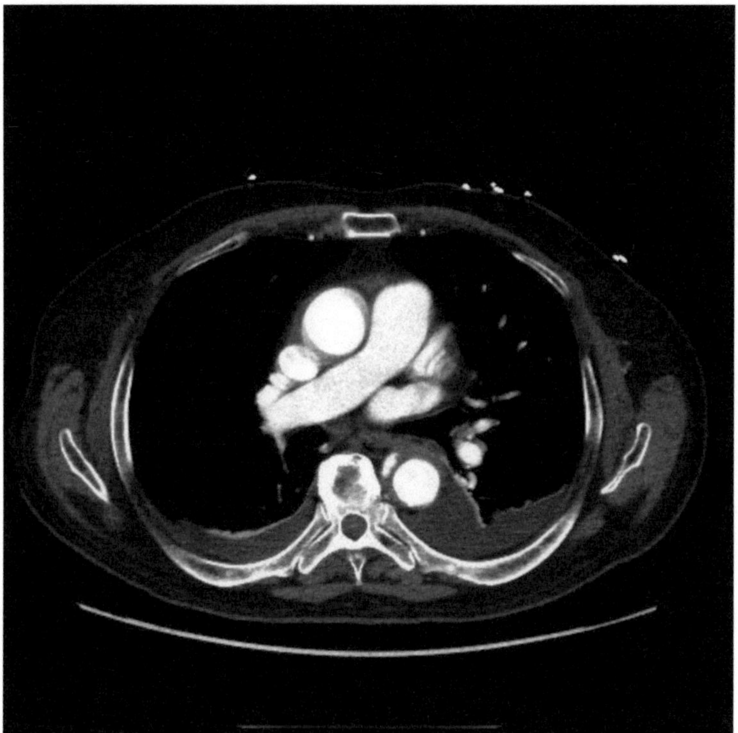

Fig. 5. Axial CT image of TAI with contrast extravasation and adjacent contained hematoma

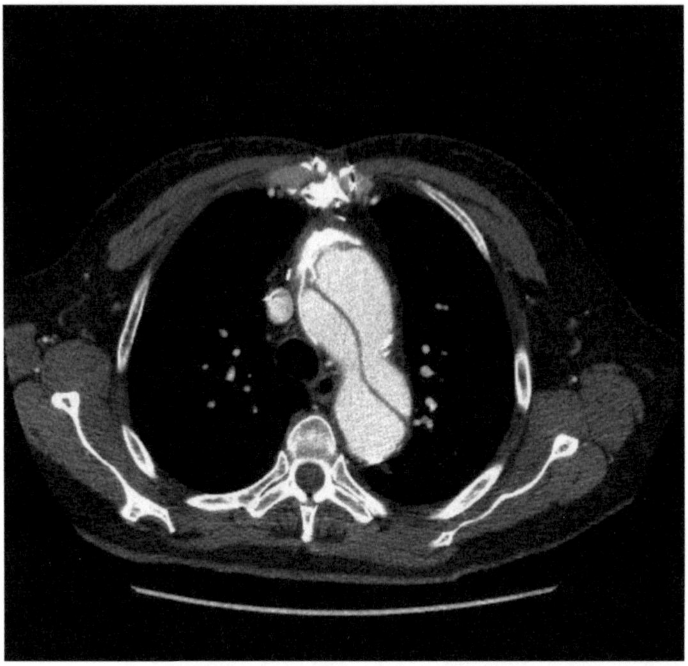

(a)

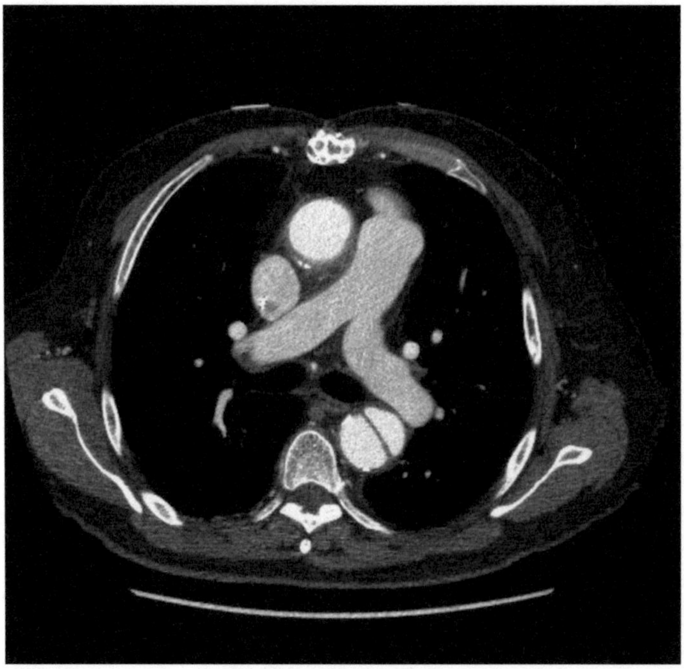

(b)

Fig. 6. Axial CT depicting aortic dissection extending from the arch (a) to the descending thoracic aorta (b)

Given these benefits some investigators have advocated abandoning chest x-ray as a screening tool in favor of CT in all patients with blunt thoracic trauma. CT's done for this purpose will reveal injuries in 5-25% of patients with normal x-rays, but will lead to a change in management in ≤ 6% of cases (Barrios, et al., 2009; Kaiser, et al., 2011; Raptopoulos, et al., 1992). Although chest x-ray may miss up to 7-8% of TAI, use of CT as a screening tool indiscriminately is unlikely to be productive or cost effective and may result in unnecessary radiation exposure with attendant increase in cancer risk (Demetriades, et al., 1998; Kaiser, et al., 2011; Melton, et al., 2004). Careful screening with chest x-ray and directed imaging in the presence of traumatic findings or in very carefully selected victims of suspicious mechanisms in the presence of previously mentioned risk factors is likely to prevent overutilization of CT and avoid missed TAI.

In contrast to blunt trauma, in the rare victims of penetrating trauma who present in hemodynamically stable condition CT has proven to be an excellent and cost effective screening examination. Patients with transthoracic or transmediastinal gunshot wounds are at risk for vascular and aerodigestive injuries. CT scan can determine which patients require surgery, or additional more invasive imaging such as esophagoscopy, esophagography or bronchoscopy. Early studies were 100% sensitive but were non-diagnostic in up to 50% of cases, more recent studies reveal conclusive results in 82.9% of cases (Hanpeter, et al., 2000; Ibirogba, et al., 2007). Equally as important is the reduction in the need for further invasive testing, in a 2007 study CT reduced the need for angiography, ultrasound and esophagography resulting in a cost reduction of 72% (Ibirogba, et al., 2007).

Unfortunately, patients who are hemodynamically unstable or require emergent surgery cannot undergo CT scanning, in these cases echocardiography may be the ideal diagnostic modality. It is portable, can be performed rapidly, is repeatable, and does not require intravenous contrast. Echocardiography can be performed via transthoracic, transesophageal or intravascular routes. Due to the low sensitivity of transthoracic echocardiography, especially in the presence of chest wall injuries transesophageal echocardiography (TEE) is the preferred method.

Characteristics of TAI on TEE include mobile intimal flaps, intraluminal mass or thrombus, and in some cases full thickness mural tear with pseudoaneurysm or mediastinal hematoma adjacent. Larger or more severe injuries can be associated with a marked enlargement of the aortic lumen and large false aneurysms (Vignon, et al., 2005). TEE can be performed in as little as 27-30 minutes with high diagnostic accuracy (Kearney, et al., 1993; Smith, et al., 1995). Sensitivity averages 98-100% (Buckmaster, et al., 1994; Goarin, et al., 2000; Kearney, et al., 1993; Smith, et al., 1995; Vignon, et al., 2001; Vignon, et al., 2005), but like most ultrasound techniques can vary widely based on operator experience, with sensitivity as low as 60-63% being reported (Patel, et al., 2003; Saletta, et al., 1995). When directly compared to angiography TEE has comparable sensitivity for surgical lesions, but has a higher sensitivity for minor lesions such as intimal flaps (Buckmaster, et al., 1994; Goarin, et al., 2000; Kearney, et al., 1993; Smith, et al., 1995; Vignon, et al., 2005). CT scan and TEE have similar diagnostic accuracy for surgical lesions, but again TEE has improved sensitivity for minor lesions (Vignon, et al., 2001). TEE can be performed safely and successfully in most patients, the failure rate in a recent meta-analysis was 1.2%, and the majority of studies report no significant procedure related complications (Buckmaster, et al., 1994; Cinnella, et al., 2004; Goarin, et al., 2000; Kearney, et al., 1993; Smith, et al., 1995; Vignon, et al., 2005).

An alternative to TEE is intravascular ultrasound. This technique involves insertion of a moderate sized catheter with an ultrasound array over a guidewire into the aorta through the femoral artery. It has excellent diagnostic accuracy, with sensitivity in the 92-100% range, and specificity nearing 100% (Azizzadeh, et al., 2011; Patel, et al., 2003). In a study comparing IVUS, TEE and angiography among patients with blunt chest trauma, IVUS outperformed both TEE and angiography with a sensitivity of 91.7%, with only one equivocal study which was found to be an intimal flap at surgery (Patel, et al., 2003).

Drawbacks of TEE include the need for specialized equipment, esophageal intubation, and operator dependence. There are also risks of esophageal injury or perforation, and airway compromise. Additionally, the 3-5cm portion of the upper ascending aorta which is obscured by interposition of the trachea between the aorta and esophagus can be a technical "blind spot" (Smith, et al., 1995). IVUS avoids this "blind spot" phenomenom, however it has similar limitations of being very operator dependent, and requiring specialized equipment. Additionally, IVUS requires arterial puncture with the attendant risk of access site complications of hematoma, fistula, pseudoaneurysm, and dissection. The risks of such local complications may be greater for IVUS than for diagnostic angiography as the sheath size required to accommodate the ultrasound probe is larger (7-8Fr) than that typically needed for diagnostic angiography (Azizzadeh, et al., 2011; Wintermark, et al., 2002). Despite the benefits of TEE and IVUS they are used in very few cases (1-4%), and appear to be decreasing in frequency, from 11.9% to 1% (Demetriades, et al., 2008b; Melton, et al., 2004). This may reflect the lack of specialty trained personnel and resultant difficulty in obtaining TEE or IVUS particularly in off hours. It may also be a result of trauma physicians lack of familiarity in performing and interpreting the results of this diagnostic modality.

MR angiography (MRA) is typically performed both before and after administration of intravenous gadolinium. In contrast to prior time-of-flight examinations contrast enhanced MRA (CE-MRA) is able to obtain images of a higher quality more often due to decreased respiratory and cardiac artifacts (Goldman. 2003). CE-MRA is also particularly well suited to 3-dimensional reconstruction which is of great value in pre-operative or pre-stent planning. Compared to traditional angiography MRA does not require arterial puncture, and is non-invasive. In comparison to CT scanning MRA has the benefit of avoiding ionizing radiation as well as iodinated contrast. MR findings consistent with TAI are similar to those of CT angiography and include intraluminal mass, flap, or luminal irregularity, as well as pseudoaneurysm, and hematoma (Wintermark, et al., 2002). CE-MRA can be used for diagnosis with a sensitivity and specificity between 98-100% (Bruckner, et al., 2006; Chirillo, et al., 1996; Fattori, et al., 1996; Khalil, et al., 2007; Mirvis&Shanmuganathan. 2000). However, CE-MRA has the drawbacks of requiring lengthy exam times outside of a monitored critical care setting, and potentially lengthy transport times. While avoiding nephrotoxicity, gadolinium is not entirely benign, and nephrogenic systemic fibrosis can occur in up to 2-5% of patients with renal insufficiency (Li, et al., 2006; Martin, et al., 2009). Lastly, CE-MRA is not available in many centers, and in hospitals where it is available, may not be operational at night, on holidays or weekends. Because of these drawbacks it is particularly ill suited to the acute trauma work up. However it has been suggested as a logical mode of follow up in the subacute and chronic phases in cases of medical management of minor injuries, or as a follow up after surgical or endovascular repair (Fattori, et al., 1996; Mirvis & Shanmuganathan. 2000; Wintermark, et al., 2002).

2.2.2 Subclavian artery

Subclavian artery injuries are primarily due to penetrating mechanisms, but are rare, affecting less than 3% of all penetrating traumas. Injuries associated with blunt trauma are even more uncommon affecting only 0.4% of patients. These injuries are highly lethal, resulting in death in up to 42% of patients prior to, or upon presentation to the hospital (Demetriades, et al., 1999). Patients often present with hypotension, hard signs of vascular injury, or compartment syndrome and are taken emergently to the operating room. In rare instances patients present in stable condition with soft signs of injury, or are asymptomatic, in these cases CT angiography can be very helpful in detecting injuries, for preoperative planning, and in some cases determining if endovascular therapy is feasible. Two studies of endovascular therapy report utilization of CTA angiography in planning stent-graft deployment, both report successful treatment of lesions, based on CT findings, but are small, and do not describe sensitivity or specificity (Castelli, et al., 2005; Hilfiker, et al., 2000). There is little to no evidence in the literature specifically studying the use of CTA angiography in subclavian artery injuries, however, several large series of CT in proximal extremity injury including the subclavian and axillary artery have found excellent sensitivity and specificity. A study of 142 CTA angiograms, including 7 subclavian artery injuries, found a sensitivity of 95.1% and specificity of 98.7% (Soto, et al., 2001). In a study of 41 stable patients with penetrating thoracic trauma CTA angiography did not miss any injuries in 9 patients who underwent both CT and traditional angiography (LeBlang & Dolich. 2000). Traditional angiography may also be utilized and was found to be helpful in operative planning in a series of 50 patients from South Africa (Sobnach, et al., 2010), and has the added benefit of providing access for possible endovascular therapy such as embolization or stent-graft deployment. Literature on the utility of ultrasound and MRI/MRA in diagnosis of subclavian artery injury following trauma is lacking. There is evidence in the vascular literature suggesting good sensitivity and specificity of ultrasound for subclavian occlusive disease. In a study of 150 controls and 33 patients with occlusive disease ultrasound was able to correctly identify lesions in 89% of right sided, and 96%of left sided lesions, with a sensitivity of 88% and specificity of 94% compared to a gold standard of digital subtraction angiography (Yurdakul, et al., 2008). However, it is unlikely that sensitivity and specificity will be as high in trauma patients in whom intravascular volume depletion, hematoma, and subcutaneous emphysema may obscure abnormalities and increase technical difficulty. In a study of penetrating trauma patients Demetriades and colleagues found that ultrasound coupled with clinical exam had a sensitivity of 91.7% and a specificity of 100% for detecting vascular injury compared to angiography and operative findings, however, this study included only 4 subclavian injuries (Demetriades, et al., 1997).

2.2.3 Iliac artery

Though uncommon overall iliac artery and vein injuries account for 11% of vascular injuries, making them one of the most common truncal vascular structures to be injured. Iliac artery injury is quite morbid resulting in a survival of only 51% (Asensio, et al., 2003; Mattox, et al., 1989). Most commonly due to penetrating trauma, iliac artery injury in patients following blunt trauma is rare occurring in only 3.5% of all patients with severe pelvic fractures, and is associated with significant morbidity (Cestero, et al., 2009; Cushman, et al., 1997). When patients are hemodynamically stable CT has become the diagnostic tool of choice for detection of vascular injury and need for further procedures (Vu, et al., 2010). Conversely, unstable patients have historically been triaged according to the results of pelvic plain x-rays and Focused Assessment with Sonography for Trauma (FAST). Patients with evidence of significant hemoperitoneum were taken for operative exploration while those with minimal or no peritoneal fluid and severe pelvic fracture, where retroperitoneal sources of hemorrhage are likely, were resuscitated and taken for angiography. However, this occasionally resulted in negative laparotomies due to the poor sensitivity/specificity of FAST, particularly in victims of penetrating trauma. There is currently growing support for the use of CT scanning in the triage of even unstable patients with pelvic trauma. A review of 545 patients with both pelvic and abdominal trauma revealed an increasing use of pre-operative/pre-angiographic CT for triage even among patients with blood pressures ≤ 90 mm Hg. This study revealed no increase in mortality as a result of CT scanning, nor was there a significant increase in time to angiography or laparotomy as a result of CT scanning. The authors did note a significantly decreased rate of negative laparotomy from 36% to 16%, as well as a success rate of angiographic intervention in 71-74% of patients with increased CT utilization (Fang, et al., 2011). CT reveals evidence of bleeding in up to 75% of cases, with arterial sources found in up to 57% of cases. However, the majority of arterial bleeds are due to injuries in branches of the internal iliac, injuries to the iliac arteries themselves are rare (Pinto, et al., 2010; Romano, et al., 2000). It has been noted that triple phase CT scanning (arterial, venous, and portal venous) may result in increased sensitivity and specificity for diagnosis of arterial injury as compared to the typical trauma scan utilizing just the portal venous phase (Vu, et al., 2010). However, even among studies utilizing single phase "trauma" scans, if newer generation multi-detector instruments are used sensitivity can be as high as 92.6% for detecting pelvic bleeding requiring intervention (Maturen, et al., 2007). It should also be kept in mind that triple phase scans will result in increased radiation exposure and slightly increased scan times.

3. Management

Open surgery with primary repair, vein patch, and interposition or bypass grafting has been the gold standard for management of all vascular injury. However, endovascular treatment has a number of advantages over open repair including decreased ischemia time as there is no need for cross-clamping of the vessel for repair, less incisional pain, decreased recovery time and length of stay, as well as avoidance of complications related to laparotomy or thoracotomy. Endovascular treatment options include stenting, coil, and chemical embolization. Embolization is best utilized for smaller vessels and areas with rich collateral circulation such as the pelvis, or long necked pseudoaneurysms. For larger vessels and those that should not be occluded, both bare stents and covered stent-grafts are good alternatives. In general bare stents (Figure 7) are utilized for injuries which are not full thickness such as intimal tears with or without thrombosis, and dissections. For full thickness injuries, with or without bleeding, covered stent-grafts are required. Most series favor the use of self-expanding devices such as the Wallstent, Wallgraft, and Fluency as they are more flexible and do not require balloon expansion, which may worsen arterial injuries (Brandt, et al., 2001; Piffaretti, et al., 2007; White, et al., 2006). Overall utilization of endovascular therapies for acute trauma is increasing. A study of the National Trauma Data Bank (NTDB) revealed a significant increase in the number of endovascular treatments from 1997 to 2003. This increase was particularly prominent in the years spanning 2000-2003, where endovascular techniques increased from 2.4% to 8.1%. This study found that patients undergoing endovascular therapy were, in general, less severely injured than those undergoing open repair. However, after correcting for injury severity score and associated injuries patients undergoing endovascular repair retained a survival advantage over their open surgery counterparts (odds ratio for death 0.18; 95% confidence interval 0.04-0.84, p=0.029). Patients with torso arterial injury, especially thoracic aortic injury appeared to benefit most from endovascular repair (Reuben, et al., 2007). Despite the advantages of endovascular therapy there are a number of concerns that must be addressed before endovascular therapy can be widely advocated including long term patency, device failure, migration, leak, and deformation rates over time; as well as long term morbidity and mortality. The long term outcomes are particularly important to determine as the majority of trauma patients are young, and may survive many decades with their endovascular prosthetics. Further, the need for anticoagulation and antiplatelet agents in the peri-procedural time period, as well as their role in the maintenance of long term patency of stents and stent-grafts has yet to be defined. Lastly, the type and timing of follow up imaging for surveillance are all unknown at this time. The majority of studies of stent graft deployment use a combination of physical

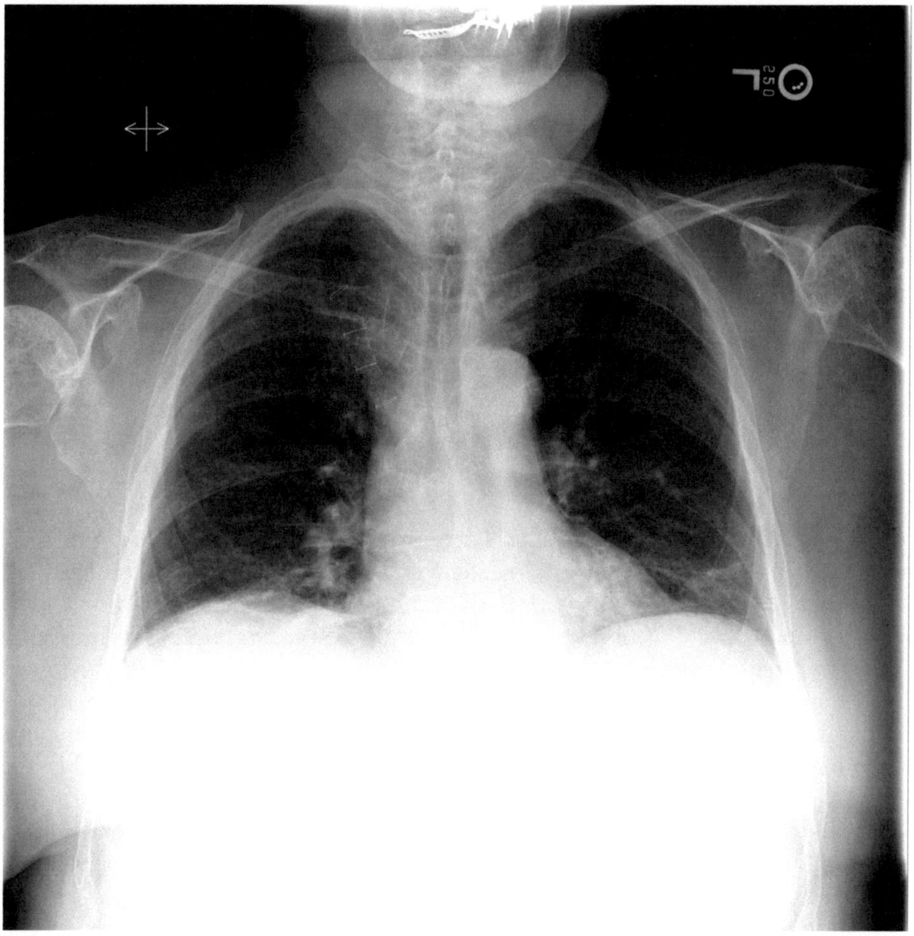

Fig. 7. Chest radiograph demonstrating bare metal stent in the right subclavian vein.

exam findings, as well as surveillance imaging for follow up. Studies use CTA, and ultrasound preferentially, no studies utilize traditional angiography as a method of surveillance, however, the optimal timing and frequency of surveillance is yet to be determined. Additionally, it is unclear if CTA will provide a significant benefit over ultrasonography in terms of sensitivity and specificity for identification of post-stent complications in locations where ultrasound is an option such as the subclavian, axillary, femoral and in certain patients iliac arteries. To surveill the arch and thoracic aorta, CT is the only non-invasive method of imaging, ultrasound requires either intravascular or transesophageal probes.

3.1 Thoracic aorta

Traditionally patients with thoracic aortic injury underwent emergent open repair, recently conservative management with blood pressure and heart rate control have allowed many patients to be temporized until open or endovascular treatment can be undertaken when the patient has been stabilized (Demetriades, et al., 2008a; Fabian, et al., 1998). Open repair is associated with significant blood loss, high mortality and morbidity, the most significant of which is paraplegia occurring in 1.6-14% of patients (Demetriades, et al., 2008a; Xenos, et al., 2008). Because of the morbidity and mortality of traditional repair, perhaps more than any other injury, the use of endovascular techniques has significantly impacted the treatment algorithm for TAI. A multicenter prospective observational study revealed significantly increased use of stent grafts for treatment of TAI (Demetriades, et al., 2008a, 2008b). There have been several retrospective case series of thoracic endovascular aortic repair (TEVAR) both with and without comparisons to open repair, however to date there have been no prospective trials. Technical success rates range from 92-100%; with complications occurring in 0-15%; leaks, when reported, range from 0-15%; and mortality ranges between 0-17.9% (Alsac, et al., 2008; Asmat, et al., 2009; Canaud, et al., 2008; Day & Buckenham. 2008; Dunham, et al., 2004; Ehrlich, et al., 2009; Garcia-Toca, et al., 2010; Moainie, et al., 2008; Oberhuber, et al., 2010; Rahimi, et al., 2010; Urgnani, et al., 2009). The leak rate may increase with time, as several studies have shown an increase in need for second intervention with follow up among TEVAR patients compared to open repair (Hershberger, et al., 2009; Lee, et al., 2011; Tang, et al., 2008). When reported the majority of leaks appear to be type I endoleaks, this is likely related to the technical difficulty in achieving a good proximal seal in the aortic arch. This difficulty is generally ascribed to the angulation of the arch, as well as the narrow aorta and difficulty with sizing stent-grafts for most young trauma patients. The majority of type I leaks are diagnosed at the time of the original procedure and treated, however, Hershberger *et al* reported 3 deaths in the literature related to failure to achieve proximal seal, highlighting the need for early detection and therapy (Hershberger, et al., 2009). Although rates of paraplegia are quoted in the literature as ranging from 0-5%, the majority of studies have no paraplegia, and three large meta-analyses found only 2 patients reported to have had paraplegia related or potentially related to TEVAR (Hershberger, et al., 2009; Tang, et al., 2008; Xenos, et al., 2008). In studies with direct comparison to open repair some studies have found no significant difference in morbidity, mortality or length of stay (Arthurs, et al., 2009; Lang, et al., 2010; Yamane, et al., 2008), while others have shown a significant decrease in mortality, blood loss, transfusion requirements, paraplegia rates, operating room times, and length of stay (Buz, et al., 2008; Moainie, et al., 2008; Rousseau, et al., 2005).

In two large meta-analyses encompassing 589 and 699 patients respectively the authors found a significant improvement in procedure related mortality and paraplegia rates among patients treated with TEVAR compared to open surgical repair. In the first meta-analysis TEVAR patients were significantly more injured, however in the second the patient demographics were roughly equivalent (Tang, et al., 2008; Xenos, et al., 2008). In a subsequent review of the literature undertaken by a panel of experts for the Society of Vascular Surgery a total of 7768 patients with TAI were identified. Compared to patients treated with medical management and open repair, patients undergoing endovascular repair had a significantly decreased mortality (46 and 19% vs. 9%). The rate of spinal cord ischemia was also decreased among TEVAR patients 9% vs. 3% (Lee, et al., 2011). Based on these findings the panel suggested that TEVAR be preferentially performed over open surgical repair or non-operative management, although based on low grade evidence (Level C).

It should be kept in mind that there have been reports of significant procedure related complications associated with TEVAR, the most common of which is iliac artery injury. Other procedure related complications include brachial artery injury and compression of the left bronchus. Additionally, when recorded the rate of stent coverage of the subclavian or carotid artery origin ranged from 50-85% (Alsac, et al., 2008; Asmat, et al., 2009; Canaud, et al., 2008; Day & Buckenham. 2008; Dunham, et al., 2004; Ehrlich, et al., 2009; Garcia-Toca, et al., 2010; Oberhuber, et al., 2010; Rahimi, et al., 2010; Urgnani, et al., 2009). Coverage of the origin of these great vessels has been associated with a risk of neurologic complication in 5.6% of patients, a rate that appears to be decreased with prophylactic re-vascularization (Hershberger, et al., 2009). Lastly long term follow up in most studies is lacking, averaging only 14-24 months (Hershberger, et al., 2009; Lee, et al., 2011; Tang, et al., 2008).

3.2 Subclavian

Because of the posterior location and intimate relationship of the subclavian artery to the brachial plexus operative exposure can be incredibly difficult, particularly in the bleeding hypotensive patient. Once localized primary repair is preferred, however tissue loss often makes this unfeasable as this vessel has very little mobility and is very friable, in these cases the vessel may be ligated or shunted. With any operative repair there is significant risk of bleeding, nerve injury, and in the case of ligation, compartment syndrome and ischemia. Operative repair is also associated with a very high mortality, up to 42% (Demetriades, et al., 1999). Because of this alternatives to open surgical repair are very attractive, and there is growing experience with covered stents for treatment of subclavian artery injuries (Figure 8, 9a, 9b, 9c). Several case series have been reported revealing mortality of 0-33%, technical success rates ranging from 67-100%, primary patency rates of 83-100%, short term complications occurring in 0-22% of patients, and long term complications ranging from 0-32% (Carrick, et al., 2010; Castelli, et al., 2005; Cohen, et al., 2008; Danetz, et al., 2005; du Toit, et al., 2008; Hilfiker, et al., 2000). Short term complications most often include access site bleeding/hematoma, infection, pseudoaneurysm and fistula. Long term complications include stent-graft stenosis, occlusion and fracture. These series are limited by relatively short term follow up and small numbers, with populations ranging from 6-57 patients, additionally the majority are limited to hemodynamically stable penetrating trauma patients, which is an uncommon presentation, and a small subset of the trauma population. A review of the literature performed by Hershberger included 23 articles describing 91 patients with subclavian artery injury treated with endovascular techniques. This review found a technical success rate of 96.7%, with a procedural complication rate of 12.1% and mortality of 3.2%. Complications included stent fracture, thrombosis, and access site pseudoaneurysm. Late complications occurred in 8.8% of patients in a mean follow up of 17 months, these included stent fracture, stenosis and occlusion (Hershberger, et al., 2009). Late stenosis and occlusions can be diagnosed with surveillance imaging or by directed investigations after patients develop symptoms. Interestingly, one study found patients with stenosis all presented with symptoms of claudication, while those with occlusion were all asymptomatic (du Toit, et al., 2008).

In most series, patients who were unstable were not considered for endovascular therapy, and in one series, the authors report one patient dying of exsanguinations in the angiography suite (Carrick, et al., 2010). Despite this, some centers with significant endovascular experience and 24 hour a day on call interventional teams have utilized stent-grafts in unstable patients with some success (Cohen, et al., 2008). Other considerations/contra-indications for endovascular repair include vessel transection, and lack of a proximal vascular fixation site. In some cases stent-graft deployment may occlude the origins of one of the subclavian artery branches, the most important of which are the vertebral and internal mammary artery. If the vertebral may be occluded it is imperative to assess if the contralateral vertebral circulation is intact, and if cerebral perfusion will be maintained after occlusion. The internal mammary may be sacrificed however, at the cost of future use for cardiac revascularization. If all of these considerations are taken into account, approximately 37% of patients presenting with subclavian artery injuries may be amenable to endovascular repair (Danetz, et al., 2005).

There is some suggestion that more flexible stents may result in better outcomes with lower rates of graft deformation or compression in comparison to stiffer devices such as the Wallgraft (du Toit, et al., 2008). This is likely to be of particular importance when treating distal lesions that may be near, or span a joint and be subject to a great deal of motion and extrinsic compression at the thoracic outlet and across the shoulder joint. While endovascular therapies most often consist of stent-graft deployment, there have been case reports of coil and thrombin embolization of pseudoaneurysms of the subclavian with good success (Lee, et al., 2010).

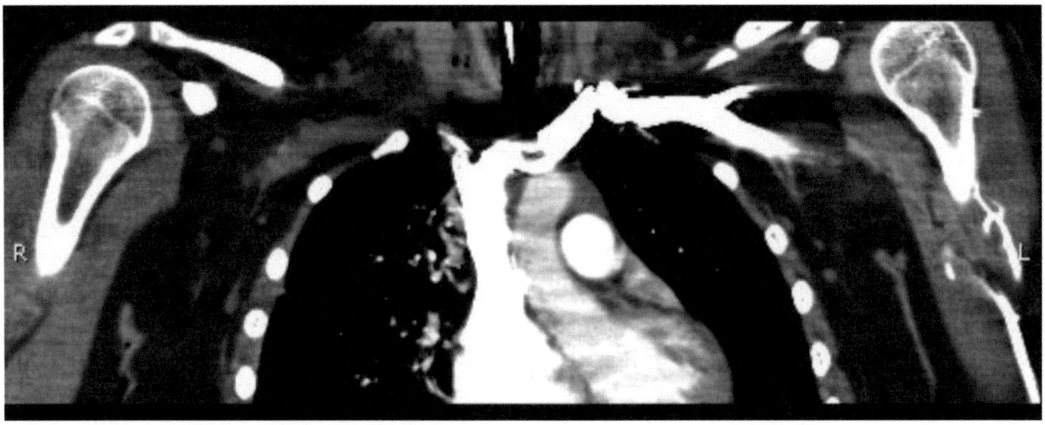

Fig. 8. Coronal CT depicting occlusion of the right subclavian artery following gunshot wound. Note the birdsbeak like tapering of the artery and surrounding subcutaneous emphysema in the neck and mediastinum.

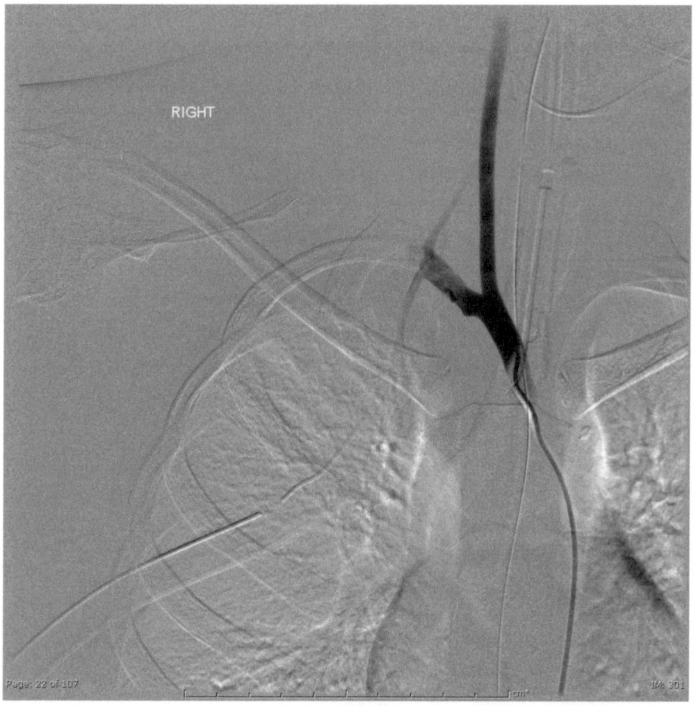

(a)

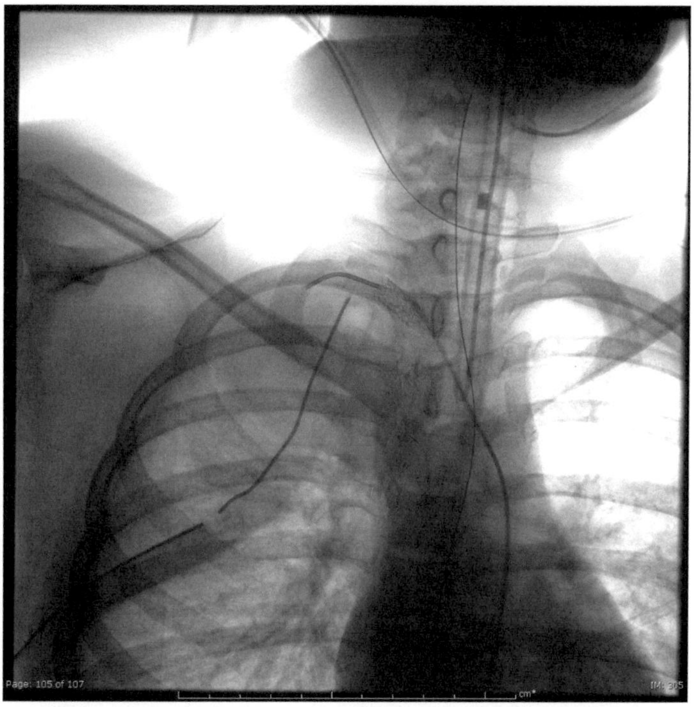

(b)

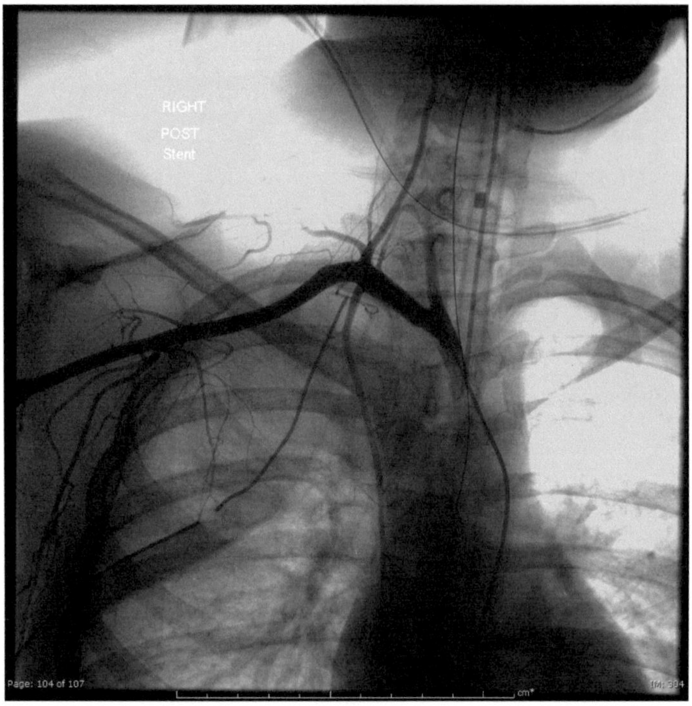

(c)

Fig. 9. Subclavian artery injury: Angiogram depicting a) occlusion at the proximal right subclavian artery similar to the CT scan b) stent deployment across the injury without contrast c) with contrast demonstrating restoration of flow and no evidence of contrast extravasation

3.3 Iliac

Iliac arterial injury has historically been known for the difficulty of its exposure particularly in the narrow male pelvis, and its repair is rife with the potential for complications and blood loss. Advances in endovascular therapies have significantly changed the treatment approach for this rare and difficult injury. In patients who are hemodynamically stable but with severe pelvic fractures or with evidence of active extravasation on CT scan, angiography and embolization is now the treatment of choice for injuries to the internal iliac artery or its branches (Cherry, et al., 2011; Reuben, et al., 2007; Velmahos, et al., 2002). In operative cases, the use of endovascular adjuncts, pre, post, or intra-operatively has been increasing in frequency (Cherry, et al., 2011). Even among patients who present with hemodynamic instability, or ongoing transfusion requirements, angiography is increasingly viewed as an acceptable primary treatment option resulting in hemodynamic stabilization and a survival rate of 72-92% (Cherry, et al., 2011; Fang, et al., 2011; Fu, et al., 2010). Studies have also investigated the role of mobile angiography with capabilities of performing angioembolization in the emergency department with good outcomes (Morozumi, et al., 2010).

Angiographic embolization of the internal iliac artery or its branches with coils or gelfoam is common and well tolerated (Costantini, et al., 2010; Velmahos, et al., 1999). Embolization is successful in arresting hemorrhage in 80-100% of cases (Fangio, et al., 2005; Velmahos, et al., 2002). Embolization can be performed with gelfoam, which is particularly suited to highly selective embolization of branch vessels. The gelfoam can be delivered easily, and is absorbed with subsequent recanalization of the vessel in a few weeks. In larger vesssels and pseudoaneurysms, coils may be required to achieve hemostasis. Gelfoam can be used to supplement the coils as well. In cases where selective angio-emoblization is not possible, or for patients in whom the risk of hemorrhage is high, but no active bleeding is seen at angiography, bilateral internal iliac artery embolization can be performed with a gelfoam slurry. The slurry is propelled by antegrade flow and fills the majority of the hypogastric circulation. While a few case reports of ischemic complications of bilateral internal iliac artery embolization exist, major complications following therapeutic or prophylactic angioembolization are rare (Christopher J. Dente, David V. Feliciano ,2008; gracias, v. reilly, p. mckenny, m. velmahos, g ,2009; Ramirez, et al., 2004; Velmahos, et al., 2000; Velmahos, et al., 2002). Re-bleeding, or continued hemorrhage following therapeutic angioembolization is rare, occurring in about 7% of cases (Boufi, et al., 2011; Gourlay, et al., 2005). However, because of the risk of re-bleeding many trauma surgeons and interventional radiologists recommend leaving the arterial access sheath in place following the first angiogram for at least 24 hours (Christopher J. Dente, David V. Feliciano ,2008; Gracias, V. Reilly, P. Mckenny, M. Velmahos, G ,2009).

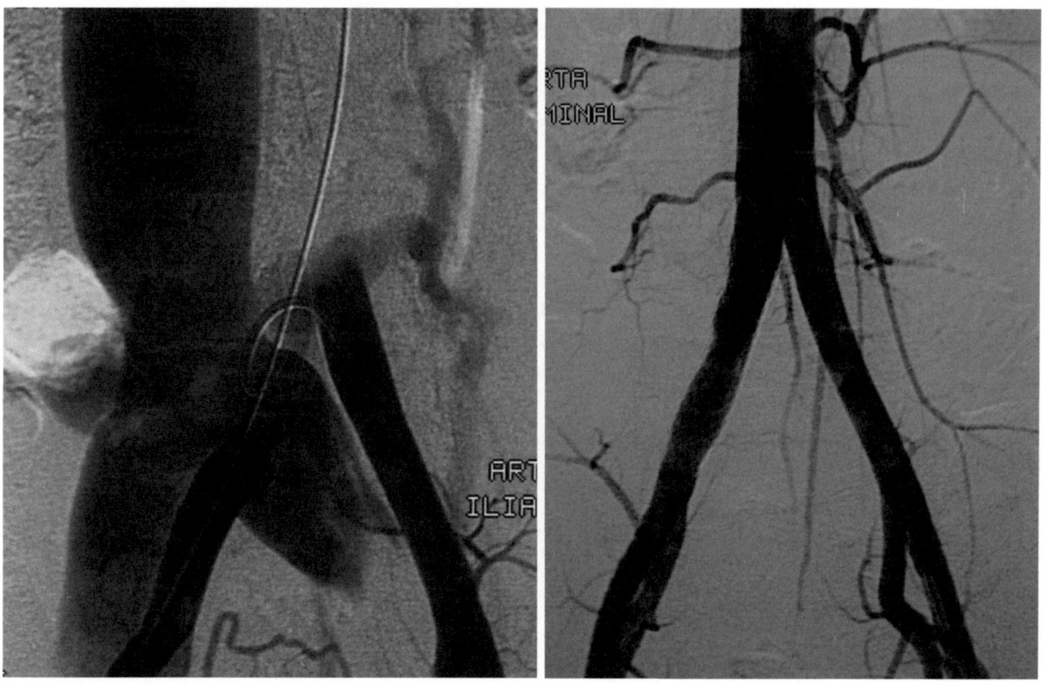

(a) (b)

Fig. 10. Aortogram depicting a) right common iliac arteriovenous fistula with immediate filling of the inferior vena cava via the fistula and b) stent graft deployed in the artery occluding flow through the fistula

Good outcomes with the placement of covered stent grafts across external and common iliac artery injuries (Figure 10) have been described, however these have been small series (Boufi, et al., 2011; Shah, et al., 2003; Starnes&Arthurs. 2006). Success rates vary from 75-100%, with complications occurring in very few patients, however, follow up was variable (Boufi, et al., 2011; Piffaretti, et al., 2007; Shah, et al., 2003). One of the larger series utilizing Wallgraft stent-grafts including 33 iliac artery injuries reports a post-procedure exclusion rate of 93.5%, a one-year exclusion rate of 91.3%, a one year primary patency rate of 76.4%, and bypass free rate of 74.3%. Complications were rare occurring in less than 10% of cases, the most common was stent-graft occlusion followed by stenosis. However, the majority of injuries treated in this study were due to iatrogenic causes, with only 13 injuries due to trauma, the majority of which were blunt (White, et al., 2006).

4. Conclusion

Vascular injury whether central or peripheral remains a challenge to the trauma surgeon. These injuries are rare and lethal, preventing even senior physicians from gaining significant experience with their management. Timely diagnosis and treatment are essential for a positive outcome, and the increasing availability and advances in imaging technology have aided in these efforts. Nowhere has this been more apparent than in the increasing utilization and accuracy of CT scanning, which is fast becoming the dominant mode of diagnosis for most vascular lesions in stable or semi-stable patients. Foreknowledge of these injuries can aid in planning incisions and operative strategy, and allows for directed therapeutic endovascular therapy in an increasing number of vascular injuries. The most common of which is the thoracic aorta. The literature to date is promising, firmly establishing that endovascular therapy is possible in an increasing number of patients, for an ever broadening range of indications. However, long term outcomes are unknown, and the optimal means, method and timing of surveillance imaging have yet to be determined.

5. References

Alsac J.M., Boura B., Desgranges P., Fabiani J.N., Becquemin J.P., Leseche G. & PARIS-VASC. (2008). Immediate endovascular repair for acute traumatic injuries of the thoracic aorta: a multicenter analysis of 28 cases. *Journal of Vascular Surgery : Official Publication, the Society for Vascular Surgery [and] International Society for Cardiovascular Surgery, North American Chapter,* 48, 6, (Dec), pp. (1369-1374), 1097-6809; 0741-5214.

Anderson S.W., Foster B.R. & Soto J.A. (2008). Upper extremity CT angiography in penetrating trauma: use of 64-section multidetector CT. *Radiology,* 249, 3, (Dec), pp. (1064-1073), 1527-1315; 0033-8419.

Arthurs Z.M., Starnes B.W., Sohn V.Y., Singh N., Martin M.J. & Andersen C.A. (2009). Functional and survival outcomes in traumatic blunt thoracic aortic injuries: An analysis of the National Trauma Databank. *Journal of Vascular Surgery : Official Publication, the Society for Vascular Surgery [and] International Society for Cardiovascular Surgery, North American Chapter,* 49, 4, (Apr), pp. (988-994), 1097-6809; 0741-5214.

Asensio J.A., Chahwan S., Hanpeter D., Demetriades D., Forno W., Gambaro E., Murray J., Velmahos G., Marengo J., Shoemaker W.C. & Berne T.V. (2000). Operative management and outcome of 302 abdominal vascular injuries. *American Journal of Surgery*, 180, 6, (Dec), pp. (528-33; discussion 533-4), 0002-9610; 0002-9610.

Asensio J.A., Britt L.D., Borzotta A., Peitzman A., Miller F.B., Mackersie R.C., Pasquale M.D., Pachter H.L., Hoyt D.B., Rodriguez J.L., Falcone R., Davis K., Anderson J.T., Ali J. & Chan L. (2001a). Multiinstitutional experience with the management of superior mesenteric artery injuries. *Journal of the American College of Surgeons*, 193, 4, (Oct), pp. (354-65; discussion 365-6), 1072-7515; 1072-7515.

Asensio J.A., Britt L.D., Borzotta A., Peitzman A., Miller F.B., Mackersie R.C., Pasquale M.D., Pachter H.L., Hoyt D.B., Rodriguez J.L., Falcone R., Davis K., Anderson J.T., Ali J. & Chan L. (2001b). Multiinstitutional experience with the management of superior mesenteric artery injuries. *Journal of the American College of Surgeons*, 193, 4, (Oct), pp. (354-65; discussion 365-6), 1072-7515; 1072-7515.

Asensio J.A., Forno W., Roldan G., Petrone P., Rojo E., Ceballos J., Wang C., Costaglioli B., Romero J., Tillou A., Carmody I., Shoemaker W.C. & Berne T.V. (2002). Visceral vascular injuries. *The Surgical Clinics of North America*, 82, 1, (Feb), pp. (1-20, xix), 0039-6109; 0039-6109.

Asensio J.A., Petrone P., Roldan G., Kuncir E., Rowe V.L., Chan L., Shoemaker W. & Berne T.V. (2003). Analysis of 185 iliac vessel injuries: risk factors and predictors of outcome. *Archives of Surgery (Chicago, Ill.: 1960)*, 138, 11, (Nov), pp. (1187-93; discussion 1193-4), 0004-0010; 0004-0010.

Asmat A., Tan L., Caleb M.G., Lee C.N. & Robless P.A. (2009). Endovascular management of traumatic thoracic aortic transection. *Asian Cardiovascular & Thoracic Annals*, 17, 5, (Oct), pp. (458-461), 1816-5370; 0218-4923.

Azizzadeh A., Valdes J., Miller C.C.,3rd, Nguyen L.L., Estrera A.L., Charlton-Ouw K., Coogan S.M., Holcomb J.B. & Safi H.J. (2011). The utility of intravascular ultrasound compared to angiography in the diagnosis of blunt traumatic aortic injury. *Journal of Vascular Surgery : Official Publication, the Society for Vascular Surgery [and] International Society for Cardiovascular Surgery, North American Chapter*, 53, 3, (Mar), pp. (608-614), 1097-6809; 0741-5214.

Barrios C., Malinoski D., Dolich M., Lekawa M., Hoyt D. & Cinat M. (2009). Utility of thoracic computed tomography after blunt trauma: when is chest radiograph enough? *The American Surgeon*, 75, 10, (Oct), pp. (966-969), 0003-1348; 0003-1348.

Bellin M.F., Jakobsen J.A., Tomassin I., Thomsen H.S., Morcos S.K., Thomsen H.S., Morcos S.K., Almen T., Aspelin P., Bellin M.F., Clauss W., Flaten H., Grenier N., Idee J.M., Jakobsen J.A., Krestin G.P., Stacul F., Webb J.A. & Contrast Media Safety Committee Of The European Society Of Urogenital Radiology. (2002). Contrast medium extravasation injury: guidelines for prevention and management. *European Radiology*, 12, 11, (Nov), pp. (2807-2812), 0938-7994; 0938-7994.

Bertrand S., Cuny S., Petit P., Trosseille X., Page Y., Guillemot H. & Drazetic P. (2008). Traumatic rupture of thoracic aorta in real-world motor vehicle crashes. *Traffic Injury Prevention*, 9, 2, (Jun), pp. (153-161), 1538-957X; 1538-9588.

Boufi M., Bordon S., Dona B., Hartung O., Sarran A., Nadeau S., Maurin C. & Alimi Y.S. (2011). Unstable patients with retroperitoneal vascular trauma: an endovascular approach. *Annals of Vascular Surgery*, 25, 3, (Apr), pp. (352-358), 1615-5947; 0890-5096.

Brandt M.M., Kazanjian S. & Wahl W.L. (2001). The utility of endovascular stents in the treatment of blunt arterial injuries. *The Journal of Trauma,* 51, 5, (Nov), pp. (901-905), 0022-5282; 0022-5282.

Bruckner B.A., DiBardino D.J., Cumbie T.C., Trinh C., Blackmon S.H., Fisher R.G., Mattox K.L. & Wall M.J. (2006). Critical evaluation of chest computed tomography scans for blunt descending thoracic aortic injury. *The Annals of Thoracic Surgery,* 81, 4, (Apr), pp. (1339-1346), 1552-6259; 0003-4975.

Buckmaster M.J., Kearney P.A., Johnson S.B., Smith M.D. & Sapin P.M. (1994). Further experience with transesophageal echocardiography in the evaluation of thoracic aortic injury. *The Journal of Trauma,* 37, 6, (Dec), pp. (989-995), 0022-5282; 0022-5282.

Buz S., Zipfel B., Mulahasanovic S., Pasic M., Weng Y. & Hetzer R. (2008). Conventional surgical repair and endovascular treatment of acute traumatic aortic rupture. *European Journal of Cardio-Thoracic Surgery : Official Journal of the European Association for Cardio-Thoracic Surgery,* 33, 2, (Feb), pp. (143-149), 1010-7940; 1010-7940.

Canaud L., Alric P., Branchereau P., Marty-Ane C. & Berthet J.P. (2008). Lessons learned from midterm follow-up of endovascular repair for traumatic rupture of the aortic isthmus. *Journal of Vascular Surgery : Official Publication, the Society for Vascular Surgery [and] International Society for Cardiovascular Surgery, North American Chapter,* 47, 4, (Apr), pp. (733-738), 0741-5214; 0741-5214.

Carrick M.M., Morrison C.A., Pham H.Q., Norman M.A., Marvin B., Lee J., Wall M.J.,Jr & Mattox K.L. (2010). Modern management of traumatic subclavian artery injuries: a single institution's experience in the evolution of endovascular repair. *American Journal of Surgery,* 199, 1, (Jan), pp. (28-34), 1879-1883; 0002-9610.

Castelli P., Caronno R., Piffaretti G., Tozzi M., Lagana D., Carrafiello G. & Cuffari S. (2005). Endovascular repair of traumatic injuries of the subclavian and axillary arteries. *Injury,* 36, 6, (Jun), pp. (778-782), 0020-1383; 0020-1383.

Cestero R.F., Plurad D., Green D., Inaba K., Putty B., Benfield R., Lam L., Talving P. & Demetriades D. (2009). Iliac artery injuries and pelvic fractures: a national trauma database analysis of associated injuries and outcomes. *The Journal of Trauma,* 67, 4, (Oct), pp. (715-718), 1529-8809; 0022-5282.

Cherry R.A., Goodspeed D.C., Lynch F.C., Delgado J. & Reid J.S. (2011). Intraoperative angioembolization in the management of pelvic-fracture related hemodynamic instability. *Journal of Trauma Management & Outcomes,* 5, 1, (May 13), pp. (6), 1752-2897; 1752-2897.

Chirillo F., Totis O., Cavarzerani A., Bruni A., Farnia A., Sarpellon M., Ius P., Valfre C. & Stritoni P. (1996). Usefulness of transthoracic and transoesophageal echocardiography in recognition and management of cardiovascular injuries after blunt chest trauma. *Heart (British Cardiac Society),* 75, 3, (Mar), pp. (301-306), 1355-6037; 1355-6037.

Christopher J. Dente, David V. Feliciano. Abdominal Vascular Injury. In: David V. Feliciano, Kenneth L. Mattox, Ernest E. Moore, ed. *Trauma.* McGraw Hill Medical: NY NY; 2008:737.

Cinnella G., Dambrosio M., Brienza N., Tullo L. & Fiore T. (2004). Transesophageal echocardiography for diagnosis of traumatic aortic injury: an appraisal of the evidence. *The Journal of Trauma,* 57, 6, (Dec), pp. (1246-1255), 0022-5282; 0022-5282.

Cohen J.E., Rajz G., Gomori J.M., Verstandig A., Berlatzky Y., Anner H., Grigoriadis S., Lylyk P., Ceratto R. & Klimov A. (2008). Urgent endovascular stent-graft placement for traumatic penetrating subclavian artery injuries. *Journal of the Neurological Sciences*, 272, 1-2, (Sep 15), pp. (151-157), 0022-510X; 0022-510X.

Collins R., Cranny G., Burch J., Aguiar-Ibanez R., Craig D., Wright K., Berry E., Gough M., Kleijnen J. & Westwood M. (2007). A systematic review of duplex ultrasound, magnetic resonance angiography and computed tomography angiography for the diagnosis and assessment of symptomatic, lower limb peripheral arterial disease. *Health Technology Assessment (Winchester, England)*, 11, 20, (May), pp. (iii-iv, xi-xiii, 1-184), 1366-5278; 1366-5278.

Costantini T.W., Bosarge P.L., Fortlage D., Bansal V. & Coimbra R. (2010). Arterial embolization for pelvic fractures after blunt trauma: are we all talk? *American Journal of Surgery*, 200, 6, (Dec), pp. (752-7; discussion 757-8), 1879-1883; 0002-9610.

Cushman J.G., Feliciano D.V., Renz B.M., Ingram W.L., Ansley J.D., Clark W.S. & Rozycki G.S. (1997). Iliac vessel injury: operative physiology related to outcome. *The Journal of Trauma*, 42, 6, (Jun), pp. (1033-1040), 0022-5282; 0022-5282.

Danetz J.S., Cassano A.D., Stoner M.C., Ivatury R.R. & Levy M.M. (2005). Feasibility of endovascular repair in penetrating axillosubclavian injuries: a retrospective review. *Journal of Vascular Surgery : Official Publication, the Society for Vascular Surgery [and] International Society for Cardiovascular Surgery, North American Chapter*, 41, 2, (Feb), pp. (246-254), 0741-5214; 0741-5214.

Day C.P. & Buckenham T.M. (2008). Outcomes of endovascular repair of acute thoracic aortic injury: interrogation of the New Zealand thoracic aortic stent database (NZ TAS). *European Journal of Vascular and Endovascular Surgery : The Official Journal of the European Society for Vascular Surgery*, 36, 5, (Nov), pp. (530-534), 1532-2165; 1078-5884.

Demetriades D., Theodorou D., Cornwell E., Berne T.V., Asensio J., Belzberg H., Velmahos G., Weaver F. & Yellin A. (1997). Evaluation of penetrating injuries of the neck: prospective study of 223 patients. *World Journal of Surgery*, 21, 1, (Jan), pp. (41-7; discussion 47-8), 0364-2313; 0364-2313.

Demetriades D., Gomez H., Velmahos G.C., Asensio J.A., Murray J., Cornwell E.E.,3rd, Alo K. & Berne T.V. (1998). Routine helical computed tomographic evaluation of the mediastinum in high-risk blunt trauma patients. *Archives of Surgery (Chicago, Ill.: 1960)*, 133, 10, (Oct), pp. (1084-1088), 0004-0010; 0004-0010.

Demetriades D., Chahwan S., Gomez H., Peng R., Velmahos G., Murray J., Asensio J. & Bongard F. (1999). Penetrating injuries to the subclavian and axillary vessels. *Journal of the American College of Surgeons*, 188, 3, (Mar), pp. (290-295), 1072-7515; 1072-7515.

Demetriades D., Velmahos G.C., Scalea T.M., Jurkovich G.J., Karmy-Jones R., Teixeira P.G., Hemmila M.R., O'Connor J.V., McKenney M.O., Moore F.O., London J., Singh M.J., Lineen E., Spaniolas K., Keel M., Sugrue M., Wahl W.L., Hill J., Wall M.J., Moore E.E., Margulies D., Malka V., Chan L.S. & American Association for the Surgery of Trauma Thoracic Aortic Injury Study Group. (2008a). Operative repair or endovascular stent graft in blunt traumatic thoracic aortic injuries: results of an American Association for the Surgery of Trauma Multicenter Study. *The Journal of Trauma*, 64, 3, (Mar), pp. (561-70; discussion 570-1), 1529-8809; 0022-5282.

Demetriades D., Velmahos G.C., Scalea T.M., Jurkovich G.J., Karmy-Jones R., Teixeira P.G., Hemmila M.R., O'Connor J.V., McKenney M.O., Moore F.O., London J., Singh M.J., Spaniolas K., Keel M., Sugrue M., Wahl W.L., Hill J., Wall M.J., Moore E.E., Lineen E., Margulies D., Malka V. & Chan L.S. (2008b). Diagnosis and treatment of blunt thoracic aortic injuries: changing perspectives. *The Journal of Trauma*, 64, 6, (Jun), pp. (1415-8; discussion 1418-9), 1529-8809; 0022-5282.

Dennis J.W., Frykberg E.R., Veldenz H.C., Huffman S. & Menawat S.S. (1998). Validation of nonoperative management of occult vascular injuries and accuracy of physical examination alone in penetrating extremity trauma: 5- to 10-year follow-up. *The Journal of Trauma*, 44, 2, (Feb), pp. (243-52; discussion 242-3), 0022-5282; 0022-5282.

Doody O., Given M.F. & Lyon S.M. (2008). Extremities--indications and techniques for treatment of extremity vascular injuries. *Injury*, 39, 11, (Nov), pp. (1295-1303), 1879-0267; 0020-1383.

du Toit D.F., Lambrechts A.V., Stark H. & Warren B.L. (2008). Long-term results of stent graft treatment of subclavian artery injuries: management of choice for stable patients? *Journal of Vascular Surgery : Official Publication, the Society for Vascular Surgery [and] International Society for Cardiovascular Surgery, North American Chapter*, 47, 4, (Apr), pp. (739-743), 0741-5214; 0741-5214.

Dunham M.B., Zygun D., Petrasek P., Kortbeek J.B., Karmy-Jones R. & Moore R.D. (2004). Endovascular stent grafts for acute blunt aortic injury. *The Journal of Trauma*, 56, 6, (Jun), pp. (1173-1178), 0022-5282; 0022-5282.

Dyer D.S., Moore E.E., Ilke D.N., McIntyre R.C., Bernstein S.M., Durham J.D., Mestek M.F., Heinig M.J., Russ P.D., Symonds D.L., Honigman B., Kumpe D.A., Roe E.J. & Eule J.,Jr. (2000). Thoracic aortic injury: how predictive is mechanism and is chest computed tomography a reliable screening tool? A prospective study of 1,561 patients. *The Journal of Trauma*, 48, 4, (Apr), pp. (673-82; discussion 682-3), 0022-5282; 0022-5282.

Ehrlich M.P., Rousseau H., Heijman R., Piquet P., Beregi J.P., Nienaber C.A., Sodeck G. & Fattori R. (2009). Early outcome of endovascular treatment of acute traumatic aortic injuries: the talent thoracic retrospective registry. *The Annals of Thoracic Surgery*, 88, 4, (Oct), pp. (1258-1263), 1552-6259; 0003-4975.

Exadaktylos A.K., Duwe J., Eckstein F., Stoupis C., Schoenfeld H., Zimmermann H. & Carrel T.P. (2005). The role of contrast-enhanced spiral CT imaging versus chest X-rays in surgical therapeutic concepts and thoracic aortic injury: a 29-year Swiss retrospective analysis of aortic surgery. *Cardiovascular Journal of South Africa : Official Journal for Southern Africa Cardiac Society [and] South African Society of Cardiac Practitioners*, 16, 3, (May-Jun), pp. (162-165), 1015-9657; 1015-9657.

Fabian T.C., Davis K.A., Gavant M.L., Croce M.A., Melton S.M., Patton J.H.,Jr, Haan C.K., Weiman D.S. & Pate J.W. (1998). Prospective study of blunt aortic injury: helical CT is diagnostic and antihypertensive therapy reduces rupture. *Annals of Surgery*, 227, 5, (May), pp. (666-76; discussion 676-7), 0003-4932; 0003-4932.

Fang J.F., Shih L.Y., Wong Y.C., Lin B.C. & Hsu Y.P. (2011). Angioembolization and laparotomy for patients with concomitant pelvic arterial hemorrhage and blunt abdominal trauma. *Langenbeck's Archives of Surgery / Deutsche Gesellschaft Fur Chirurgie*, 396, 2, (Feb), pp. (243-250), 1435-2451; 1435-2443.

Fangio P., Asehnoune K., Edouard A., Smail N. & Benhamou D. (2005). Early embolization and vasopressor administration for management of life-threatening hemorrhage from pelvic fracture. *The Journal of Trauma,* 58, 5, (May), pp. (978-84; discussion 984), 0022-5282; 0022-5282.

Fanucci E., Fiaschetti V., Rotili A., Floris R. & Simonetti G. (2007). Whole body 16-row multislice CT in emergency room: effects of different protocols on scanning time, image quality and radiation exposure. *Emergency Radiology,* 13, 5, (Feb), pp. (251-257), 1070-3004; 1070-3004.

Fattori R., Celletti F., Bertaccini P., Galli R., Pacini D., Pierangeli A. & Gavelli G. (1996). Delayed surgery of traumatic aortic rupture. Role of magnetic resonance imaging. *Circulation,* 94, 11, (Dec 1), pp. (2865-2870), 0009-7322; 0009-7322.

Feliciano D.V., Moore F.A., Moore E.E., West M., Davis J., Cocanour C.S., Kozar R.A. & McIntyre R.C. (2011). Evaulation and management of peripheral vascular injury. Part 1. Western Trauma Association/Critical Decision in Trauma. 70, 6, (June 2011), pp. (1551),.

Fisher R.G., Chasen M.H. & Lamki N. (1994). Diagnosis of injuries of the aorta and brachiocephalic arteries caused by blunt chest trauma: CT vs aortography. *AJR.American Journal of Roentgenology,* 162, 5, (May), pp. (1047-1052), 0361-803X; 0361-803X.

Fitzharris M., Franklyn M., Frampton R., Yang K., Morris A. & Fildes B. (2004). Thoracic aortic injury in motor vehicle crashes: the effect of impact direction, side of body struck, and seat belt use. *The Journal of Trauma,* 57, 3, (Sep), pp. (582-590), 0022-5282; 0022-5282.

Flamm S.D. (2007). Cross-sectional imaging studies: what can we learn and what do we need to know? *Seminars in Vascular Surgery,* 20, 2, (Jun), pp. (108-114), 0895-7967; 0895-7967.

Fleiter T.R. & Mervis S. (2007). The role of 3D-CTA in the assessment of peripheral vascular lesions in trauma patients. *European Journal of Radiology,* 64, 1, (Oct), pp. (92-102), 0720-048X; 0720-048X.

Fruhwirth J., Pascher O., Hauser H. & Amann W. (1996). Local vascular complications after iatrogenic femoral artery puncture. *Wiener Klinische Wochenschrift,* 108, 7, pp. (196-200), 0043-5325; 0043-5325.

Frykberg E.R., Dennis J.W., Bishop K., Laneve L. & Alexander R.H. (1991). The reliability of physical examination in the evaluation of penetrating extremity trauma for vascular injury: results at one year. *The Journal of Trauma,* 31, 4, (Apr), pp. (502-511), 0022-5282; 0022-5282.

Fu C.Y., Wang Y.C., Wu S.C., Chen R.J., Hsieh C.H., Huang H.C., Huang J.C., Lu C.W. & Huang Y.C. (2010). Angioembolization provides benefits in patients with concomitant unstable pelvic fracture and unstable hemodynamics. *The American Journal of Emergency Medicine,* (Dec 13), 1532-8171; 0735-6757.

Garcia-Toca M., Naughton P.A., Matsumura J.S., Morasch M.D., Kibbe M.R., Rodriguez H.E., Pearce W.H. & Eskandari M.K. (2010). Endovascular repair of blunt traumatic thoracic aortic injuries: seven-year single-center experience. *Archives of Surgery (Chicago, Ill.: 1960),* 145, 7, (Jul), pp. (679-683), 1538-3644; 0004-0010.

Goarin J.P., Cluzel P., Gosgnach M., Lamine K., Coriat P. & Riou B. (2000). Evaluation of transesophageal echocardiography for diagnosis of traumatic aortic injury. *Anesthesiology,* 93, 6, (Dec), pp. (1373-1377), 0003-3022; 0003-3022.

Goldman J.P. (2003). New techniques and applications for magnetic resonance angiography. *The Mount Sinai Journal of Medicine, New York,* 70, 6, (Nov), pp. (375-385), 0027-2507; 0027-2507.

Gonzalez R.P. & Falimirski M.E. (1999). The utility of physical examination in proximity penetrating extremity trauma. *The American Surgeon,* 65, 8, (Aug), pp. (784-789), 0003-1348; 0003-1348.

Gourlay D., Hoffer E., Routt M. & Bulger E. (2005). Pelvic angiography for recurrent traumatic pelvic arterial hemorrhage. *The Journal of Trauma,* 59, 5, (Nov), pp. (1168-73; discussion 1173-4), 0022-5282; 0022-5282.

Gracias, V. Reilly, P. Mckenny, M. Velmahos, G. (Ed.). (2009). *Acute Care Surgery: A Guide for General Surgeons.* McGraw-Hill.

Hanpeter D.E., Demetriades D., Asensio J.A., Berne T.V., Velmahos G. & Murray J. (2000). Helical computed tomographic scan in the evaluation of mediastinal gunshot wounds. *The Journal of Trauma,* 49, 4, (Oct), pp. (689-94; discussion 694-5), 0022-5282; 0022-5282.

Haveman J.W., Gansevoort R.T., Bongaerts A.H. & Nijsten M.W. (2006). Low incidence of nephropathy in surgical ICU patients receiving intravenous contrast: a retrospective analysis. *Intensive Care Medicine,* 32, 8, (Aug), pp. (1199-1205), 0342-4642; 0342-4642.

Hershberger R.C., Aulivola B., Murphy M. & Luchette F.A. (2009). Endovascular grafts for treatment of traumatic injury to the aortic arch and great vessels. *The Journal of Trauma,* 67, 3, (Sep), pp. (660-671), 1529-8809; 0022-5282.

Hilfiker P.R., Razavi M.K., Kee S.T., Sze D.Y., Semba C.P. & Dake M.D. (2000). Stent-graft therapy for subclavian artery aneurysms and fistulas: single-center mid-term results. *Journal of Vascular and Interventional Radiology : JVIR,* 11, 5, (May), pp. (578-584), 1051-0443; 1051-0443.

Hood D.B., Weaver F.A. & Yellin A.E. (1998). Changing perspectives in the diagnosis of peripheral vascular trauma. *Seminars in Vascular Surgery,* 11, 4, (Dec), pp. (255-260), 0895-7967; 0895-7967.

Hoyt D.B., Coimbra R., Potenza B.M. & Rappold J.F. (2001). Anatomic exposures for vascular injuries. *The Surgical Clinics of North America,* 81, 6, (Dec), pp. (1299-330, xii), 0039-6109; 0039-6109.

Ibirogba S., Nicol A.J. & Navsaria P.H. (2007). Screening helical computed tomographic scanning in haemodynamic stable patients with transmediastinal gunshot wounds. *Injury,* 38, 1, (Jan), pp. (48-52), 0020-1383; 0020-1383.

Inaba K., Potzman J., Munera F., McKenney M., Munoz R., Rivas L., Dunham M. & DuBose J. (2006). Multi-slice CT angiography for arterial evaluation in the injured lower extremity. *The Journal of Trauma,* 60, 3, (Mar), pp. (502-6; discussion 506-7), 0022-5282; 0022-5282.

Itani K.M., Burch J.M., Spjut-Patrinely V., Richardson R., Martin R.R. & Mattox K.L. (1992). Emergency center arteriography. *The Journal of Trauma,* 32, 3, (Mar), pp. (302-6; discussion 306-7), 0022-5282; 0022-5282.

Kaiser M.L., Whealon M.D., Barrios C.,Jr, Dobson S.C., Malinoski D.J., Dolich M.O., Lekawa M.E., Hoyt D.B. & Cinat M.E. (2011). Risk factors for traumatic injury findings on thoracic computed tomography among patients with blunt trauma having a normal chest radiograph. *Archives of Surgery (Chicago, Ill.: 1960),* 146, 4, (Apr), pp. (459-463), 1538-3644; 0004-0010.

Kearney P.A., Smith D.W., Johnson S.B., Barker D.E., Smith M.D. & Sapin P.M. (1993). Use of transesophageal echocardiography in the evaluation of traumatic aortic injury. *The Journal of Trauma,* 34, 5, (May), pp. (696-701; discussion 701-3), 0022-5282; 0022-5282.

Khalil A., Helmy T. & Porembka D.T. (2007). Aortic pathology: aortic trauma, debris, dissection, and aneurysm. *Critical Care Medicine,* 35, 8 Suppl, (Aug), pp. (S392-400), 0090-3493; 0090-3493.

Lang J.L., Minei J.P., Modrall J.G., Clagett G.P. & Valentine R.J. (2010). The limitations of thoracic endovascular aortic repair in altering the natural history of blunt aortic injury. *Journal of Vascular Surgery : Official Publication, the Society for Vascular Surgery [and] International Society for Cardiovascular Surgery, North American Chapter,* 52, 2, (Aug), pp. (290-7; discussion 297), 1097-6809; 0741-5214.

LeBlang S.D. & Dolich M.O. (2000). Imaging of penetrating thoracic trauma. *Journal of Thoracic Imaging,* 15, 2, (Apr), pp. (128-135), 0883-5993; 0883-5993.

Lee G.S., Brawley J. & Hung R. (2010). Complex subclavian artery pseudoaneurysm causing failure of endovascular stent repair with salvage by percutaneous thrombin injection. *Journal of Vascular Surgery : Official Publication, the Society for Vascular Surgery [and] International Society for Cardiovascular Surgery, North American Chapter,* 52, 4, (Oct), pp. (1058-1060), 1097-6809; 0741-5214.

Lee W.A., Matsumura J.S., Mitchell R.S., Farber M.A., Greenberg R.K., Azizzadeh A., Murad M.H. & Fairman R.M. (2011). Endovascular repair of traumatic thoracic aortic injury: clinical practice guidelines of the Society for Vascular Surgery. *Journal of Vascular Surgery : Official Publication, the Society for Vascular Surgery [and] International Society for Cardiovascular Surgery, North American Chapter,* 53, 1, (Jan), pp. (187-192), 1097-6809; 0741-5214.

Lencioni R., Fattori R., Morana G. & Stacul F. (2010). Contrast-induced nephropathy in patients undergoing computed tomography (CONNECT) - a clinical problem in daily practice? A multicenter observational study. *Acta Radiologica (Stockholm, Sweden : 1987),* 51, 7, (Sep), pp. (741-750), 1600-0455; 0284-1851.

Levy B.A., Zlowodzki M.P., Graves M. & Cole P.A. (2005). Screening for extermity arterial injury with the arterial pressure index. *The American Journal of Emergency Medicine,* 23, 5, (Sep), pp. (689-695), 0735-6757; 0735-6757.

Li A., Wong C.S., Wong M.K., Lee C.M. & Au Yeung M.C. (2006). Acute adverse reactions to magnetic resonance contrast media--gadolinium chelates. *The British Journal of Radiology,* 79, 941, (May), pp. (368-371), 0007-1285; 0007-1285.

Loupatatzis C., Schindera S., Gralla J., Hoppe H., Bittner J., Schroder R., Srivastav S. & Bonel H.M. (2008). Whole-body computed tomography for multiple traumas using a triphasic injection protocol. *European Radiology,* 18, 6, (Jun), pp. (1206-1214), 0938-7994; 0938-7994.

Martin D.R., Semelka R.C., Chapman A., Peters H., Finn P.J., Kalb B. & Thomsen H. (2009). Nephrogenic systemic fibrosis versus contrast-induced nephropathy: risks and benefits of contrast-enhanced MR and CT in renally impaired patients. *Journal of*

Magnetic Resonance Imaging : JMRI, 30, 6, (Dec), pp. (1350-1356), 1522-2586; 1053-1807.

Mattox K.L., Feliciano D.V., Burch J., Beall A.C.,Jr, Jordan G.L.,Jr & De Bakey M.E. (1989). Five thousand seven hundred sixty cardiovascular injuries in 4459 patients. Epidemiologic evolution 1958 to 1987. *Annals of Surgery*, 209, 6, (Jun), pp. (698-705; discussion 706-7), 0003-4932; 0003-4932.

Maturen K.E., Adusumilli S., Blane C.E., Arbabi S., Williams D.M., Fitzgerald J.T. & Vine A.A. (2007). Contrast-enhanced CT accurately detects hemorrhage in torso trauma: direct comparison with angiography. *The Journal of Trauma*, 62, 3, (Mar), pp. (740-745), 0022-5282; 0022-5282.

Melton S.M., Kerby J.D., McGiffin D., McGwin G., Smith J.K., Oser R.F., Cross J.M., Windham S.T., Moran S.G., Hsia J. & Rue L.W.,3rd. (2004). The evolution of chest computed tomography for the definitive diagnosis of blunt aortic injury: a single-center experience. *The Journal of Trauma*, 56, 2, (Feb), pp. (243-250), 0022-5282; 0022-5282.

Meyerson S.L., Feldman T., Desai T.R., Leef J., Schwartz L.B. & McKinsey J.F. (2002). Angiographic access site complications in the era of arterial closure devices. *Vascular and Endovascular Surgery*, 36, 2, (Mar-Apr), pp. (137-144), 1538-5744; 1538-5744.

Mirvis S.E., Bidwell J.K., Buddemeyer E.U., Diaconis J.N., Pais S.O., Whitley J.E. & Goldstein L.D. (1987). Value of chest radiography in excluding traumatic aortic rupture. *Radiology*, 163, 2, (May), pp. (487-493), 0033-8419; 0033-8419.

Mirvis S.E. & Shanmuganathan K. (2000). MR imaging of thoracic trauma. *Magnetic Resonance Imaging Clinics of North America*, 8, 1, (Feb), pp. (91-104), 1064-9689; 1064-9689.

Mirvis S.E. & Shanmuganathan K. (2007). Diagnosis of blunt traumatic aortic injury 2007: still a nemesis. *European Journal of Radiology*, 64, 1, (Oct), pp. (27-40), 0720-048X; 0720-048X.

Moainie S.L., Neschis D.G., Gammie J.S., Brown J.M., Poston R.S., Scalea T.M. & Griffith B.P. (2008). Endovascular stenting for traumatic aortic injury: an emerging new standard of care. *The Annals of Thoracic Surgery*, 85, 5, (May), pp. (1625-9; discussion 1629-30), 1552-6259; 0003-4975.

Modrall J.G., Weaver F.A. & Yellin A.E. (1998). Diagnosis and management of penetrating vascular trauma and the injured extremity. *Emergency Medicine Clinics of North America*, 16, 1, (Feb), pp. (129-144), 0733-8627; 0733-8627.

Morcos S.K. (2005). Review article: Acute serious and fatal reactions to contrast media: our current understanding. *The British Journal of Radiology*, 78, 932, (Aug), pp. (686-693), 0007-1285; 0007-1285.

Morozumi J., Homma H., Ohta S., Noda M., Oda J., Mishima S. & Yukioka T. (2010). Impact of mobile angiography in the emergency department for controlling pelvic fracture hemorrhage with hemodynamic instability. *The Journal of Trauma*, 68, 1, (Jan), pp. (90-95), 1529-8809; 0022-5282.

Neschis D.G., Scalea T.M., Flinn W.R. & Griffith B.P. (2008). Blunt aortic injury. *The New England Journal of Medicine*, 359, 16, (Oct 16), pp. (1708-1716), 1533-4406; 0028-4793.

Nguyen D., Platon A., Shanmuganathan K., Mirvis S.E., Becker C.D. & Poletti P.A. (2009). Evaluation of a single-pass continuous whole-body 16-MDCT protocol for patients with polytrauma. *AJR.American Journal of Roentgenology,* 192, 1, (Jan), pp. (3-10), 1546-3141; 0361-803X.

Oberhuber A., Erhard L., Orend K.H. & Sunder-Plassmann L. (2010). Ten years of endovascular treatment of traumatic aortic transection--a single centre experience. *The Thoracic and Cardiovascular Surgeon,* 58, 3, (Apr), pp. (143-147), 1439-1902; 0171-6425.

O'Conor C.E. (2004). Diagnosing traumatic rupture of the thoracic aorta in the emergency department. *Emergency Medicine Journal : EMJ,* 21, 4, (Jul), pp. (414-419), 1472-0213; 1472-0205.

O'Gorman R.B., Feliciano D.V., Bitondo C.G., Mattox K.L., Burch J.M. & Jordan G.L.,Jr. (1984). Emergency center arteriography in the evaluation of suspected peripheral vascular injuries. *Archives of Surgery (Chicago, Ill.: 1960),* 119, 5, (May), pp. (568-573), 0004-0010; 0004-0010.

Patel N.H., Hahn D. & Comess K.A. (2003). Blunt chest trauma victims: role of intravascular ultrasound and transesophageal echocardiography in cases of abnormal thoracic aortogram. *The Journal of Trauma,* 55, 2, (Aug), pp. (330-337), 0022-5282; 0022-5282.

Peng P.D., Spain D.A., Tataria M., Hellinger J.C., Rubin G.D. & Brundage S.I. (2008). CT angiography effectively evaluates extremity vascular trauma. *The American Surgeon,* 74, 2, (Feb), pp. (103-107), 0003-1348; 0003-1348.

Piffaretti G., Tozzi M., Lomazzi C., Rivolta N., Caronno R., Lagana D., Carrafiello G. & Castelli P. (2007). Endovascular treatment for traumatic injuries of the peripheral arteries following blunt trauma. *Injury,* 38, 9, (Sep), pp. (1091-1097), 0020-1383; 0020-1383.

Pinto A., Niola R., Tortora G., Ponticiello G., Russo G., Di Nuzzo L., Gagliardi N., Scaglione M., Merola S., Stavolo C., Maglione F. & Romano L. (2010). Role of multidetector-row CT in assessing the source of arterial haemorrhage in patients with pelvic vascular trauma. Comparison with angiography. *La Radiologia Medica,* 115, 4, (Jun), pp. (648-667), 1826-6983; 0033-8362.

Ptak T., Rhea J.T. & Novelline R.A. (2003). Radiation dose is reduced with a single-pass whole-body multi-detector row CT trauma protocol compared with a conventional segmented method: initial experience. *Radiology,* 229, 3, (Dec), pp. (902-905), 0033-8419; 0033-8419.

Pucelikova T., Dangas G. & Mehran R. (2008). Contrast-induced nephropathy. *Catheterization and Cardiovascular Interventions : Official Journal of the Society for Cardiac Angiography & Interventions,* 71, 1, (Jan 1), pp. (62-72), 1522-726X; 1522-1946.

Rahimi S.A., Darling R.C.,3rd, Mehta M., Roddy S.P., Taggert J.B. & Sternbach Y. (2010). Endovascular repair of thoracic aortic traumatic transections is a safe method in patients with complicated injuries. *Journal of Vascular Surgery : Official Publication, the Society for Vascular Surgery [and] International Society for Cardiovascular Surgery, North American Chapter,* 52, 4, (Oct), pp. (891-896), 1097-6809; 0741-5214.

Ramirez J.I., Velmahos G.C., Best C.R., Chan L.S. & Demetriades D. (2004). Male sexual function after bilateral internal iliac artery embolization for pelvic fracture. *The Journal of Trauma,* 56, 4, (Apr), pp. (734-9; discussion 739-41), 0022-5282; 0022-5282.

Raptopoulos V., Sheiman R.G., Phillips D.A., Davidoff A. & Silva W.E. (1992). Traumatic aortic tear: screening with chest CT. *Radiology,* 182, 3, (Mar), pp. (667-673), 0033-8419; 0033-8419.

Rashid A.H., Brieva J.L. & Stokes B. (2009). Incidence of contrast-induced nephropathy in intensive care patients undergoing computerised tomography and prevalence of risk factors. *Anaesthesia and Intensive Care,* 37, 6, (Nov), pp. (968-975), 0310-057X; 0310-057X.

Reuben B.C., Whitten M.G., Sarfati M. & Kraiss L.W. (2007). Increasing use of endovascular therapy in acute arterial injuries: analysis of the National Trauma Data Bank. *Journal of Vascular Surgery : Official Publication, the Society for Vascular Surgery [and] International Society for Cardiovascular Surgery, North American Chapter,* 46, 6, (Dec), pp. (1222-1226), 0741-5214; 0741-5214.

Rieger M., Mallouhi A., Tauscher T., Lutz M. & Jaschke W.R. (2006). Traumatic arterial injuries of the extremities: initial evaluation with MDCT angiography. *AJR.American Journal of Roentgenology,* 186, 3, (Mar), pp. (656-664), 0361-803X; 0361-803X.

Romano L., Pinto A., De Lutio Di Castelguidone E., Scaglione M., Giovine S., Sacco M. & Pinto F. (2000). Spiral computed tomography in the assessment of vascular lesions of the pelvis due to blunt trauma. *La Radiologia Medica,* 100, 1-2, (Jul-Aug), pp. (29-32), 0033-8362; 0033-8362.

Rousseau H., Dambrin C., Marcheix B., Richeux L., Mazerolles M., Cron C., Watkinson A., Mugniot A., Soula P., Chabbert V., Canevet G., Roux D., Massabuau P., Meites G., Tran Van T. & Otal P. (2005). Acute traumatic aortic rupture: a comparison of surgical and stent-graft repair. *The Journal of Thoracic and Cardiovascular Surgery,* 129, 5, (May), pp. (1050-1055), 0022-5223; 0022-5223.

Sadjadi J., Cureton E.L., Dozier K.C., Kwan R.O. & Victorino G.P. (2009). Expedited treatment of lower extremity gunshot wounds. *Journal of the American College of Surgeons,* 209, 6, (Dec), pp. (740-745), 1879-1190; 1072-7515.

Saletta S., Lederman E., Fein S., Singh A., Kuehler D.H. & Fortune J.B. (1995). Transesophageal echocardiography for the initial evaluation of the widened mediastinum in trauma patients. *The Journal of Trauma,* 39, 1, (Jul), pp. (137-41; discussion 141-2), 0022-5282; 0022-5282.

Seamon M.J., Smoger D., Torres D.M., Pathak A.S., Gaughan J.P., Santora T.A., Cohen G. & Goldberg A.J. (2009). A prospective validation of a current practice: the detection of extremity vascular injury with CT angiography. *The Journal of Trauma,* 67, 2, (Aug), pp. (238-43; discussion 243-4), 1529-8809; 0022-5282.

Shah S.H., Ledgerwood A.M. & Lucas C.E. (2003). Successful endovascular stenting for common iliac artery injury associated with pelvic fracture. *The Journal of Trauma,* 55, 2, (Aug), pp. (383-385), 0022-5282; 0022-5282.

Smith M.D., Cassidy J.M., Souther S., Morris E.J., Sapin P.M., Johnson S.B. & Kearney P.A. (1995). Transesophageal echocardiography in the diagnosis of traumatic rupture of the aorta. *The New England Journal of Medicine,* 332, 6, (Feb 9), pp. (356-362), 0028-4793; 0028-4793.

Sobnach S., Nicol A.J., Nathire H., Edu S., Kahn D. & Navsaria P.H. (2010). An analysis of 50 surgically managed penetrating subclavian artery injuries. *European Journal of Vascular and Endovascular Surgery : The Official Journal of the European Society for Vascular Surgery,* 39, 2, (Feb), pp. (155-159), 1532-2165; 1078-5884.

Soto J.A., Munera F., Morales C., Lopera J.E., Holguin D., Guarin O., Castrillon G., Sanabria A. & Garcia G. (2001). Focal arterial injuries of the proximal extremities: helical CT arteriography as the initial method of diagnosis. *Radiology,* 218, 1, (Jan), pp. (188-194), 0033-8419; 0033-8419.

Starnes B.W. & Arthurs Z.M. (2006). Endovascular management of vascular trauma. *Perspectives in Vascular Surgery and Endovascular Therapy,* 18, 2, (Jun), pp. (114-129), 1531-0035; 1521-5768.

Tang G.L., Tehrani H.Y., Usman A., Katariya K., Otero C., Perez E. & Eskandari M.K. (2008). Reduced mortality, paraplegia, and stroke with stent graft repair of blunt aortic transections: a modern meta-analysis. *Journal of Vascular Surgery : Official Publication, the Society for Vascular Surgery [and] International Society for Cardiovascular Surgery, North American Chapter,* 47, 3, (Mar), pp. (671-675), 0741-5214; 0741-5214.

Tizon-Marcos H. & Barbeau G.R. (2008). Incidence of compartment syndrome of the arm in a large series of transradial approach for coronary procedures. *Journal of Interventional Cardiology,* 21, 5, (Oct), pp. (380-384), 1540-8183; 0896-4327.

Ungar T.C., Wolf S.J., Haukoos J.S., Dyer D.S. & Moore E.E. (2006). Derivation of a clinical decision rule to exclude thoracic aortic imaging in patients with blunt chest trauma after motor vehicle collisions. *The Journal of Trauma,* 61, 5, (Nov), pp. (1150-1155), 0022-5282; 0022-5282.

Urgnani F., Lerut P., Da Rocha M., Adriani D., Leon F. & Riambau V. (2009). Endovascular treatment of acute traumatic thoracic aortic injuries: a retrospective analysis of 20 cases. *The Journal of Thoracic and Cardiovascular Surgery,* 138, 5, (Nov), pp. (1129-1138), 1097-685X; 0022-5223.

Velmahos G.C., Demetriades D., Chahwan S., Gomez H., Hanks S.E., Murray J.A., Asensio J.A. & Berne T.V. (1999). Angiographic embolization for arrest of bleeding after penetrating trauma to the abdomen. *American Journal of Surgery,* 178, 5, (Nov), pp. (367-373), 0002-9610; 0002-9610.

Velmahos G.C., Chahwan S., Hanks S.E., Murray J.A., Berne T.V., Asensio J. & Demetriades D. (2000). Angiographic embolization of bilateral internal iliac arteries to control life-threatening hemorrhage after blunt trauma to the pelvis. *The American Surgeon,* 66, 9, (Sep), pp. (858-862), 0003-1348; 0003-1348.

Velmahos G.C., Toutouzas K.G., Vassiliu P., Sarkisyan G., Chan L.S., Hanks S.H., Berne T.V. & Demetriades D. (2002). A prospective study on the safety and efficacy of angiographic embolization for pelvic and visceral injuries. *The Journal of Trauma,* 53, 2, (Aug), pp. (303-8; discussion 308), 0022-5282; 0022-5282.

Vignon P., Boncoeur M.P., Francois B., Rambaud G., Maubon A. & Gastinne H. (2001). Comparison of multiplane transesophageal echocardiography and contrast-enhanced helical CT in the diagnosis of blunt traumatic cardiovascular injuries. *Anesthesiology,* 94, 4, (Apr), pp. (615-22; discussion 5A), 0003-3022; 0003-3022.

Vignon P., Martaille J.F., Francois B., Rambaud G. & Gastinne H. (2005). Transesophageal echocardiography and therapeutic management of patients sustaining blunt aortic injuries. *The Journal of Trauma,* 58, 6, (Jun), pp. (1150-1158), 0022-5282; 0022-5282.

Vu M., Anderson S.W., Shah N., Soto J.A. & Rhea J.T. (2010). CT of blunt abdominal and pelvic vascular injury. *Emergency Radiology,* 17, 1, (Jan), pp. (21-29), 1438-1435; 1070-3004.

Wang C.L., Cohan R.H., Ellis J.H., Adusumilli S. & Dunnick N.R. (2007). Frequency, management, and outcome of extravasation of nonionic iodinated contrast medium in 69,657 intravenous injections. *Radiology,* 243, 1, (Apr), pp. (80-87), 0033-8419; 0033-8419.

Weaver F.A., Yellin A.E., Bauer M., Oberg J., Ghalambor N., Emmanuel R.P., Applebaum R.M., Pentecost M.J. & Shorr R.M. (1990). Is arterial proximity a valid indication for arteriography in penetrating extremity trauma? A prospective analysis. *Archives of Surgery (Chicago, Ill.: 1960)*, 125, 10, (Oct), pp. (1256-1260), 0004-0010; 0004-0010.

White P.W., Gillespie D.L., Feurstein I., Aidinian G., Phinney S., Cox M.W., Adams E. & Fox C.J. (2010). Sixty-four slice multidetector computed tomographic angiography in the evaluation of vascular trauma. *The Journal of Trauma*, 68, 1, (Jan), pp. (96-102), 1529-8809; 0022-5282.

White R., Krajcer Z., Johnson M., Williams D., Bacharach M. & O'Malley E. (2006). Results of a multicenter trial for the treatment of traumatic vascular injury with a covered stent. *The Journal of Trauma*, 60, 6, (Jun), pp. (1189-95; discussion 1195-6), 0022-5282; 0022-5282.

Willmann J.K. & Wildermuth S. (2005). Multidetector-row CT angiography of upper- and lower-extremity peripheral arteries. *European Radiology*, 15 Suppl 4, (Nov), pp. (D3-9), 0938-7994; 0938-7994.

Wintermark M., Wicky S. & Schnyder P. (2002). Imaging of acute traumatic injuries of the thoracic aorta. *European Radiology*, 12, 2, (Feb), pp. (431-442), 0938-7994; 0938-7994.

Wong H., Gotway M.B., Sasson A.D. & Jeffrey R.B. (2004). Periaortic hematoma at diaphragmatic crura at helical CT: sign of blunt aortic injury in patients with mediastinal hematoma. *Radiology*, 231, 1, (Apr), pp. (185-189), 0033-8419; 0033-8419.

Woodring J.H. & Dillon M.L. (1984). Radiographic manifestations of mediastinal hemorrhage from blunt chest trauma. *The Annals of Thoracic Surgery*, 37, 2, (Feb), pp. (171-178), 0003-4975; 0003-4975.

Woodring J.H. (1990). The normal mediastinum in blunt traumatic rupture of the thoracic aorta and brachiocephalic arteries. *The Journal of Emergency Medicine*, 8, 4, (Jul-Aug), pp. (467-476), 0736-4679; 0736-4679.

Xenos E.S., Abedi N.N., Davenport D.L., Minion D.J., Hamdallah O., Sorial E.E. & Endean E.D. (2008). Meta-analysis of endovascular vs open repair for traumatic descending thoracic aortic rupture. *Journal of Vascular Surgery : Official Publication, the Society for Vascular Surgery [and] International Society for Cardiovascular Surgery, North American Chapter*, 48, 5, (Nov), pp. (1343-1351), 1097-6809; 0741-5214.

Yamane B.H., Tefera G., Hoch J.R., Turnipseed W.D. & Acher C.W. (2008). Blunt thoracic aortic injury: open or stent graft repair? *Surgery*, 144, 4, (Oct), pp. (575-80; discussion 580-2), 1532-7361; 0039-6060.

Yaquinto J.J., Harms S.E., Siemers P.T., Flamig D.P., Griffey R.H. & Foreman M.L. (1992). Arterial injury from penetrating trauma: evaluation with single-acquisition fat-suppressed MR imaging. *AJR.American Journal of Roentgenology*, 158, 3, (Mar), pp. (631-633), 0361-803X; 0361-803X.

Yurdakul M., Tola M. & Uslu O.S. (2008). Color Doppler ultrasonography in occlusive diseases of the brachiocephalic and proximal subclavian arteries. *Journal of Ultrasound in Medicine : Official Journal of the American Institute of Ultrasound in Medicine*, 27, 7, (Jul), pp. (1065-1070), 0278-4297; 0278-4297.

3

Eversion Carotid Endarterectomy in Patients with Near-Total Internal Carotid Artery Occlusion – Diagnostic Modalities, Indications and Surgical Technique

Đorđe Radak and Slobodan Tanasković
„Dedinje" Cardiovascular Institute, Vascular surgery Clinic, Belgrade, Serbia

1. Introduction

There is a general agreement that symptomatic patients with high-grade stenosis of internal carotid artery (ICA) should be treated with either surgery or percutaneous intervention.[1,2] On the other hand, there is considerable controversy with respect to the approach to the patients with near total ICA occlusion. These patients are considered to be at lower risk for transient ischemic attack (TIA), stroke, and death than patients with a lesser degree of stenosis. [3] There are no prospective randomized clinical trials dealing with this issue, and the available data mostly originate from the post-hoc analysis of the large trials performed in the late 1990s. The results of these studies are conflicting and provide little benefit in clinical decision making. [4,5] Therefore, the aim of the present study was to prospectively evaluate clinical effects of eversion carotid endarterectomy (ECEA) versus best medical treatment of symptomatic patients with near total ICA occlusion.

2. Methods

2.1 Patients

From January 2003 to December 2006, a total of 359 patients with near total ICA occlusion were referred to Dedinje Cardiovascular Institute for evaluation and therapy. Patients were excluded from the study if they were asymptomatic (32 patients), had occlusion of the contralateral ICA (8 patients), or were considered to have unacceptably high surgical risk due to associated comorbidities (10 patients). Therefore, the final study group consisted of 309 patients. Symptoms were identified as TIA and stroke. In order to enter the study patients had to be symptomatic for 12 months or less. Since near total occlusion is not that often seen in our population, randomization was difficult so patients were nonrandomly divided in group A (259 patients), who underwent ECEA surgery, and group B (50 patients), who refused surgery. Inclusion criteria were near total ICA occlusion and previous neurological ischemic events (TIA, stroke...). A high proportion of patients who refused surgery was due to the fact that all patients were thoroughly informed about the conflicting data regarding the potential surgical benefit. Patients in group B received best medical treatment based on the opinion of the attending vascular surgeon and/or angiologist. This study conforms with the principles outlined in the Declaration of Helsinki and all patients signed a written informed consent. Likewise, this study was approved by institutional review board (IRB).

2.2 Diagnostic techniques

Initial diagnostic technique of choice was Duplex ultrasonographic scan of the carotid arteries. Diagnosis of near total ICA occlusion was made if 95% to 99% stenosis was found and if there was either obvious diameter reduction of ICA compared with opposite ICA, or ICA diameter reduction compared with ipsilateral external carotid artery. (Figure 1) For the ICA stenosis degree assessment we used ECST [1] criteria. Additionally, near total occlusion was diagnosed if peak systolic velocity ICA was greater than 230 cm/s, end-diastolic velocity ICA was greater than 100 cm/s, and ICA/common carotid artery (CCA) ratio was greater than 4. When diagnosis based only on ultrasonography was in question, arterial angiography (9 patients) or 64-slice computer tomography (21 patients) was performed. (Figures 2 and 3) Severity of stenosis of contralateral ICA was also assessed by Duplex scan at the time of the initial examination.

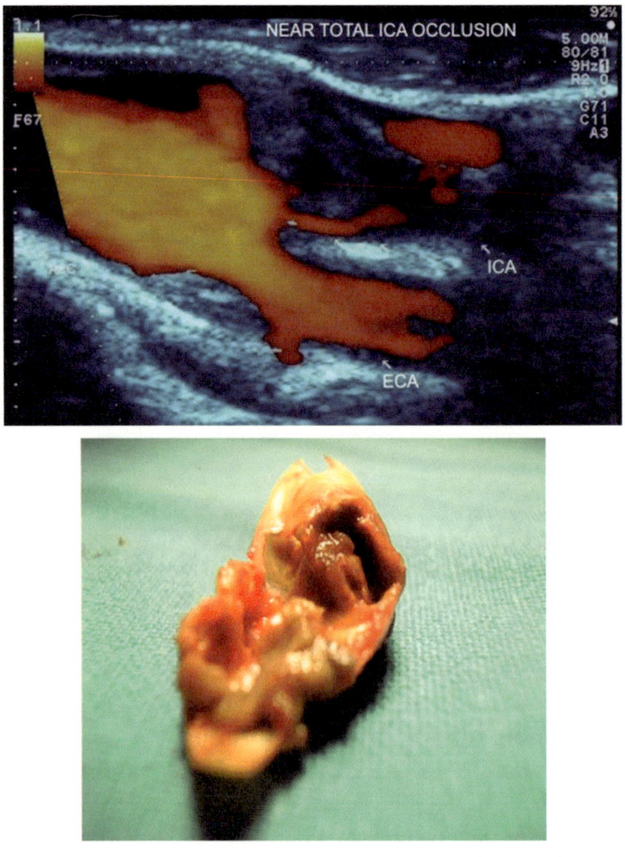

Fig. 1. Ultrasonography of near total ICA occlusion (top) confirmed by intraoperative findings (bottom)

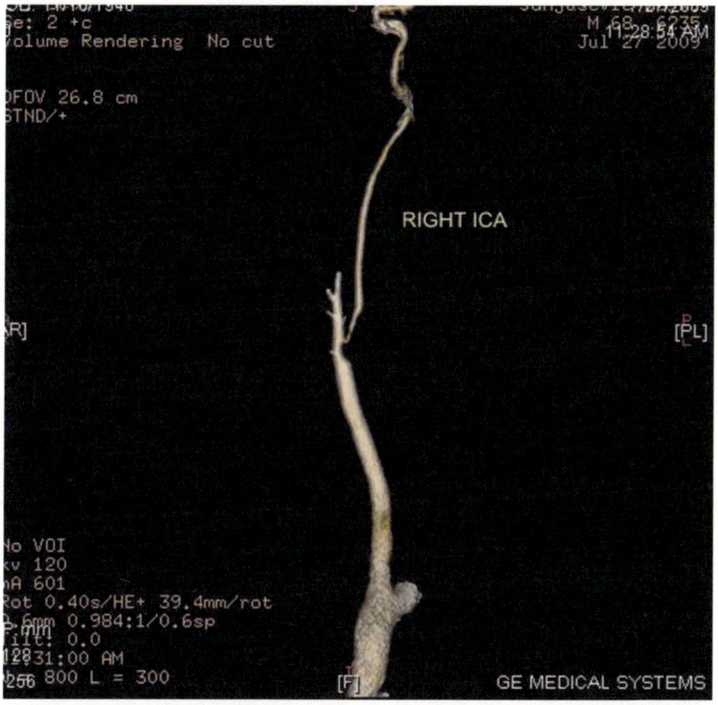

Fig. 2. Multilsice CT angiography. Right ICA near total occlusion

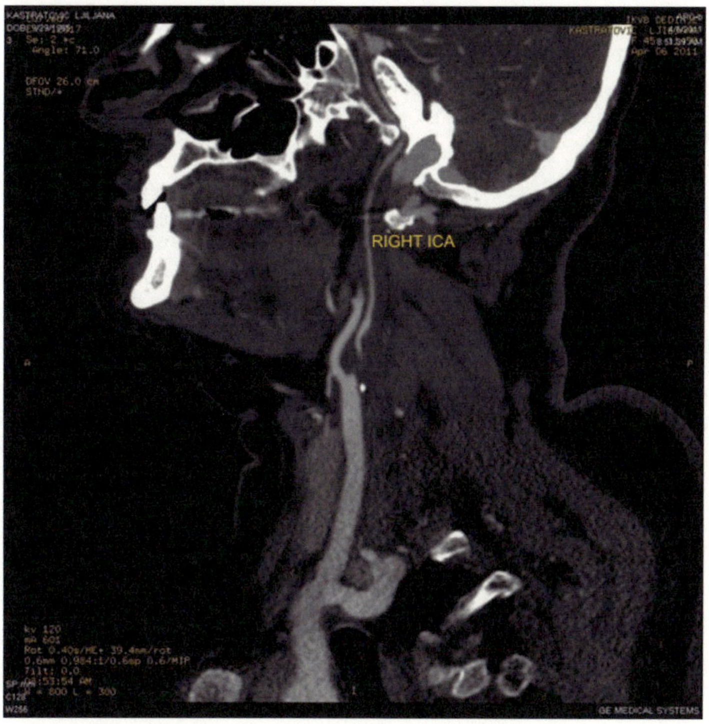

Fig. 3. Multislice CT angiography. Near total ICA occlusion

2.3 Eversion carotid endarterectomy and postoperative treatment

Good surgical technique is the determing factor for achieving good quality results of carotid endarterectomy. Any technical error (intimal or medial flap, the stricture of suture line, artery injury following clamping, inadequate resection of carotid artery elongation, thrombosis within arterial wall, intraoperative embolisation or brain ischemia, etc...) may manifest in early and/or late complications. Systemic factors (hipercoagulability, etc...) are rarely to blame for the occurrence of complications. Eversion carotid endarterectomy reduces the possibility of technical errors.

Eversion carotid endarterectomy includes:

- carotid artery resection at the bifurcation level
- atherosclerotic plaque removal by eversion technique (Figures 4 and 5)
- anatomic reimplantation of internal carotid artery (Figures 6 and 7)

Advantages of eversion endarterectomy are: shorter clamping time, anatomical reconstruction of carotid bifurcation, shorter and transverse placed suture line. Implantation of foreign material (patch) is not required. Resection of carotid artery elongation (kinking, coiling) is far simpler. However, many vascular surgeons still hesitate to accept this surgical technique and expand the standard repertoire of carotid artery reconstruction. Preoperative diagnosis and indications for eversion carotid endartectomy are no different than for standard endarterectomy.

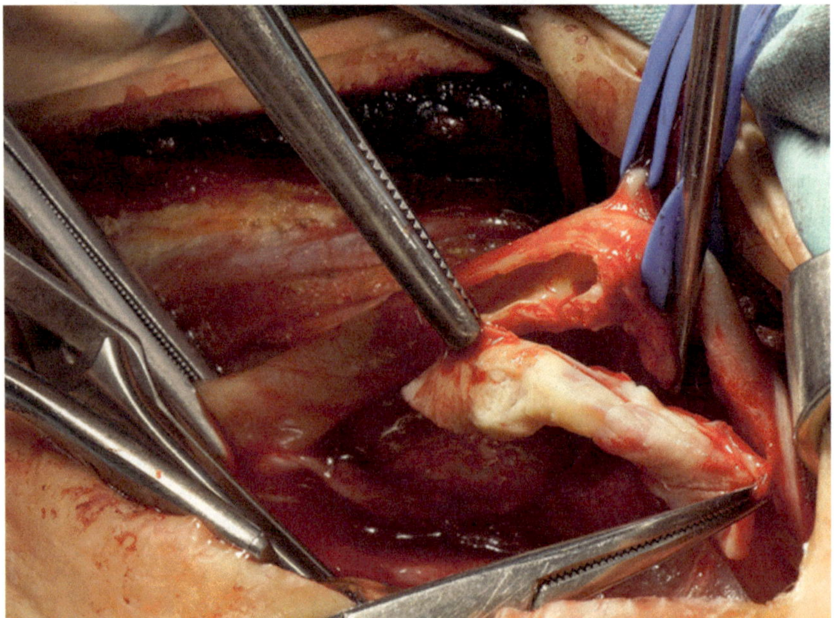

Fig. 4. Atherosclerotic plaque removal by eversion technique

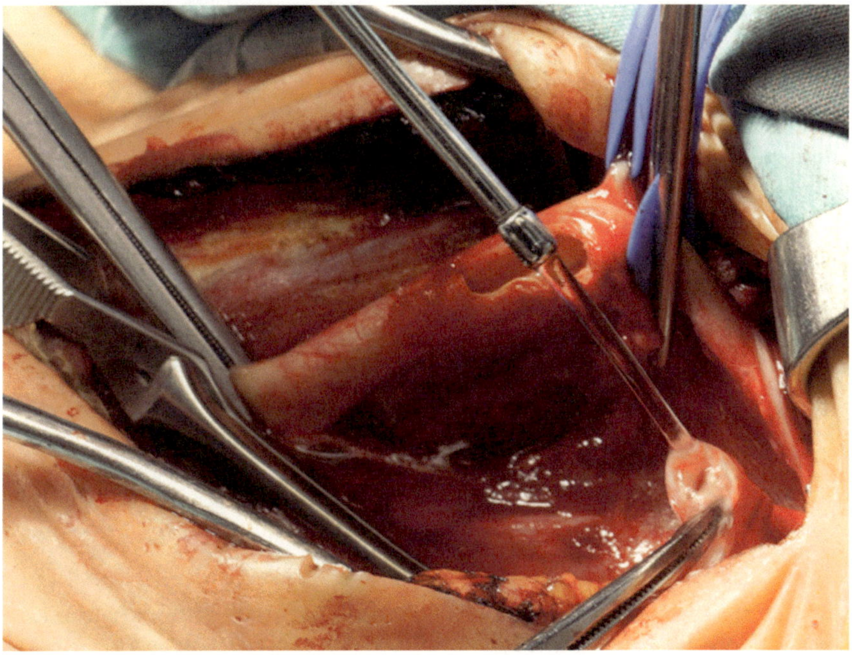

Fig. 5. Distal endarterectomy verification

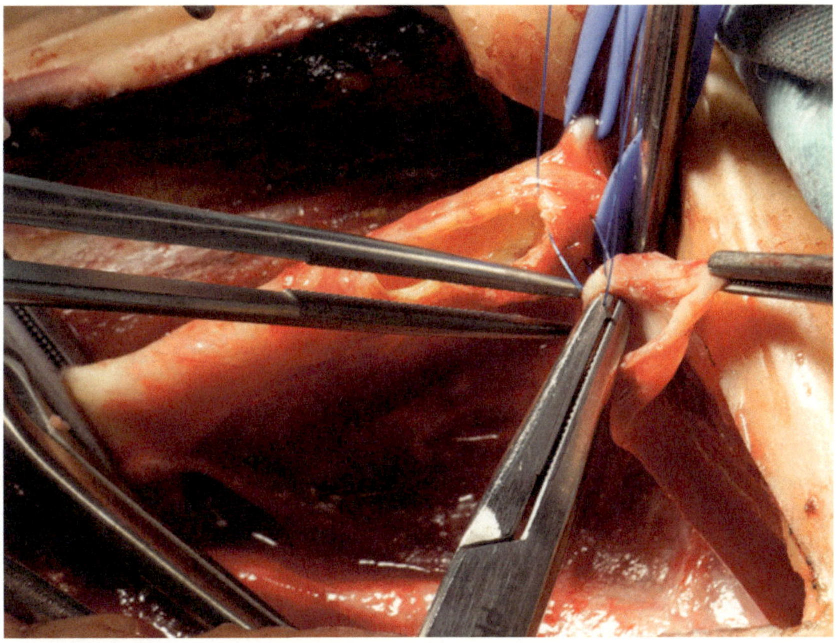

Fig. 6. Beginning of anastomosis creation

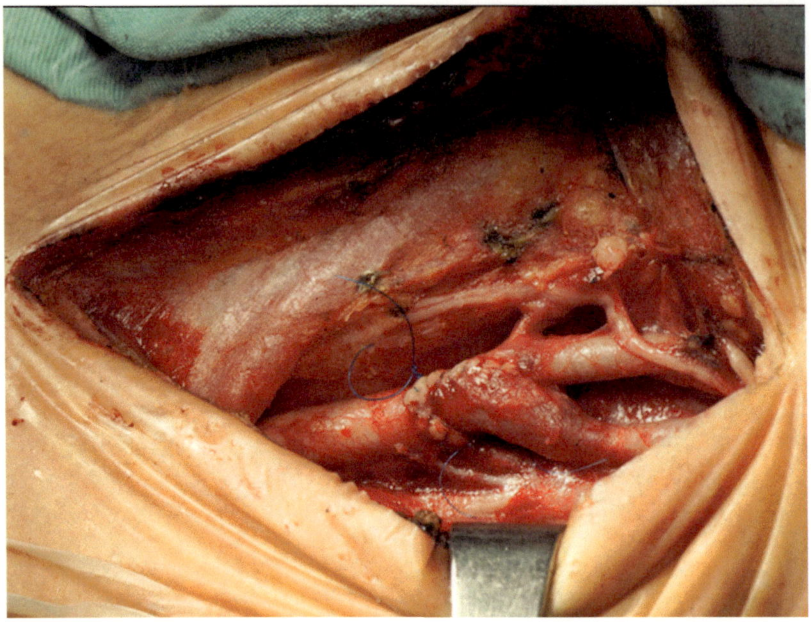

Fig. 7. Preserved morphological and hemodynamic characteristics after anatomical reimplantation of internal carotid artery

All patients who were surgically treated underwent ECEA under general anesthesia, without shunting and without intraoperative monitoring of cerebral functions. If postoperative course was uneventful, patients were discharged from hospital by the third postoperative day.

2.4 Medications

Patients who were taking standard antiplatelet therapy (aspirin and/or clopidogrel) were taken off these drugs at least 2 days before the operation, as this is a routine practice in our institution to minimize operative and perioperative bleeding. All patients were discharged on either aspirin or clopidogrel or both medications. These drugs were continued upon discharge. Other cardiovascular medications (b-blockers, inhibitors of angiotensinconverting enzyme, angiotensin receptor blockers, diuretics, and/or statins) in both groups of patients were prescribed if clinically indicated.

2.5 Follow-up

Follow-up consisted of detailed history and physical examination at 1, 3, 6, and 12 months. Patients were followed for ipsilateral stroke, TIA, and neurologic mortality. Duplex ultrasonographic scan of the carotid arteries was repeated at 12 months. After this period patients were sent for regular control examinations to the competent surgeon.

2.6 Statistical analysis

All data were collected prospectively as a part of our institution's database. Data are expressed as mean ± standard deviation. T-Test and chi-squared tests were used for comparisons between the subgroups for continuous and categorical variables, respectively (a probability value of $p<0.05$ was considered significant). Kaplan-Meier analysis was performed to assess differences in event-free survival between the groups.

3. Results

	Group A (n=259)	Group B (n=50)	*p* value
Sex (male)	184 (71%)	34 (68%)	0.79
Age (yr), mean±SD	64 ± 8	65 ± 10	0.44
Stroke	100 (39%)	17 (34%)	0.64
TIA	159 (61%)	33 (66%)	0.64
Hypertension	199 (76%)	40 (80%)	0.76
Hyperlipoproteinaemia	144 (55%)	36 (72%)	0.049
Diabetes	68 (26%)	15 (30%)	0.70
Smoking	77 (30%)	34 (68%)	<0.001
CAD	50 (19%)	11 (22%)	0.80
PVD	61 (23%)	12 (24%)	0.90

CAD - coronary artery disease; PVD - peripheral vascular disease; TIA - transitory ischemic attack.

Table 1. Baseline demographic and clinical data

Table 1 depicts basic demographic and clinical data. Briefly, there was no difference between the groups with respect to age, sex, symptoms, and risk factors for atherosclerosis except for the smoking and hyperlipoproteinemia. Importantly, there was also no difference in incidence of peripheral vascular and coronary artery disease between the groups. There were no intra- and perioperative deaths and strokes in patients who were subjected to surgery. TIA was noted in 4 (1.5%) of these patients. There were no differences between the groups with respect to medications on discharge. The majority of patients were on aspirin and statins, but clopidogrel was prescribed rarely (Table 2).

	Group A (n=259)	Group B (n=50)	*p* value
B-blockers	160 (61%)	28 (56%)	0.54
ACEi/ARB	201 (77%)	36 (72%)	0.49
Statins	212 (81%)	40 (80%)	0.91
Aspirin	245 (94%)	46 (92%)	0.69
Clopidogrel	20 (7%)	5 (10%)	0.76

ACEI - angiotensin-converting enzyme inhibitor; ARB - angiotensin receptor blocker.

Table 2. Medications on discharge

Cumulative 12-month incidence of TIA, ipsilateral stroke, and neurologic mortality in both groups is shown in Table 3.

	Group A (n=259)	Group B (n=50)	RR (95% CI)	*p* value
TIA	13 (5%)	12 (24%)	1.14 (1.02-1.18)	<0.001
Stroke	4 (1.5%)	7 (14%)	1.24 (1.06-1.46)	<0.001
Death	4 (1.5%)	4 (8%)	.07 (0.98-1.16)	0.034

CI - confidence interval; RR - risk reduction; TIA - transitory ischemic attack.

Table 3. Cumulative incidence of TIA, ipsilateral stroke, and neurologic mortality at 12 months

It is evident that patients who underwent ECEA had lower incidence of all three events at 12 months than did patients who received medical therapy. Follow-up data were available for 255 (98%) of surgically treated and 50 (100%) for medically treated patients.

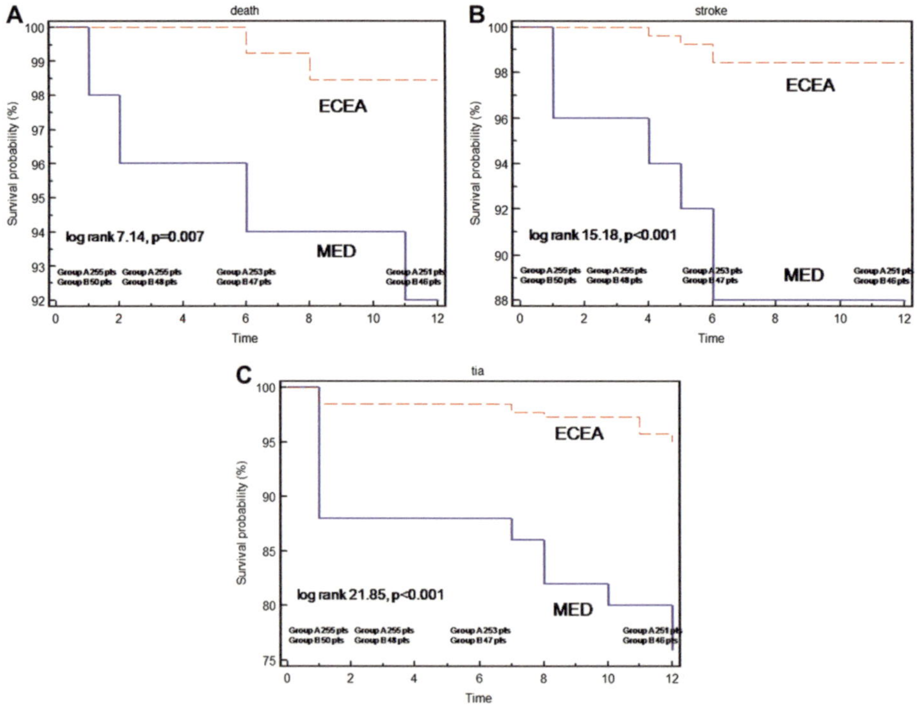

ECEA - eversion carotid endarterectomy; MED - medical treatment; TIA - transient ischemic attack.

Fig. 8. Kaplan-Meier curves for (A) neurologic death, (B) ipsilateral stroke, and (C) TIA for surgically and medically treated patients.

Figures 8, A-C depict Kaplan-Meier curves for death, ipsilateral stroke, and TIA for surgically and medically treated patients, respectively, which demonstrate better 12-month outcome for surgical patients with respect to all three variables.

Duplex ultrasonographic scan of the carotid arteries was performed after 12 months in 220 (84%) patients in group A and 40 (80%) patients in group B. Restenosis of the operated ICA was noted in 7 (3%) patients, and progression of near to total occlusion was seen in 15 (37%)

patients in group B. Stroke/TIA was noted in 12 patients in group B who progressed to total occlusion; conversely, stroke/TIA was also noted in 2 patients who did not progress to total occlusion.

4. Discussion

Since 1991, when first ECEA was performed at our institution, this surgical technique gradually replaced longitudinal arteriotomy as the treatment of choice in patients with carotid atherosclerosis. [6-8] One of the major reasons why ECEA is a technique of choice at our institution is shorter clamping time (12.4 ± 3.1 min). [7,9] This fact made shunting unnecessary, which resulted in nearly total abandoning of shunt use in recent years (0.5% of all patients). [7] The choice of anesthetic management for carotid surgery is still controversial. [10-12] The vast majority of operations in our series were performed under general anesthesia, whereby we have not registered disadvantages of this procedure in relation to the outcome.

Eversion carotid endarterectomy showed satisfactory results in near total ICA occlusion treatment as well. Our data indicate that recently (within12 months) symptomatic patients with near total ICA occlusion who underwent ECEA have better prognosis over 12-month follow-up compared with medically treated patients in terms of increased neurologic mortality and morbidity. The prevalence of near total occlusion is uncertain and it has been estimated in the range of 0.5-10% of all patients undergoing surgery. [13] The issue of management of patients with near total ICA occlusion is highly controversial as it has been suggested that patients with reduced ICA lumen diameter distal to severe symptomatic stenosis are at low risk of ischemic stroke. [14] Currently, there are no randomized clinical trials that would address this important problem.

Data that are currently available mostly originate from post-hoc analysis of NASCET and ESCT studies. [15,16] For the problem to be worse, these post-hoc analyses produced conflicting results. Analysis from the NASCET trial identified 106 symptomatic patients with near total occlusion of ICA and concluded that carotid endarterectomy is beneficial and not more dangerous than in patients with 70-94% stenosis, provided that the procedure is performed by experienced surgeons with low complication rate.

Of the 48 patients with near occlusion treated with CEA, 3 (6.3%) had perioperative strokes, and only 1 of 58 patients (1.7%) with near occlusion treated medically had a stroke in the first month. For medically treated patients with near occlusion, the 1-year stroke risk was 11.1%. A comparison of treatment differences indicated that surgery reduces the risk of stroke at 1 year by approximately one-half ($p < 0.001$) in patients with near ICA occlusion. [4]

In contrast, a report after reanalysis of the final results of the ECST trial concluded that surgery was of little benefit in symptomatic patients with near total occlusion. This study included 125 patients with near occlusion, of whom 78 were treated surgically and 47 medically. Perioperative stroke was noted in 3 (3.8%) patients, and there were no perioperative deaths. [5] Finally, when these patients were pooled together, 3-year risks of ipsilateral stroke for 114 medically treated patients with near occlusion was 15.1% versus 10.9% for 148 surgically treated (absolute risk reduction 4.2%; $p < 0.33$), indicating no clear benefit of surgery for near total occlusion. [17]

Since the incidences of stroke and death in medically treated patients were similar in our patients as in previously reported trials, it can be assumed that the difference in the outcome was drawn from low perioperative and 12-month mortality and morbidity in our group of surgically treated patients. To our knowledge, this is the largest reported group of operated patients with near total ICA occlusion.

It is not entirely clear why the outcome in our patients was more favorable than in NASCET and ESCT trials but the following may be operative. All patients were operated in one center using ECEA technique. It is noteworthy that all of our surgeons, both senior and junior, are dedicated vascular surgeons with comprehensive training in ECEA.

Furthermore, our center is a high-volume center for ECEA, with over 700 surgeries per year. [6-8] This surely contributes to good surgical results, as it has been shown that high-volume surgeons (more than 60 surgeries per year) have fewer surgical complications [18] and that the results of carotid endarterectomy are better if performed exclusively by vascular surgeons. [19] Furthermore, it appears that the choice of surgical technique may also play a role as it has been suggested that ECEA may be associated with lower risk of arterial occlusion and restenosis than longitudinal arteriotomy. [20]

NASCET and ESCT trials were done more than 15 years ago in an era when the concomitant use of vasculoprotective medications was less well established. Therefore, it can also be assumed that the widespread use of statins, antiplatelet therapy, and angiotensin-converting enzyme inhibitors/angiotensin receptor blockers had modulated atherosclerotic process in our patients. Since the use of medication was similar between the groups, it can be postulated that improved hemodynamics and lower baseline incidence of smoking and hyperlipoproteinemia in medically treated patients may also play a role. Patient population between our and previous trials was also somewhat different, as our study included only recently (within 12 months) symptomatic patients who are regarded to be at higher risk for future neurologic events. [1,2] This may further emphasize the need for surgery and/or tailored medical treatment in high-risk patient population.

Diagnosis of near total ICA occlusion can be challenging, but our experience is in keeping with previous reports that Duplex ultrasonography should be the initial diagnostic test, which can be supplemented by other imaging techniques when the diagnosis is in doubt. [21] The major drawback of our study is that this is a nonrandomized trial. The general policy in our institution is that all symptomatic patients with significant carotid atherosclerotic disease should be operated on, and it was deemed unethical to refuse surgery to a significant number of patients despite conflicting prior evidence.

All patients were thoroughly informed about the potential surgical risk and benefits and the final decision was made according to their preferences. However, two groups were well matched with respect to sex, age, symptoms, and demographic characteristics and we believe that valid comparisons can be made.

The other potential drawback is that we did not assess the presence of collateral circulation, since it has been shown that the 2-year risk of TIAs, hemispheric stroke, and disabling or fatal strokes was reduced in the presence of collaterals on cerebral angiography in medically treated patients, [22] which can further refine risk stratification in patients with near total ICA occlusion.

5. Conclusion

Our data indicate that recently (within 12 months) symptomatic patients with near total ICA occlusion who underwent ECEA have lower incidence of TIA, ipsilateral stroke, and neurologic death during follow-up than medically treated patients. It appears that, at least in high-volume centers, ECEA should be favored over medical treatment for the management of these patients.

6. References

[1] North American Symptomatic Carotid Endarterectomy Trialists Collaborative Group. The final results of the NASCET trial. N Engl J Med 1998;339:1415-1425.
[2] European Carotid Surgery Trialists Collaborative Group. Randomised trial of carotid endarterectomy for recently symptomatic stenosis: final results of the MRC European Carotid Surgery Trial (ECST). Lancet 1998;351:1379-1387.
[3] Paciaroni M, Eliasziw M, Sharpe BLS, Meldrum H, et al. Long-term clinical and angiographic outcomes in symptomatic patients with 70% to 99% carotid artery stenosis. Stroke 2000;31:2037-2042.
[4] Morgenstern LB, Fox AJ, Sharpe BL, et al. The risks and benefits of carotid endarterectomy in patients with near occlusion of the carotid artery. Neurology 1997;48:911-915.
[5] Rothwell PM, Gutnikov SA, Warlow CP. The European Carotid Surgery Trialists' Collaboration. Reanalysis of the final results of the European Carotid Surgery Trial. Stroke 2003;34:514-523.
[6] Radak D, Radevic B, Sternic N, et al. Single center experience on eversion versus standard carotid endarterectomy: a prospective non-randomized study. Cardiovasc Surg 2000;8:422–8.
[7] Radak Dj, Ilijevski N, Nenezic D, Popov P, Vucurevic G, Gajin P, Jocic D, Kolar J, Radak S, Sagic D, Matic P, Milicic M, Otasevic P. Temporal trends in eversion carotid endarterectomy for carotid atherosclerosis: single-center experience with 5,034 Patients. Vascular 2007;15:205-210.
[8] Radak Dj, Tanasković S, Ilijevski N, Davidović L, Kolar J, Radak S, Otašević P. Eversion carotid endarterectomy versus best medical treatment in symptomatic patients with near total internal carotid occlusion: A prospective nonrandomized trial. Ann Vasc Surg Nov 2009; 185-189.
[9] Green RM, Greenberg R, Illig K, et al. Eversion endarterectomy of the carotid artery: technical considerations and recurrent stenosis. J Vasc Surg 2000;32:1052–61.
[10] McCarthy RJ, Nasr MK, McAteer P, Horrocks M. Physiological advantages of cerebral flow during carotid endarterectomy under local anesthesia: a randomized clinical trial. Eur J Vasc Endovasc Surg 2002;22:215–21.
[11] Kasprzak PM, Altmeppen J, Angerer M, et al. General versus locoregional anesthesia in carotid surgery: a prospective randomized trial. Vasa 2006;35:232–8.
[12] Rerkasem K, Bond R, Rothwell PM. Local versus general anaesthesia for carotid endarterectomy. Cochrane Database Syst Rev 2004;(2):CD000126.
[13] Barnett HJ, Meldrum HE, Eliasziw M. North American Symptomatic Carotid Endarterectomy Trial (NASCET) Collaborators. The appropriate use of carotid endarterectomy. C.M.A.J. 2002;166:1169-1179.

[14] Rothwell PM, Warlow CP. Low risk of ischemic stroke in patients with reduced internal carotid artery lumen diameter distal to severe symptomatic stenosis. Cerebral protection due to low poststenotic flow? Stroke 2000;31:622-630.
[15] North American Symptomatic Carotid Endarterectomy Trial (NASCET) Investigations. Clinical alert: benefit of carotid endarterectomy for patients with high-grade stenosis if the internal carotid artery. Stroke 1991;22:816-817.
[16] European Carotid Surgery Trialists, Collaborative Group. MRC European Carotid Surgery Trial: interim results for symptomatic patients with severe (70-99%) or with mild (0-29%) stenosis. Lancet 1991;337:1235-1243.
[17] Fox AJ, Eliasziw M, Rothwell PM, et al. Identification, prognosis, and management of patients with carotid artery near occlusion. Am J Neuroradiol 2005;26:2086-2094.
[18] Pearce WH, Parker MA, Feinglass J, et al. The importance of surgeon volume and training in outcomes for vascular surgical procedures. J Vasc Surg 1999;29:768-776.
[19] Hannan EL, Popp JA, Feustel P, et al. Association of surgical specialty and processes of care with patient outcomes for carotid endarterectomy. Stroke 2001;32:2890-2897.
[20] Cao P, De Rango P, Zannetti S. Eversion versus conventional carotid endarterectomy: a systematic review. Eur J Vasc Endovasc Surg 2002;23:195-201.
[21] Furst G, Saleh A, Wenserski F, et al. Reliability and validity of noninvasive imaging of internal carotid artery pseudoocclusion. Stroke 1999;30:1444-1449.
[22] Henderson RD, Eliasziw M, Fox AJ, et al. Angiographically defined collateral circulation and risk of stroke in patients with severe carotid artery stenosis. Stroke 2000;31:128-132.

4

Vascular Complications After Renal Transplantation

Taylan Ozgur Sezer and Cuneyt Hoscoskun
*Department of General Surgery and Transplantation Unit,
Ege University School of Medicine, Izmir,
Turkey*

1. Introduction

Renal transplantation has become the treatment of choice for end-stage renal disease due to advances in surgical techniques, perioperative management, and immunosuppressive regimens. Surgical techniques for kidney transplantation were first described in 1951 by Kuss et al. and have since changed very little. The most common surgical procedure is extraperitoneal transplantation in the right iliac fossa, with end-to-side to the external iliac artery or end-to-end anastomosis to the internal iliac artery, and end-to-side anastomosis to the external iliac vein.

The overall incidence of vascular complications following kidney transplantation is low, especially when compared to other solid organ transplantation of such organs as the liver or pancreas. The incidence of vascular complications following renal transplantation ranges from 3% to 15%.[1] Arterial complications occur more frequently and are more dangerous than venous. Both arterial and venous thromboses tend to occur within the first few days of transplantation. Improvements in immunosuppressive therapy have led to a 1-year post transplantation acute rejection incidence rate of <20%. The incidence of graft loss due to acute and chronic rejection is decreasing; however, the incidence of early allograft loss due to acute vascular complications has remained constant, accounting for a proportionally higher percentage of early loss. Reducing the incidence of vascular complications depends to a great extent on the careful evaluation of the recipient, the donor kidney, and the surgical technique used for implantation.

1.1 Transplantation region

As a general rule, left kidney is implanted in the right iliac fossa, whereas right kidney is implanted in the left iliac fossa. Using this technique the urinary collecting system is medially located, facilitating easy access to the ureter and possible percutaneous kidney biopsy; however, because left donor nephrectomy is commonly performed and the right iliac veins are more superficial, kidneys are implanted in the right retroperitoneal iliac fossa. The left iliac fossa is reserved primarily for pancreas transplantation candidates, patients with previous transplants, and those with vascular problems. In patients undergoing simultaneous pancreas and renal transplantation, or in those with a history of surgery in both iliac regions intraperitoneal transplantation should be performed.

1.2 Which kidney to choose – left or right?

Right and left kidney transplant outcomes are similar;[2] however, given a choice surgeons prefer the left kidney because the left renal vein is longer and less fragile, and anastomosis to the recipient right external iliac vein, which is situated superficial, is easier. Right kidney transplantation leads to more stretching of the anastomosis site because the right renal vein is short. On the other hand, a long renal artery may lead to a kink. In transplantation of kidneys with multiple renal arteries the contralateral kidney should be used because the duration of surgery is long, and hot and cold ischemia negatively affect graft survival.

1.3 Preparation of the allograft

Donor kidneys should be prepared on the back table before implantation in the recipient, whether obtained from a deceased or a living donor. Arterial anomalies, atheromatous plaques, thromboses, and intimal flaps that may be overlooked during explantation or donor nephrectomy. In such cases the duration of hot or cold ischemia will be kept to a minimum due to preparation performed on the back table.

In living donor transplantation accessory superior pole or inferior pole arteries that may have escaped detection during back table preparation may become evident with cold perfusion; however; in transplants performed with deceased organs prepared with in situ perfusion, accessory arteries may be overlooked. The tissue surrounding the donor renal artery and vein should be mobilized without extreme dissection. Hemostasis should be maintained using cauterization to separate the perirenal fat tissue and tying or clipping the small venous structures, which will decrease the volume of bleeding during reperfusion.

In deceased kidney transplantation the second flushing at the back table after explantation helps clean away remnant venous blood and facilitates detection of veins that may have been previously overlooked. Furthermore, flushing kidneys twice reduced the primary non-function rate.[3] In donors with multiple arteries, 2 arteries should be unified as a single artery via trouser-like stenting, if possible (artery diameter >3 mm), and used as a single anastomosis in the recipient (Figure 1a). The smaller graft artery can be anastomosed end-to-side to the larger one (Figure 1b). Alternately, there can be 2 separate anastomoses performed on the internal iliac and external iliac arteries (Figure 1c).

Superior pole arteries with a diameter <1 mm and an ischemic surface <1 cm^2 can be ligated. Even if the surface appears pink with reperfusion following superior pole artery ligation, there will be a small ischemic area in deep region due to the nature of the renal artery system. As the inferior pole artery might also nourish the ureter, it is more difficult to sacrifice, and because of the area it nourishes there is the potential for ureterovesical anastomosis leakage, ureteral necrosis, and urinary fistula. The inferior pole artery should be anastomosed end-to-side to the renal artery, and in cases in which the iliac artery is extremely atherosclerotic it should be anastomosed to the inferior epigastric artery in an end-to-end fashion.

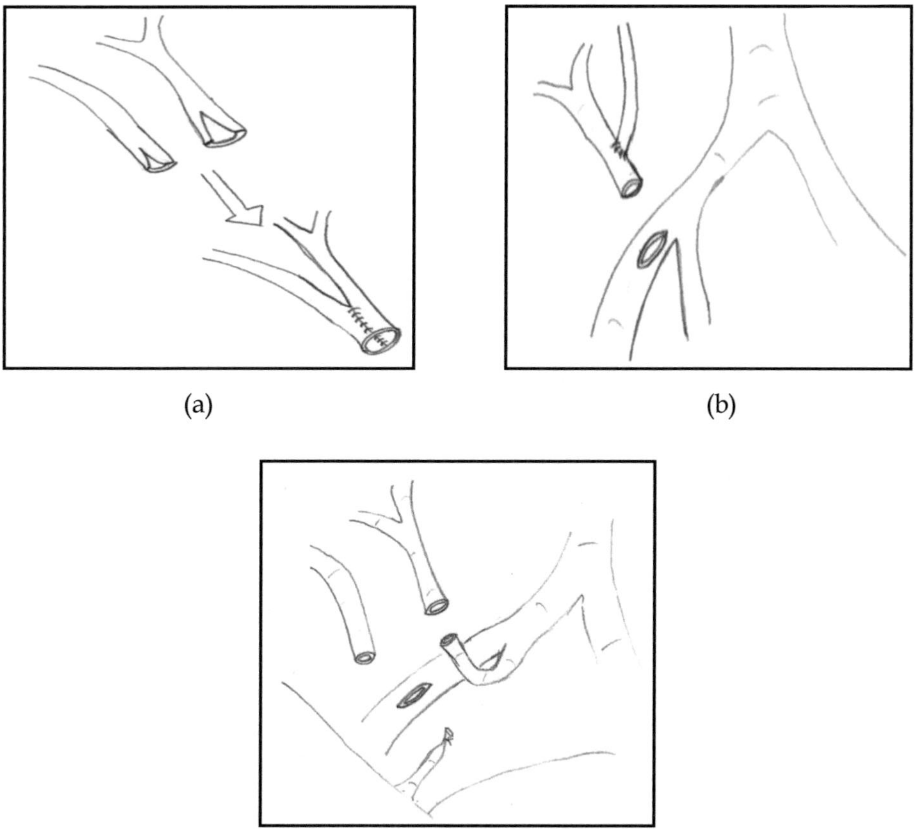

(a) (b) (c)

Fig. 1. There are multipl alternatives in artery anastomosis. **a.** Anastomosis of donor renal arteries before transplantation. **b.** Donor accessory renal artery can be anastomosed to main renal artery. **c.** Two renal arteries can be anastomosed to the internal iliac artery and external iliac artery.

1.4 Venous anastomosis

In living donor transplantation if the donor does not have multiple renal arteries or collecting system anomalies the left kidney should be used, because the left renal vein is longer. In deceased renal transplantation choice of side is unimportant. The left kidney is preferred primarily because the right renal vein is shorter and the right renal vein wall is thinner than the left. Vein anastomosis should be performed prior to artery anastomosis. The most common technique is end-to-side anastomosis between the renal vein and external iliac vein (Figure 2); when this cannot be performed other techniques can be used. If the renal vein is short the internal iliac vein can be ligated to achieve mobility, followed by end-to-side anastomosis to the external iliac vein. When the branches of the external iliac vein are occluded and the vena cava is functional, end-to-side anastomosis to the vena cava can be performed. When there is a short renal vein in cadaver transplants, venoplasty can be performed to extend the renal vein that is explanted along with vena cava.

After the iliac vein's anastomosis site is determined a venous clamp is situated horizontally and venotomy is performed. To prevent stitching from the opposite wall 5/0 stitches are placed in all 4 quadrants of the iliac vein. It is stitched continuously with 5/0 non-absorbable material. Another technique is situation of venous clamp horizontally. Venotomy is performed in accordance with the diameter of renal vein that will be anostomosed. Following the posterior wall, anterior wall anostomoses is performed with continue suture technique. In this tecnique, from outside to inside at distal corner of iliac venotomy and from inside to outside at distal corner of renal vein, folllowing posterior wall, anterior wall is erected continuously with the 6 / 0 polypropylene suture material. Surgeons must closely monitor the tension of the anastomosis and look for kinks (Figure 2).

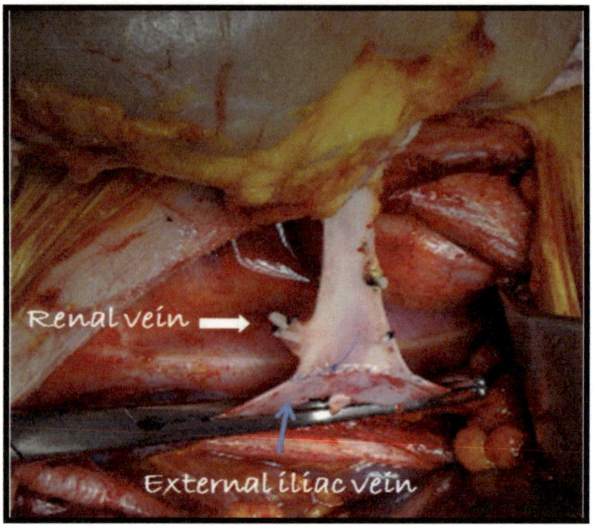

Fig. 2. End-to-side anastomosis of renal vein to the external iliac vein.

1.5 Arterial anastomosis

The renal arteries typically originate from the sides of the abdominal aorta, 1-2 cm distal of the superior mesenteric artery from the level of second lumbar vertebra. Normally, a single renal artery crosses the crura of the diaphragm and provides branches to the adrenal gland, kidneys, and ureters. Anatomical variation is more frequent than expected. Celiac truncus, superior mesenteric artery, phrenic artery, aortic bifurcation, common iliac artery, and even contralateral renal artery origin have been reported. Variations can be misleading during explantation and result in accidents during dissection. Renal arteries can be multiple (2-4 arteries) and in cadaver explantation they should always be removed from the aorta with a patch. Multiple arteries tend to be bilateral. The right renal artery is located behind the vena cava and is longer than the left (right: 0.8-8.0 cm; left: 0.5-6 cm). Renal artery diameter differs in males and females and is approximately 6.4-7.8 mm.

In 20% of cases the left kidney has multiple renal arteries.[4] An accessory superior pole renal artery <1 mm can be fastened; however, for arteries with a diameter similar to the common renal artery anastomosis should be performed. When there a 2 renal arteries both can be anastomosed to the external iliac artery end-to-side, one can be anastomosed end-to-end to the internal iliac artery and the other end-to-side to the external iliac artery, or the common renal artery can be anastomosed to the external iliac artery end-to-side and the inferior pole artery can be anastomosed to the inferior epigastric artery end-to-end. When the appropriate technique is used the vascular complication rate of multiple renal artery transplantation is similar to that of single renal artery transplantation.[5]

In order to decrease postoperative lymphocele lymphatic channels surrounding the artery should be fastened and dissected as little as the anastomosis area. Arterial anastomosis is commonly performed in an end-to-side to the external iliac artery; however, in the right kidney, end-to-end anastomosis to the internal iliac artery can be performed. In such cases the contralateral internal iliac artery must not be fastened. Arterial dissection should be performed with vigilance because in marginal donors there could be arterial plaques.

When dissection is completed the artery clamp should be positioned horizontally in a region without arterial plaques. Because the right kidney artery is long, it can be shortened to prevent formation of a kink. In left kidney transplantation anastomosis can be performed end-to-end to the internal iliac artery because the left renal artery is short. For large-diameter arteries anastomosis should be performed in a continuous fashion with 6/0 non-absorbable material and for small-diameter arteries it should be performed one-by-one with 7/0 non-absorbable material (Figure 3). In a similar fashion, anastomosis is performed using an aortic patch in deceased transplants.

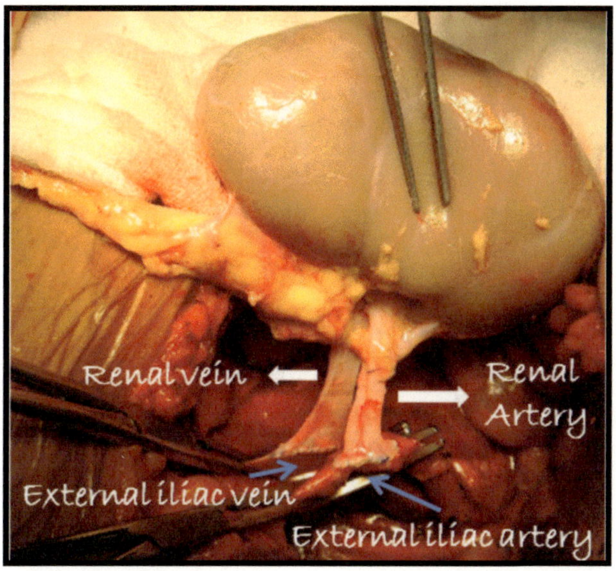

Fig. 3. Anastomosis of renal artery end-to-side to the external iliac artery.

1.6 Reperfusion

The duration of arterial and venous anastomosis should not exceed 40 min. Anastomosis exceeding 40 min increases the risk of primary non-function. Before vascular clamps are opened it should be determined if there is air in the artery; when there is, heparinized solution should be injected. Additional clamps should be placed proximal to those that were used during anastomosis and then the other clamps those used during anastomosis can be opened (Figure 4). The anastomosis region should be monitored for signs of bleeding. Bleeding usually results from a tributary vein or venous anastomosis line that is thinned due to extreme traction. If there is bleeding the site should be repaired using 5/0 or 6/0 non-absorbable sutures. After hemostasis is achieved systemic blood pressure is increased, and then the artery clamps are opened, followed by the vein clamps. When all is as it should be the renal parenchyma becomes pink and urine outflow occurs within a matter of minutes. If this is not observed, possible causes should be reviewed. For example, in marginal donor or

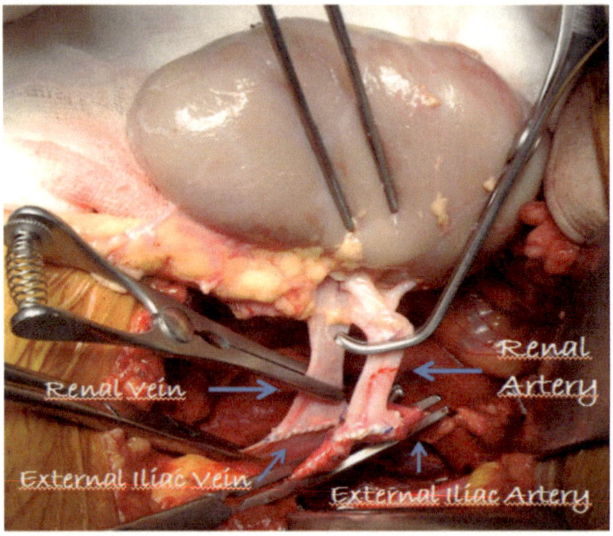

(a)

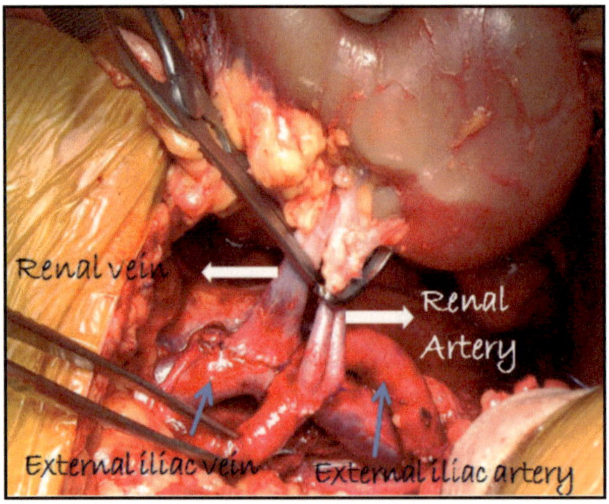

(b)

Fig. 4. **a.** Additional clamps can be placed proximal to the anastomosis. **b.** Before opening the clamps hemostasis must be cheched.

deceased transplants blotchy areas in the kidneys may be observed due to prolonged cold ischemia and the kidneys may not be totally perfused. Surgeons must first look for a kink in the renal artery and then for pulsation of the iliac artery proximal to the anastomosis line. If there is no obvious cause the artery should be clamped distally and injected with papaverine.

After arterial and venous anastomosis, ureteral anastomosis is completed via ureteroneocystostomy or ureteroureterostomy. When the kidney is implanted in the iliac fossa, care should be taken to ascertain that the artery, vein, and ureter are correctly positioned and that there is no kink.

2. Vascular thrombosis

2.1 Renal vein thrombosis

Renal vein thrombosis (RVT) is usually seen during the first post transplantation week in 0.3%-6.1% of patients.[6] Sudden oliguria, hematuria, pain in the transplantation region, life-threatening rupture and bleeding are clinical signs of this complication. Risk factors include surgical technique, hypercoagulopathy, right kidney transplantation, kidney transplantation in the left iliac fossa, lymphoceles, and vascular compression due to hematoma or hypovolemia. Venous thrombosis due to a short renal vein is seen more frequently in right kidney transplants.[7] In the late posttransplantation phase the risk factors are recurrent or de novo membranous nephropathy, iliofemoral vein thrombosis, thrombophilic disorders, and CMV infection.[8,9] With ultrasonography (US) one can observe a swollen or hypoechoic graft, a ruptured area in the cortex, lack of renal venous or arterial flow, and reverse arterial diastolic flow. Even though these findings are consistent with RVT they can be seen in cases of vascular rejection and in such cases magnetic resonance (MR) angiography can be performed for differential diagnosis.

The prognosis of RVT is poor. Acute thrombosis usually results in permanent graft loss. If RVT is suspected during the early postsurgical period additional surgery should be performed to save the graft. During such surgery the kidney should be extracted and reperfused, and should be re-implanted in the retroperitoneum after the iliac fossa is widened or implanted in the abdomen. Anastomosis should be proximal to the first anastomosis. In most center prophylactic low-dose subcutaneous heparin, sodium, or aspirin is used during the early postoperative period.[10] Late-phase thromboses secondary to iliofemoral vein thrombosis, de novo membranous nephropathy, and thrombophilic disorders are extremely rare; percutaneous interventions are commonly used to treath such complications.

2.2 Renal artery thrombosis

2.2.1 Etiology

Arterial thrombosis occurs in <1% of renal transplant patiens.[11,12] The first sign of arterial thrombosis is a sudden decrease in urine outflow; physicians should be aware that in cases in which the native kidney is producing urine and there is a delay in graft function, this early sign could be masked. The most common causes of renal artery thrombosis are technical. During nephrectomy in living donors or cadavers an intimal flap in the renal artery, occlusion due to atherom plaque in the recipient internal iliac artery or renal artery ostium, and torsion or kinking of the anastomosis can result in thrombosis. Other more rare causes include immunological reactions, hypercoagulopathy, cryoglobulin and anti-phospholipid antibodies associated with hypercoagulopathy and observed in active lupus erythrematosus patients, and thrombogenic drugs such as cyclosporin and monoclonal antibody OKT-3.[10,13]

2.2.2 Diagnosis

In all patients prerenal and post-renal causes of thrombosis should be investigated before transplantation. Hypovolemia due to prerenal reasons or hypoperfusion resulting from congestive heart disease should be excluded. Obstruction should be excluded by inserting a foley catheter. Moreover, the vascular tree should be evaluated for thrombosis. Color Doppler US is a useful investigative tool that not only shows renal artery and vein flow, but also facilitates calculation of the intraparenchymal resistance index. Angiography, which is useful for evaluating renal artery stenosis, is seldom used for investigating thrombosis. Between the onset of arterial thrombosis and its diagnosis infarcts and necrosis can develop. Most cases eventually undergo nephrectomy as a result. Allograft loss due to thrombosis rarely occurs, but its consequences are serious.

2.2.3 Treatment and prevention

Treatment of thrombosis is urgent exploration of the renal artery. In most cases the time from diagnosis to surgery is so long that necrosis occurs and nephrectomy is required. During exploration if the anastomosis line and cortical perfusion are observed to be normal Doppler US investigation and intraoperative renal biopsy should be performed. Allograft loss due to thrombosis is rare, but serious. Epidemiologic research shows that thrombotic risk factors are divided into 2 groups: those that can be modified (dialysis, drugs, and surgery) and those that cannot be modified: (age, diabetes mellitus, and vascular anomalies). It was also reported that in the first postoperative month the risk of thrombosis is higher in patients that undergo preoperative peritoneal dialysis and retansplant.[14]

Acetylsalicylic acid, low molecular weight heparin, and unfractionated heparin are used to prevent vascular thrombosis. It is reported that heparin, warfarin, and acetylsalicylic acid given in the early postoperative period decreases the vascular thrombosis rate, but increases the bleeding rate.[15-17] These studies were retrospective case-control studies and the reliability, efficacy, and optimal utilization time of such agents that prevent allograft thrombosis as acetylsalicylic acid and heparin can only be ascertained by large, multicenter randomized studies.

2.2.4 Prevention strategies

1. The most common cause of thrombosis is surgical technique. Attention should be paid to the anastomosis technique and vascular dissection; in particular, the intimal layer must not be damaged.
2. Acute tubular necrosis, one of the causes of vascular thrombosis, may be prevented by minimizing the duration of hot and cold ischemia.
3. Early diagnosis of vascular or antibody-mediated rejection, and treatment reduces the risk of both endothelial and vascular thrombosis.

4. In patients with a high risk of thrombosis low molecular weight heparin, warfarin, or acetylsalicylic acid should be administered during the early postoperative period.

3. Renal artery stenosis

The most important vascular complication during the late postsurgical period is renal artery stenosis, which has an incidence rate of 2%-8%, but has also been reported to be as high as 23%.[18,19] Its signs are poor renal function test results, sudden onset of resistant hypertension, and life-threatening congestive heart failure.[20] Most patients are investigated due to an initial diagnosis of rejection. Some patients with renal artery stenosis are asymptomatic. In asymptomatic renal transplant recipients renal artery stenosis is 12.4% based on routine Doppler screening, versus 2.4% in symptomatic patients.[21] Renal artery stenosis occurs in the anastomosis region most frequently between post transplant month 3 and year 2, although it can be pre- or post-anastomosis in origin. The incidence of renal artery stenosis is higher in cases of end-to-end anastomosis.

There are 3 types of renal artery stenosis: anastomotic, diffuse post-anastomotic, and widespread restriction in the distal arterial bed. The etiology of the anastomotic type is the restriction effect of the suture, and injury to donor vessels during nephrectomy. Intimal flaps in the vessel wall and subintimal dissection lead to intimal injury and hyperplasia. A kink in the artery or angulation when the kidney is being implanted leads to turbulent flow and stenosis in the anastomosis. The diffuse post-anastomotic type of stenosis can affect different regions of the artery (multiple stenosis), as well as the entire artery (diffuse stenosis). De novo (previously present) atherosclerosis in donor vessels can cause diffuse stenosis in the long term under the influence of immunosuppressive agents. The third type of stenosis—widespread stenosis in the distal arterial bed—usually occurs due to immune-mediated endothelial injury. Cytomegalovirus (CMV) leads to renal artery stenosis due to endothelial injury via proliferation in smooth muscle cells.

Renal artery stenosis during the late post transplant period is most often seen in kidneys with multiple renal arteries. The stenosis rate (0%) for anastomoses performed via the aortic patch technique is much lower than that (5%) observed in anastomoses performed via techniques other than the patch.[22] The aortic patch is specific to cadaveric transplantation.

3.1 Diagnosis

Doppler US, CT angiography, MR angiography, and angiographic imaging methods can be used to diagnose renal artery stenosis; however, angiography is the gold standard. Doppler US is routinely used to evaluate transplanted kidney parenchyma and vascular structures, and must be performed by experienced personel in order to achieve optimum results. In Doppler US, peak systolic velocity >2.5 m s^{-1} in the stenotic region is significant for renal artery stenosis. In a region close to the anastomosis site an iliac artery peak systolic velocity to renal artery velocity ratio >2 suggests stenosis.[23] Patients suspected to have stenosis based on Doppler US should be evaluated with CT angiography, which provides valuable information about the location and extent of renal artery stenosis. Before CT angiography adequate hidration and N-acetylcysteine should be given in order to prevent contrast-induced nephropathy. Definitive diagnosis of renal artery stenosis is made based on renal angiography.

3.2 Treatment

Treatment of renal artery stenosis can be conservative (in cases in which graft perfusion is normal) or revascularization (surgery or percutaneous transluminal angioplasty [PTA]) can be performed. If stenosis is ≤60%, renal function is normal, and arterial hypertension is manageable with medical therapy, patients can be followed-up with Doppler US. In cases in which medical therapy is inadequate PTA (with or without stenting) is the treatment of choice (Figure 5). In cases with stenosis of the hilar region or distal renal bed, PTA is the preferred treatment option. Success rate of PTA/stenting was 60%-94%, the complication rate was 0.8%-3%, and 1 year post procedure 85% of stents remained unoccluded.[24,25]

Permanent treatment of renal artery stenosis is surgery. PTA is not the treatment of choice in patients with renal artery stenosis due to arterial kinks or atherosclerotic diseases; in such patients surgical intervention should be performed. Surgery involves removal of the stenotic segment and re-anastomosis to the external iliac artery or anastomosis to the internal iliac artery using the saphenous vein. In cases of post-anastomotic stenosis the bypass grafting technique is used via autogenous graft. The surgical success rate varies between 63% and 92%,[26] and in 10%-12% of patients restenosis occurs within the first 8-9 months following surgery.[27]

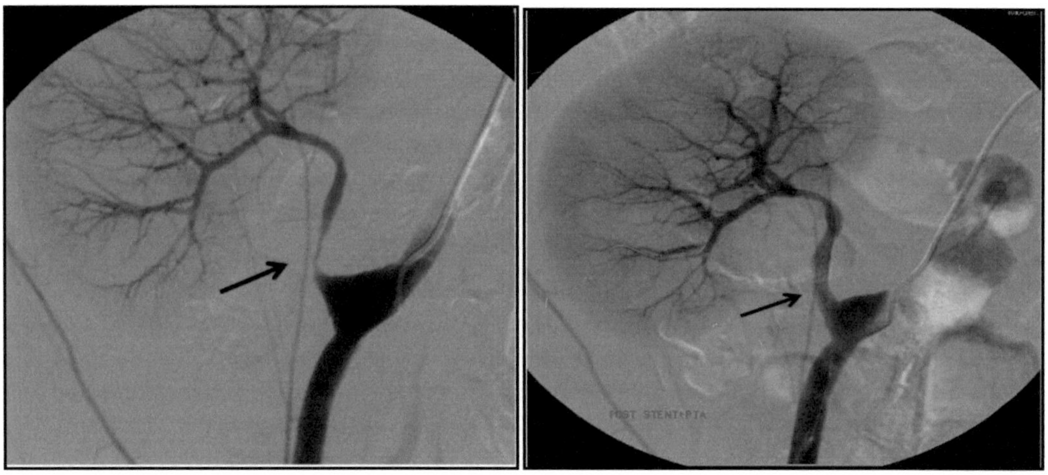

(a) (b)

Fig. 5. **a.** Conventional angiography shows stenosis of the renal artery in a kidney transplant patient (arrow) **b**. Post-PTA conventional angiography shows successful stent implantation at the renal artery stenotic segment (arrow).

4. Summary

Renal transplantation is the treatment of choice for end-stage renal disease. Despite medical and surgical advances, vascular complications after kidney transplantation remain an important clinical problem that may increase morbidity, hospitalization and costs. Vascular complications in renal transplantation are not uncommon and may often lead to allograft loss. The most common vascular complications are renal artery stenosis, renal artery thrombosis and renal vein thrombosis. Transplant renal artery and vein thrombosis have an early onset and a dramatic clinical manifestation and usually lead to allograft loss. These complications may compromise graft function and cause significant morbidity. Therefore, knowledge of the incidence, clinical manifestations and management of vascular complications is necessary for all kidney transplant surgeons.

5. References

[1] Kobayashi K, Censullo ML, Rossman LL, et al: Interventional radiologic management of renal transplant dysfunction: indications, limitations, and technical considerations. Radiographics 27:1109, 2007.

[2] Paul J. Phelan, William Shields, Patrick O'Kelly et al. Left versus right deceased donor renal allograft outcome Transpl Int. 2009;22(12):1159-63.

[3] Parrott NR, Forsythe JL, Matthews JN, et al: Late perfusion: a simple remedy for renal allograft primary nonfunction. Transplantation 49:913-915, 1990.

[4] J.K. Hwang, S.D. Kim, S.C. Park,The Long-Term Outcomes of Transplantation of Kidneys With Multiple Renal Arteries. *Transplantation Proceedings,* 42, 4053–4057 (2010).

[5] Hwang JK, Kim SD, Park SC, Choi BS, Kim JI, Yang CW, Kim YS, Moon IS. The long-term outcomes of transplantation of kidneys with multiple renal arteries. Transplant Proc. 2010 Dec;42(10):4053-7.

[6] Obed A, Uihlein DC, Zorger N, et al: Severe renal vein stenosis of a kidney transplant with beneficial clinical course after successful percutaneous stenting. Am J Transplant. 8:2173, 2008.

[7] Takahashi M, Humke U, Girndt M, Kramann B, Uder M. Early posttransplantation renal allograft perfusion failure due to dissection: diagnosis and interventional treatment. AJR Am J Roentgenol 2003; 180: 759–763.

[8] Kazory A, Ducloux D, Coaquette A, Manzoni P, Chalopin JM. Cytomegalovirus-associated venous thromboembolism in renal transplant recipients: a report of 7 cases. Transplantation 2004;77:597–599.

[9] Hausmann MJ, Vorobiov M, Zlotnik M, Rogachev B, Tomer A. Increased coagulation factor levels leading to allograft renal vein thrombosis. Clin Nephrol 2004;61:222–224.

[10] Irish A. Hypercoagulability in renal transplant recipients. Identifying patients at risk of renal allograft thrombosis and evaluating strategies for prevention. Am J Cardiovasc Drugs. 2004;4(3):139-49.

[11] M.L. Melamed, H.S. Kim and B.G. Jaar et al., Combined percutaneous mechanical and chemical thrombectomy for renal vein thrombosis in kidney transplant recipients, Am J Transplant 5 (2005), p. 621.

[12] Obed, D.C. Uihlein and N. Zorger et al., Severe renal vein stenosis of a kidney transplant with beneficial clinical course after successful percutaneous stenting, Am J Transplant (2008), p. 2173.

[13] Bombeli T, Muller M, Straub PW, Haeberli A. Cyclosporine - induced detachment of vascular endothelial cells initiates the intrinsic coagulation system in plasma and whole blood. J Lab Clin Med 1996; 127:621 - 634.

[14] R. Palomar, P. Morales, E. Rodrigo et al. Venous Graft Thrombosis in Patients on Peritoneal Dialysis Before Transplantation Transplantation Proceedings, 39, 2128–2130 (2007).

[15] Humar A, Key N, Ramcharan T, Payne WD, Sutherland DER, Matas AJ. Kidney transplants after initial graft loss to vascular thrombosis. Clin Transplant 2001: 15: 6–10.
[16] Paul E. Morrissey, Pedro J. Ramirez, Reginald Y. Gohh. et all. Management of Thrombophilia in Renal Transplant Patients American Journal of Transplantation 2002; 2: 872–876
[17] Boughey JC, Bowen PA 2nd, Gifford RR Renal transplantation in patients with hypercoagulable states. J S C Med Assoc. 2003 Dec;99 (12):372-4.)
[18] Osman Y, Shokeir A, Ali - el - Dein B, et al. Vascular complications after live donor renal transplantation: study of risk factors and effects on graft and patient survival. J Urol 2003; 169: 859 - 862.
[19] Patel NH, Jindal RM, Wilkin T, et al: Renal arterial stenosis in renal allografts: retrospective study of predisposing factors and outcome after percutaneous transluminal angioplasty. Radiology 219:663, 2001.
[20] Garovic VD, Textor SC: Renovascular hypertension and ischemic nephropathy. Circulation 112:1362-1374, 2005.
[21] Wong W, Fynn SP, Higgings RM, et al. Transplant renal artery stenosis in 77 patients: does it have an immunological cause? Transplantation 61: 1996;215–219.
[22] Fung LC, McLorie GA, Khoury AE, Churchill BM. Donor aortic cuff reduces the rate of anastomotic arterial stenosis in pediatric renal transplantation. J Urol 1995;154: 909–91.
[23] Cosgrove D, Chan K. Renal transplants: What ultrasound can and cannot do. Ultrasound Quarterly 2008;24:77-87.
[24] Peregrin JH, Stríbrná J, Lácha J, et al: Long-term follow-up of renal transplant patients with renal artery stenosis treated by percutaneous angioplasty. Eur J Radiol 66:512, 2008
[25] Patel NH, Jindal RM, Wilkin T, et al: Renal arterial stenosis in renal allografts: retrospective study of predisposing factors and outcome after percutaneous transluminal angioplasty. Radiology 219:663, 2001.
[26] Benoit G, Moukarzel M, Hiesse C, et al: Transplant renal artery stenosis: experience and comparative results between surgery and angioplasty. Transpl Int 3:137, 1990.
[27] Aktas, F. Boyvat, S. Sevmis. at al.Analysis of Vascular Complications After Renal Transplantation. Transplantation Proceedings, 43, 557–561 (2011).

5

Progressive Endolaparoscopic Vascular Training in a Computerized Enhanced Instrumentation Based on Outcome Measurements

Bernardo Martinez and George Pradeesh
Medical Director Vascular Robotic Program,
The Toledo Hospital, The Toledo Clinic, Inc.
USA

1. Introduction

Our commitment in minimally invasive vascular surgery began in 1982, when we designed our endoscope, attached to a micro video camera to make the Endoscopic transaxillary first rib and cervical bands resection safer.

During the next decade we evolved with the rapid technological development of minimally invasive surgery.

In 1996, the French Canadian Dr. Ives Dion was the first to create a solid animate Laboratory training toward the approach of full laparoscopic human aortic reconstruction.

In 1997 we modified Dr. Dion's animate model into the following aspects:

- Create the Transperitoneal approach.
- Aortic graft with two anastomosis.
- Introduction of computerized enhanced instrumentation or Robotic technology.

During the next five years, 1997-2001 few Centers around the world were divided among "robotic" vs. "Non Robotic" in pursuing the tremendous technical effort to conquer the human aortic reconstruction.

In 2002 a Dutch-American team effort (Dr. Wisselink-Dr. Gracia) conquered for the first time the Robotic Full Laparoscopic Aortic Reconstruction using the Zeus Robotic System (Computer Motion). Our first Full Laparoscopic Aortic Graft was done in 2005, and our first Robotic Assisted Aortic Graft was done in 2007.

The objective in this chapter is to describe our own training methods, not only for a vascular surgeon interested in robotic technology, but also to other specialties; this is a very friendly and cost effective approach to solve the dilemma of "steep learning curve" for vascular surgeons. In addition, resolves the credential institutional process for every specialty involved in robotic surgery.

2. Modular robotic training program

This program was created in 2004 based upon our own self training and training other individuals of different specialties since 1997.

3. Basic concept

The Robotic Surgeon, regardless of his/her specialty needs to perform three basic tasks:

1. Tissue manipulation or dissection
2. To cut tissue
3. To suture tissue or graft materials

These tasks change in intensity depending upon the surgical procedure. Specialties like vascular surgery, cardiac surgery in which the suturing task is critically important for the functional outcome of the procedure. Not only the quality, but the speed is very important. It literally separates vascular surgery from other specialties in which there is less suturing demand. We worked with Dr. James Rosser (2000-2002) adopting his own exercises of "Top Gun" Laparoscopic School of training to the robotic technology.

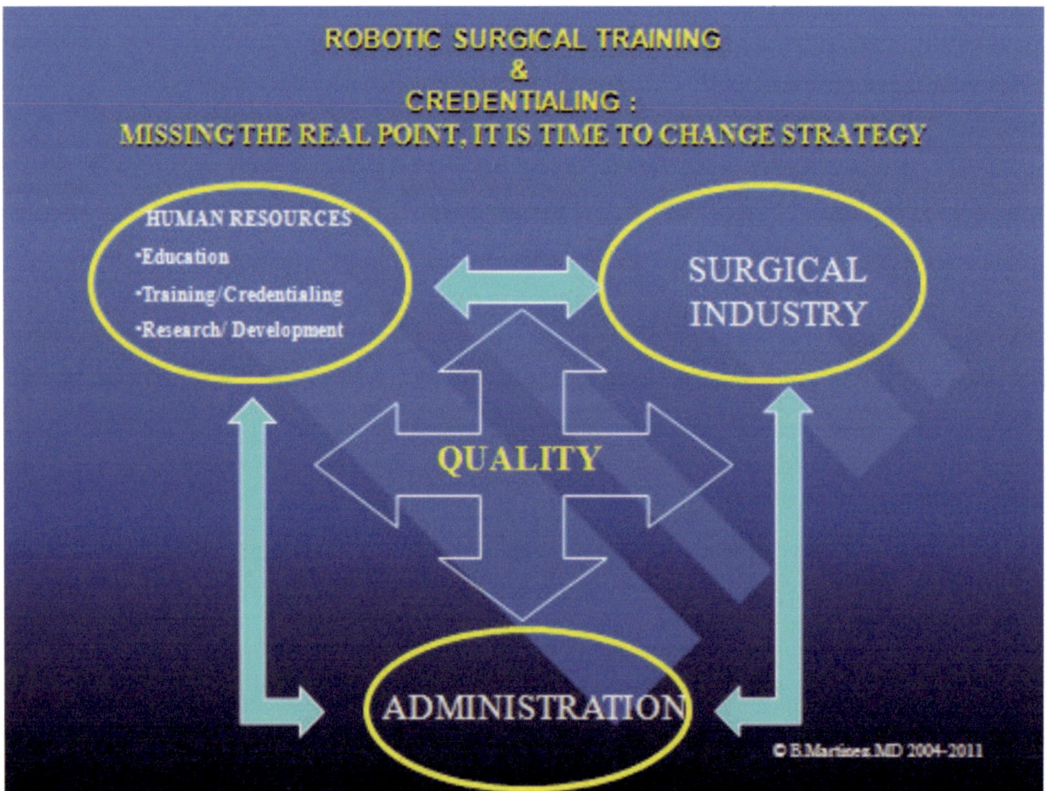

Fig. 1. Robotic Surgical Training & Credential

4. Delivery quality

The robotic trainee is not going to deliver good quality, unless there is clear support from the Institutional Administration. Full commitment for a dedicated space and human resources to support the execution of this program. Delivering quality in surgical procedures is saving economic resources for the Institution. **(Fig. 1)**

5. Learning new set of skills

The trainee (student-resident-junior or senior surgeon) is facing a real dilemma in terms of selecting the time, the opportunities, the cost and most importantly, how to put this package together in a very difficult economic era.

The individual has to learn a new set of motor sensory skills involving BRAIN-EYES-HAND-FEET functional coordination, including the function of the voice. This learning process falls into these four areas. **(Fig. 2)**

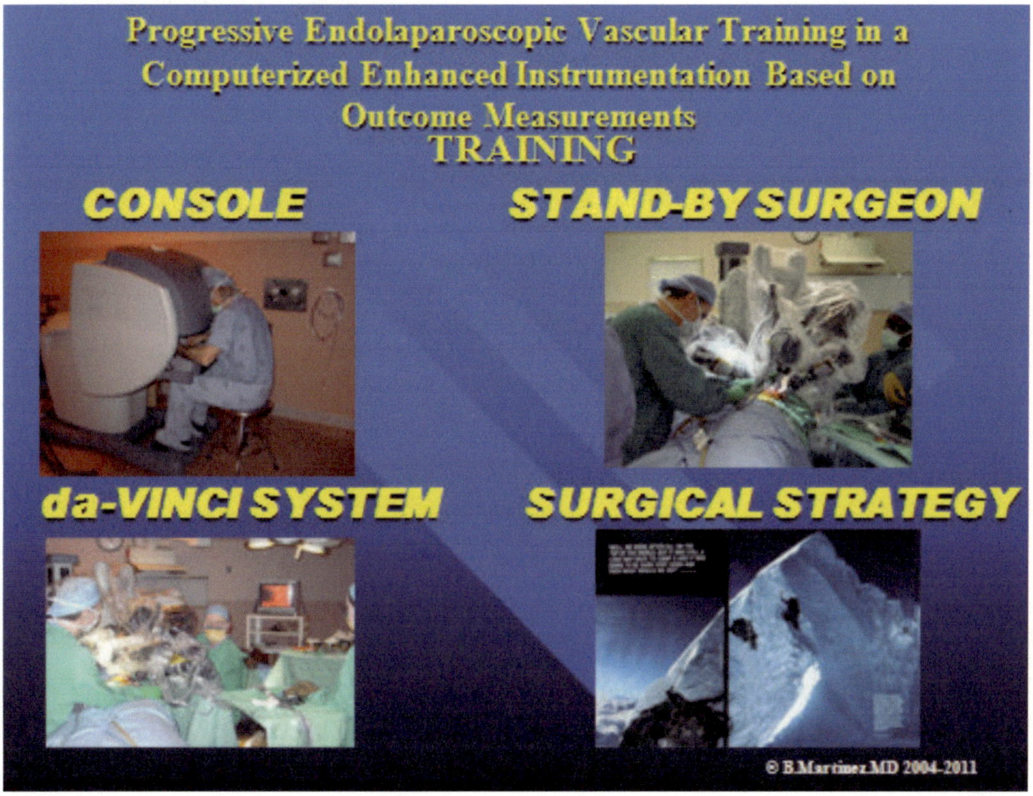

Fig. 2. Progressive Endolaparoscopic Vascular Training

1. Console: the trainee must spend time performing the exercises and measuring his/her performance.
2. Stand-By: the surgeon at the side of the patient is very important, sometimes more than the console surgeon in the execution of certain portion of the procedure.

3. Robotic System: The full potential of the equipment and its limitation must be know.
4. Classroom Debriefing: very similar to Aerial Combat, classroom didactic discussions are required in order to improve the performance of the Team. And avoidance of potential mistakes.

We took the "Rosser Cobra Rope" and the "Rosser Intracorporial suturing" to simulate tissue manipulation and tissue reconstruction functions designing our own "Cutting Exercise" technique. These are the "keys" of the entire learning process. We teach and demonstrate these exercises in individual and group sessions. When we see the immediate learning process, we then teach suturing anastomosis. **(Fig. 3)**

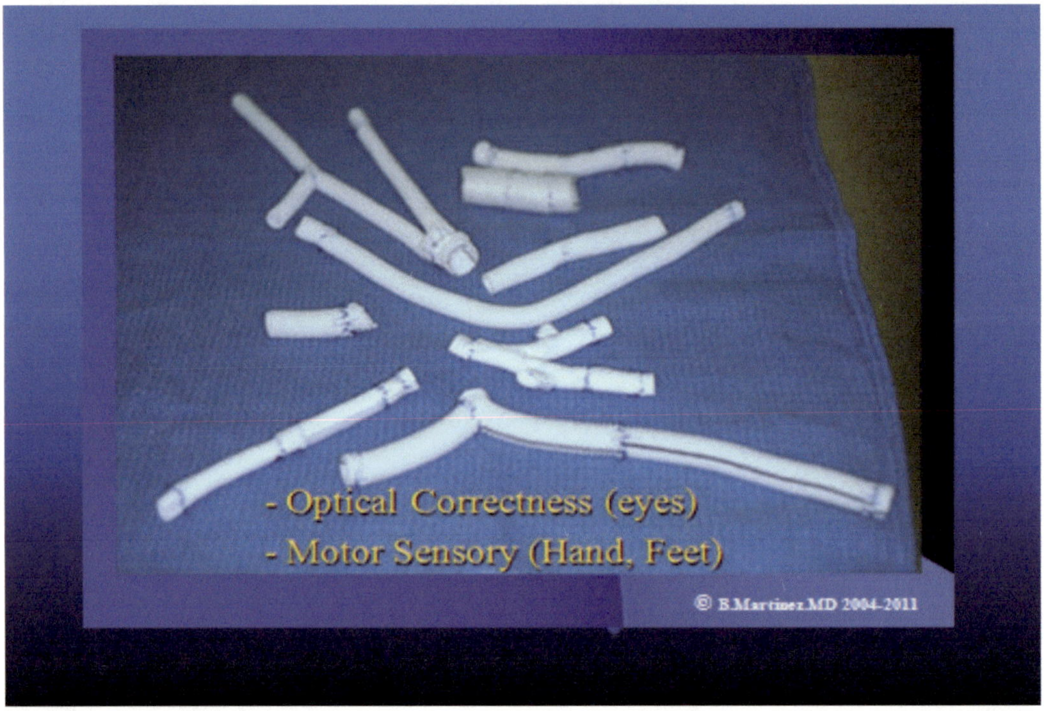

Fig. 3. Suture Anastomosis

As friendly and competitive as these exercises would be we bring the trainee slowly into a new area of measuring outcome performance for the training and credentialing process.

This computerized enhanced instrumentation training program has three different modules based upon performance. **(Fig. 4)**

1. Basic Laparoscopic, very similar to Rosser's criteria.
2. Basic Robotics
3. Advance Robotics

There are hours of minimally dry laboratory practice that are required. At the end of each module the trainee must perform "on examination": in order to pass and move to the next module of higher technical skills. The modules can be taken in separate periods of time or in a solid one time block.

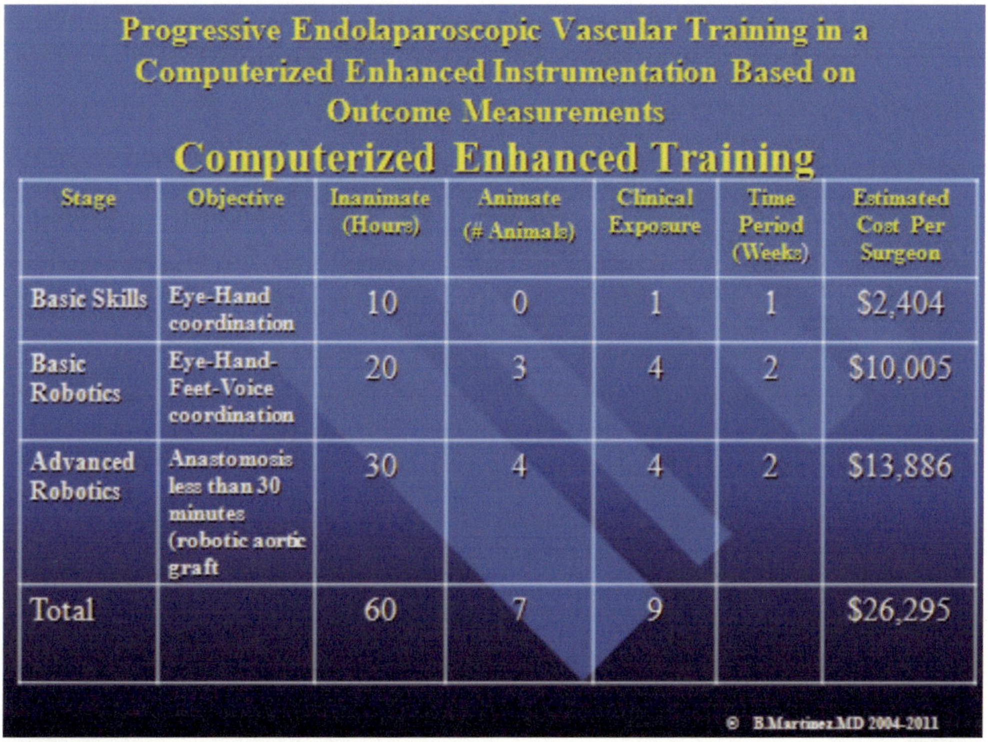

Stage	Objective	Inanimate (Hours)	Animate (# Animals)	Clinical Exposure	Time Period (Weeks)	Estimated Cost Per Surgeon
Basic Skills	Eye-Hand coordination	10	0	1	1	$2,404
Basic Robotics	Eye-Hand-Feet-Voice coordination	20	3	4	2	$10,005
Advanced Robotics	Anastomosis less than 30 minutes (robotic aortic graft	30	4	4	2	$13,886
Total		60	7	9		$26,295

Fig. 4. Computerized Enhanced Training

Animated laboratory exposure is critically important in the robotic learning process. These are a progression of tasks, as skills are developed for a maximum cost benefit. The progressive learning task involves:

1. Port placement.
2. Engagements and disengagements of the robotic system. Then performing Transperitoneal aortic dissection, clamping application of the aorta. Finally, it is the Aortic graft implant repeating two suture anastomosis.

The "graduation" or final examination is to perform a fully endolaparoscopic robotically assisted aortic graft implant in less than 200 minutes of total operative time and maximum of 72 minutes of aortic cross clamping time, delivering good anastomosis products .

The cost analysis shown was made in 2004. This was based upon our laboratory cost and it was compared with other models around the world. Significant variability exists among different institutions.

6. Clinical exposure

During the course of training the exposure of clinical material and surgery demonstrations are absolutely critical requirements. Our philosophy was that "safety" is the main priority. We worked with U.S. Food and Drug Administration during the clinical application of robotic technology in humans, we created our own aortic protocol. We obtained the investigational device exemption required for new technology. **(Table 1)**

Description	Robotic da Vinci®	Robotic da Vinci® Predetermined	AESOP® Assisted
Femoral grafts	4		
Iliac grafts	4		
Aortic grafts	4	2	45
Endoleaks type II	5		
Retroperitoneal	4		
Thoracic Outlet Syndrome	195		91
Sympathectomies	6		
Total	224		

Table 1. Total robotic Clinical Exposure

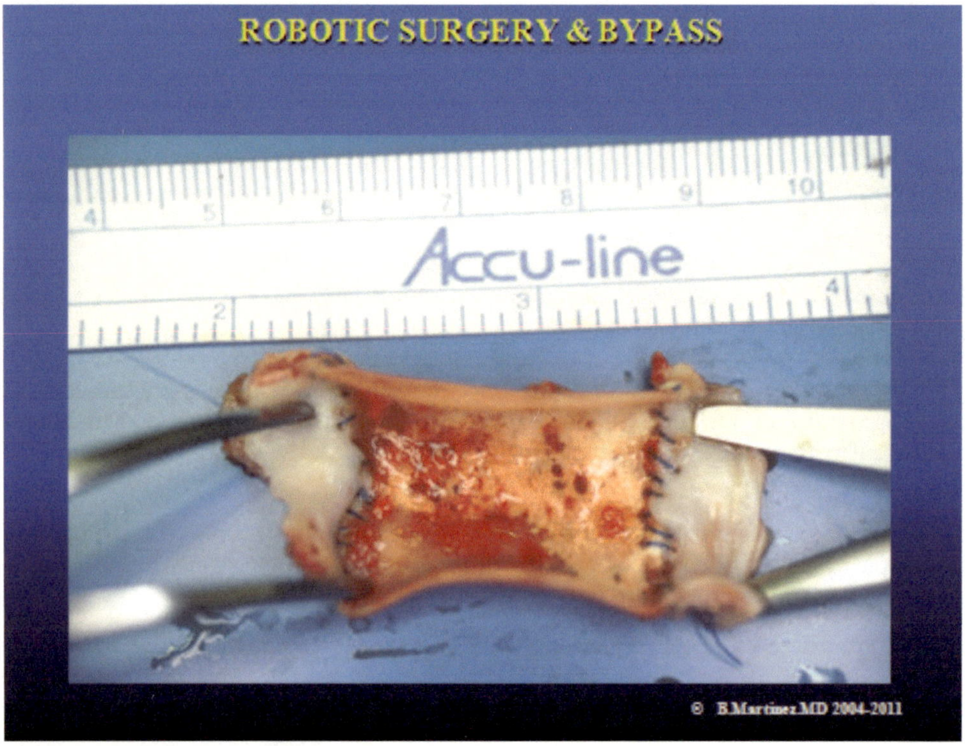

Fig. 5. Porcine Infrarenal Aortic Graft

7. Results

7.1 Trainees

During 2002-2008 fifty five trainees passed through out our laboratory of training program. Twenty nine (29%) percent were local-regional surgeons. Forty nine (49%) were residents and twenty two (22%) were visitors out of state and out of USA. **(Fig. 6)**

The following conclusions were revealed:

We found that visitor surgeons were the most successful and having the least difficulties in the establishment of robotic technology in their respective geographic locations.
We felt that our dry laboratory training program was not optimized and significant potential for improvement exists.

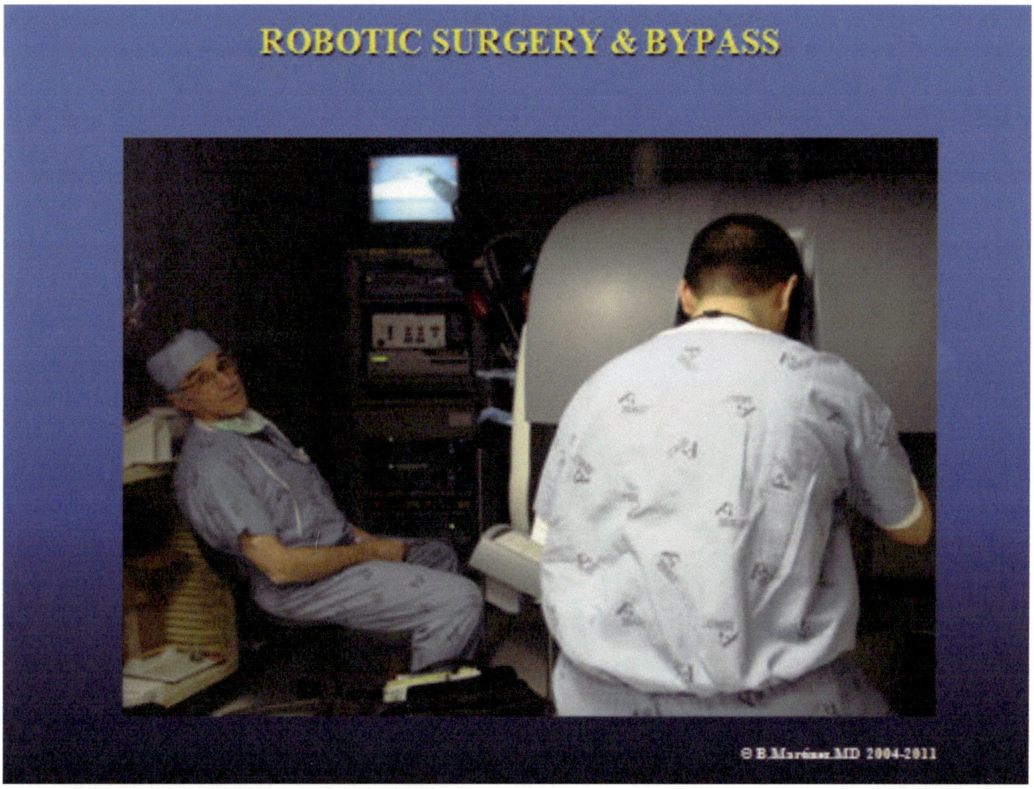

Fig. 6. Trainee in session

7.2 Laboratory model

Our laboratory training and research model has been 50 porcine models since 1997. Today we have completed 224 applications of the da Vinci® robotic in vascular surgical patients. In addition, there are 45 aortic surgical reconstruction and 91 transaxillary first rib and cervical bands resection using the first generation of robotic technology Aesop®/Hermes (1998-2002).

7.3 Aortic robotic reconstruction

Our human Aortic Robotic Reconstruction can be divided in two stages:

1. Pre da Vinci® Group (1998-2007)

Forty five patients underwent Laparoscopic Aortic Reconstruction for occlusive (29=64%) aneurysmal disease (7=16%) and combined aneurysmal and occlusive disease (9=20%).

The procedures were executed using Aesop®-Hermes robotic arm voice activated. Endoscopic Vein Harvesting instrumentation.

Thirty two patients (32/45=71%) were laparoscopic assisted (incision <9cm length) **(Fig. 7)**, twelve patients (12/45=27%) were hybrid laparoscopic assisted (incision 9-16cm) **(Fig. 8)** and one patient (1/45=2.2%) full laparoscopic. **(Fig. 9)** There was one mortality (1/45=2.2%) due to non-stone cholecystitis.

In this Pre da Vinci® group, no bleeding, non spinal cord ischemia, no thrombosis was observed. Complexity of these procedures indicates that (25/45=56%) required concomitan additional procedures like, aortic or and femoral endarterectomies and femopopliteal reconstruction.

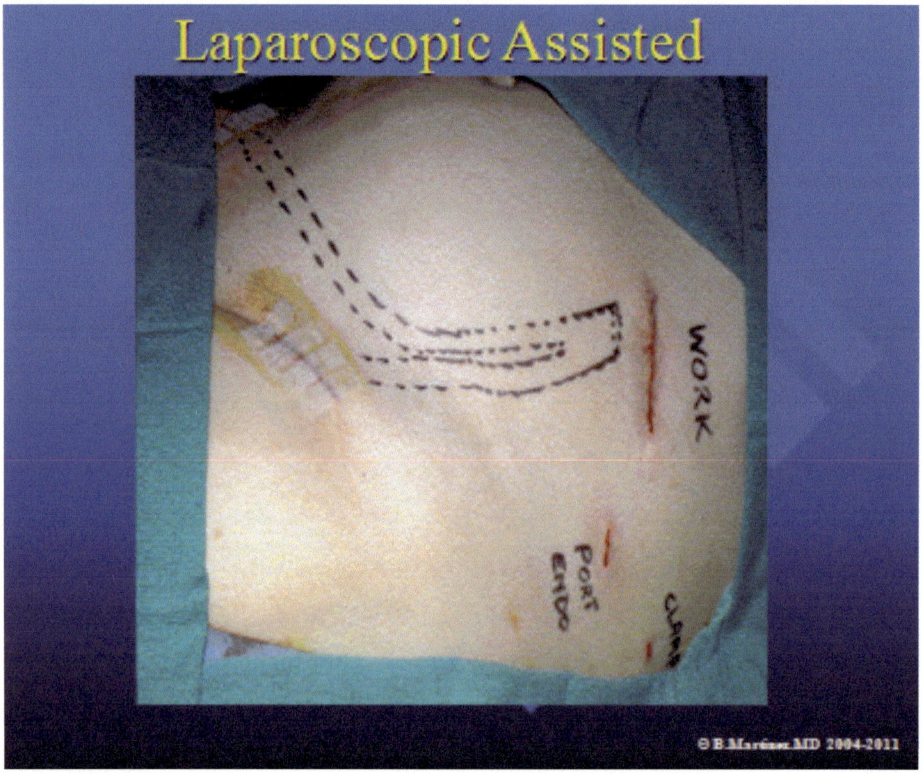

Fig. 7. Laparoscopic Assisted for Occlusive Disease (<9cm).

2. da Vinci® Group (2007-2008)

Six patients underwent aortic reconstruction for atherosclerotic occlusive disease under the U.S. Food and Drug Administration guideline protocol. Three patients had full laparoscopic robotic reconstruction. Two patients had "pre-determined" conversion to minilaparotomy. One patient with hostile bowel and one patient had "unplanned" conversion due to hostile tunnel

All patients survived without major complications. All patients are alive, having functional grafts and one patient required aortic anastomotic covered stent to protect myointimal hyperplasia postoperative. Additionally, we have performed in eight patients' illio femoral graft robotically assisted. **(Fig. 10)**

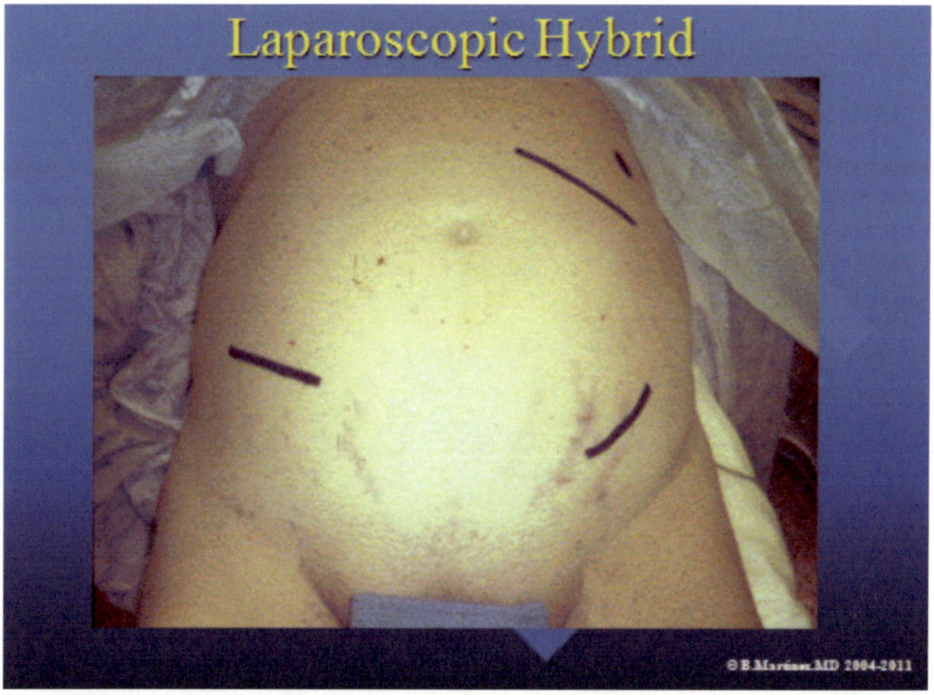

Fig. 8. Laparoscopic Hybrid for Aneurysmal Disease (<16cm).

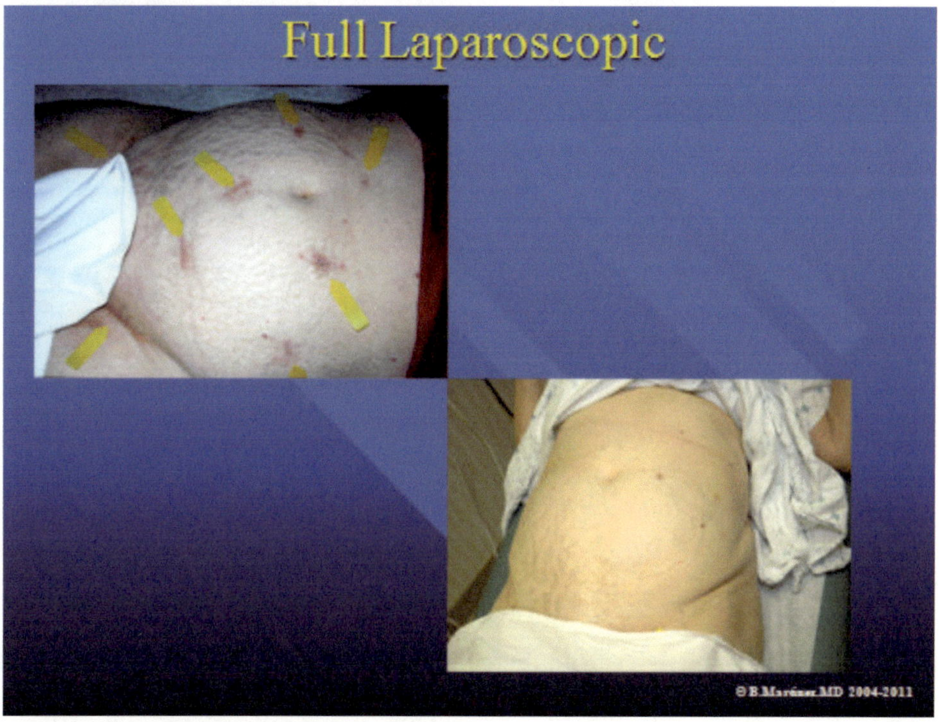

Fig. 9. Full Laparoscopic for Occlusive Disease.

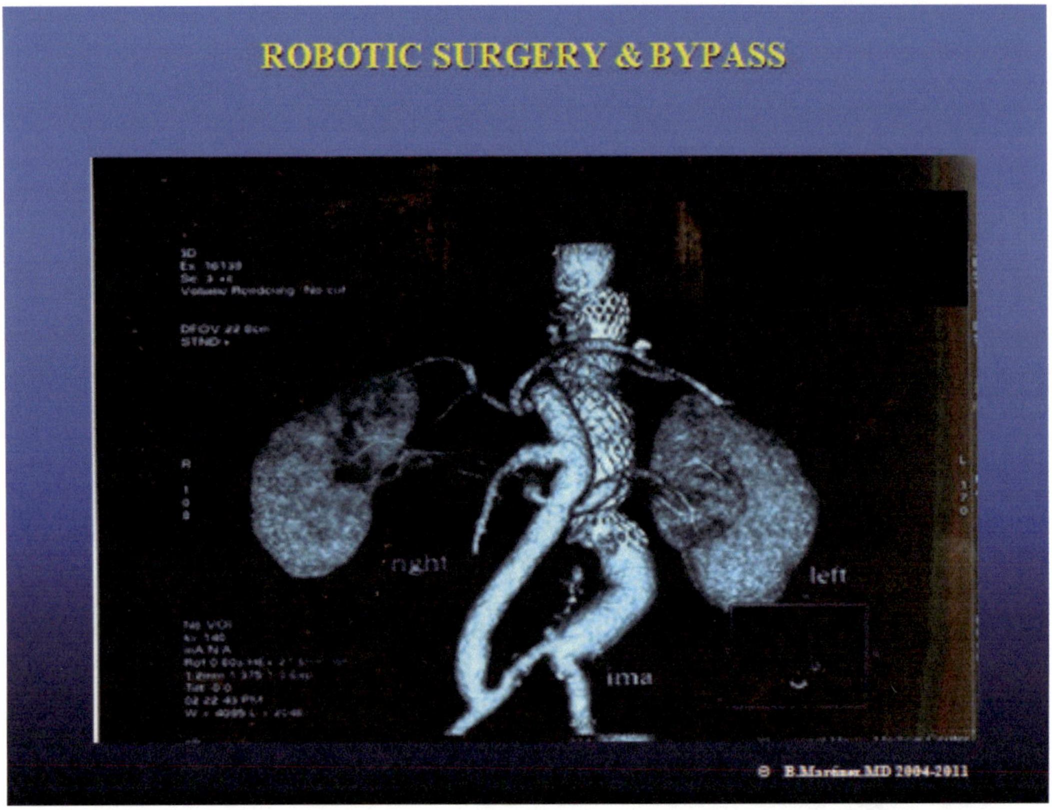

Fig. 10. Iliac to birenal-superior mesenteric and celiac graft-debranching-rebranching and aortic stenting for suprarenal aortic aneurysm. Iliac anastomosis created by full laparoscopic robotic assistance.

8. Vascular surgical approaches-new concept

Currently Vascular surgeons are most often offering to our patients, either conventional or endovascular surgical procedures- Laparoscopic Aortic Surgery is not widely accepted.

In our opinion, Laparoscopic Aortic Surgery whether it is performed using robotic technology or not, represents the "Logical Bridge" between endovascular and conventional vascular approaches.

Under the concept that we are treating the atherosclerotic occlusive and degenerative aneurysmal disease of the Infra Renal Aorta. We are at a critical evolutionary moment in which endovascular therapy is taking a primary role. However Leaders in vascular surgery, for the most part, are ignoring robotic technology as an alternative of minimally invasive vascular surgery.

Unfortunately there is a dilemma about the training and the adoption of Robotic technology.

Therefore, those vascular surgeons, without robotic training are indicating conventional surgery, whether endovascular approaches are difficult or have already failed.

Robotic Laparoscopic techniques, with their ability to "Bridge" endovascular and conventional vascular traditional surgery, are overlooked in addition to it's capability to "Rescue" endovascular procedures from complications such as "Endoleak."

9. Conclusion

Why robotics in vascular surgery? We wrote in 2004. "Because just as robotic or computer technology revolutionized "safety" in the automotive industry. This technology has the potential to revolutionize patient "safety" in surgery in the 21st century.

We have developed a very solid and comprehensive robotic training laboratory model. It allows us to demonstrate that we have delivered "safely" this technology to our patients in thoracic outlet syndrome and infrarenal aortic surgery.

The robotic vascular technology and endovascular therapy are reciprocal complementary techniques to offer minimal invasive alternatives to our patients.

The potential of robotic vascular surgery to expand in other areas (suprarenal aorta, visceral arterial reconstruction and retroperitoneal pathology) open the doors for a tremendous opportunity for training which if it is done properly as we presented, the cutting edge technology will be delivered with quality with substantial savings and economic resources for medical organizations.

10. Acknowledgment

We would like to acknowledge Ms. Tamra D. Jared , COF,CCT for her contribution to this publication.

11. References

Abaza R, Wiegand CS, Martinez BD. Laparoscopic aortorenal bypass in an acute porcine model under warm ischemia: Case reports 5 feasibility study and resident training module. J Endourol 2007;21:645-651.

Coggia M, Di Centa I, Javerliat I, Colacchio G, Goeau-Brissonniere O. Total laparoscopic aortic surgery: transperitoneal left retrorenal approach. Eur J Vasc Endovasc Surg 2004;28:619-622.

Diks J, Nio D, Jongkind V, Cuesta MA, Rauwerda JA, Wisselink W. Robot-assisted laparoscopic surgery of the infrarenal aorta: the early learning curve. Surg Endosc 2007;21:1760-1763 erratum in Surg. Endosc. 2007;21:2118-2119.

Dion YM, Katkhouda N, Rouleau C, Aucoin A. Laparoscopyassisted aortobifemoral bypass. Surg Laparosc Endosc 1993;3:425-429.

Hoff JT. Research by academic surgeons. Am J Surg 2003;1 85: 13-15.

Nio D, Diks J, Linsen MA, et al. Robot-assisted laparoscopic aortobifemoral blpass for aortoiliac occlusive disease: early clinical experience. Eur J Vasc Endovasc Surg 2005;29: 586-590.

Martinez BD, Zarins CI, Daunt DA, et ai. A porcine model for endolaparoscopic abdominal aortic repair and endoscopic training. J.S.L.S. 2003;7:129-136.

Martinez BD, Wiegand CS, Evans P, Gerhardinger A, Mendez J. Computer-assisted instrumentation during endoscopictransaxillary first rib resection for thoracic outlet syndrome: a safe aiternate approach. Vascular 2OO5;13:327 -335.

Martinez BD, Wiegand CS, Mendez J. Performance measurements in endolaparoscopic infrarenal aortic graft implantation using computer-enhanced instrumentation: a laboratory model for training. J.S.L.S. 2007; 11:326-335.

Martinez BD, Gerhardinger A, Thoracic Outlet Syndrome: Endoscopic Transaxillary First Rib Approach- 23 Years Experience (1985-2008) T.J. Fogarty, R.A. White (eds.). Peripheral Endovascular Interventions. DOI 10.1007/978-1-4419-1387-6_29. 425-430.

Ruurda JP, Wisselink w, Cuesta MA, Verhagen HJM, Broeders IA. Robot-assisted versus standard videoscopic aortic replacement: a comparative study in pigs. Eur J Vasc Endovasc Srtrg 2OO4;27 :50 I - 505.

Schreiber MA, Diferding J, Esposito TJ. Research: questions and answers from academic trauma surgeons. J Trauma 2008;64:1113-1118.

Stadler P, Sebesta P, Vitasek P, Matous P, El Samman I. A modified technique of transperitoneal direct approach for totally laparoscopic aortoiliac surgery. Eur J Vasc Endovasc Surg 2006; 31:266-269.

Wisselink W, Cuesta MA, Gracia C, Rauwerda JA. Robotassisted laparoscopic aortobifemoral bypass for aortoiliac occlusive disease: a report of two cases. J Vasc Surg 2OO2;36: 1079-1082.

Part 2

Endovascular Surgery

6

Emergency TEVAR for Complicated Acute Type B Aortic Dissection

Y. Kurimoto, Y. Asai and T. Higami
Sapporo Medical University
Japan

1. Introduction

Non-complicated type B aortic dissection has been managed by conservative treatment at least in the acute phase. However, complicated acute type B aortic dissection, such as rupture or visceral ischemia secondary to malperfusion, has required emergency open surgical management. Despite recent advance of open surgery and perioperative managements, early results of emergency surgery has been reported to be still unsatisfactory with high mortality rate of 30 - 40 % and morbidity (Fattori R, et al., 2008, Svensson LG, et al., 2008). Since more than a decade ago, percutaneous trans-catheter intervention has contributed as an emergency treatment in order to salvage ischemic visceral organs including leg ischemia secondary to acute aortic dissection (Midulla M, et al., 2011). However, bare stent placement at occluded artery or catheter fenestration of intimal flap to ameliorate organ ischemia do not change a situation of dissected aorta itself.

From the point of view as a mechanism of complications secondary to type B aortic dissection, stent-grafting to close an primary entry at the descending thoracic aorta seems rationale, especially in the acute phase, because most complications secondary to acute aortic dissection are caused by an increased blood flow in a false lumen. Recently, the attempt of an application of elective thoracic endovascular aortic repair (TEVAR) for non-complicated acute type B aortic dissection to close a primary entry during relatively early phase to improve long-term results have been reported. A benefit of TEVAR for non-complicated type was currently not confirmed. Furthermore, procedure-related complications made early results of TEVAR even worse than those of conservative management (Nienaber CA, et al., 2009). Although INSTEAD trial was not able to show a usefulness of TEVAR in the acute phase for patients with non-complicated acute type B aortic dissection, it showed that the thrombo-occlusion rate of a false lumen in the descending thoracic aorta was more than 90 % when a primary entry was closed by a stent graft in the early phase. This evidence suggests that TEVAR can manage lethal complications secondary to acute type B aortic dissection with a high success rate. In such a critical situation of complicated acute type B aortic dissection, the procedure-related complication rate which INSTEAD trial reported, might be considered to be negligible. Currently, a non-randomised clinical trial entitiled "Evaluation of the clinical performance of the Valiant Thoracic Stent Graft with the captivia delivery system (Valiant Captivia) for the treatment of acute, complicated type B aortic dissections" has been going to confirm a safety and an effectiveness of emergency TEVAR for acute complicated type B aortic dissection since 2010. This study will provide a promising early and mid-term results of emergency TEVAR for acute aortic dissection by 2017.

There are some questions regarding TEVAR for aortic dissection, especially in the acute phase. A proximal bare stent of stent graft to increase a graft stability and radial force of proxiaml end of stent graft probablly should increase a risk of new intimal tear at the aortic arch or the ascending aorta, which causes retrograde type A aortic dissection as a potentially lethal complication. Although we have no experience of retrograde type A aortic dissection following 21 emergency TEVAR for complicated acute aortic dissection, Schoder et al. reporetd that retrograde IIIb aortic dissection as a TEVAR-related complication was experienced in 2 cases (11.8 %) out of 17 cases with complicated acute type B aortic dissection (Schoder M, et al., 2006). An appropriate length of stent graft, a desirable site of a proximal landing zone and a best type of stent grafts for dissection are still unknown.

In this chapter, an application and reported results of emergency TEVAR for ruptured type B aortic dissection and visceral ischemia including leg ischemia due to obstruction of aortic branches are explained considering our 10-year experiences.

2. Ruptured acute type B aortic dissection

Despite an improved surgical technique and perioperative care, the early mortality rate of conventional open repair for ruptured acute type B aortic dissection are 30 – 40 % (Sachs T, et al., 2010, Zeeshan A, et al., 2010). Because clinical status of patients with rupture is already in a critical condition before surgery, a less-invasive initial treatment should be desirable, such as TEAVR. Emergency TEVAR is performed to close a primary entry in order to reduce a blood flow in a ruptured false lumen. Considering possible distal re-entries of ruptured acute type B aortic dissection, an expected success rate by emergency TEVAR should be different between DeBakey type IIIa (localized dissection) and DeBakey type IIIb (extended dissection). It is possible to cover all dissected aorta in type IIIa, which means that all entries including possible re-entries can be closed by stent-grafts. On the other hand, it is impossible to stop retrograde blood flow into a ruptured false lumen in the descending thoracic aorta through re-entries in the abdominal aorta or the iliac artery in cases of type IIIb. Although a 1st report of application of emegency TEVAR for ruptured acute aortic dissection was in 1996 (Dake MD, et al., 1999), there is few reports in which exact results of emergency TEVAR for ruptured acute type B aortic dissection were discribed depending on each type of localized DeBakey type IIIa or extended type IIIb dissection (Steuer J, et al., 2011). Previous reports described that early mortality rates following emergency TEVAR for ruptured acute B including both type IIIa and IIIb aortic dissection were 16 – 33% (Feezor RJ, et al., 2009, White RA, et al., 2011). Considering above mentioned background of different characters in each type of localized or extended dissection, it is hard to understand the real mean of reported early mortality rates of emergency TEVAR for ruptured acute type B aortic dissection without categolizing type IIIa or IIIb.

In a clinical setting, we sometimes experience that patients with rupture have to be transferred to the operating room without sufficient preoperative image studies. However, when considering TEAVR as an initial management for acute aortic dissection, preoperative image examination should be necessary, such as computed tomography (CT) with contrast medium. Moreover, although TEVAR for complicated acute aortic dissection is emergency, at least, multiplanar reconstruction CT images should be ready to decide an appropriate proximal landing zone preoperatively (Fig. 1). When patients are hemodynamically stable, construction of volume rendering CT images are recommended for successful TEVAR even though it is time-consuming (Fig. 2). Intra-vascular ultrasound (IVUS) is very useful to confirm a position of guide wire in a true or false lumen (Fig. 3), a location of targeted dissected aorta and a condition of a false lumen before and after TEVAR (Fig. 4) during operation. For type IIIa aortic dissection, trans-esophageal echo (TEE) can be an alternative to IVUS because dissected aorta is limited in the thoracic cavity.

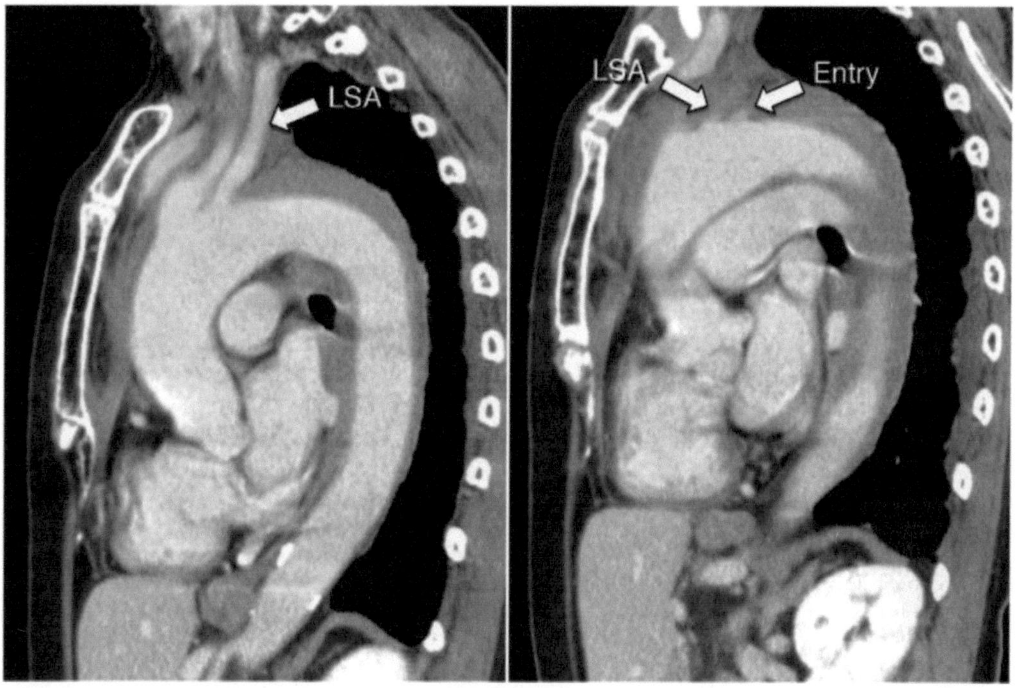

A 72-year-old woman was given a diagnosis of ruptured acute type B aortic dissection by CT. Despite a thrombosed false lumen, the patient was transferred to the operating room considering mediastinal hematoma. The patient suffered from hemorrhagic shock before an induction of general anesthesia due to re-rupture. MPR images were useful to determine an appropriate position and a length of stent grafts. The hand-made fenestrated stent graft was placed from zone 0 with a simple coverage of the left subclavian artery and preserving the brachiocephalic and left carotid arteries.

Fig. 1. Multiplanar reconstruction (MPR) computed tomography (CT) images of ruptured acute type B aortic dissection.

Complete coverage of whole dissected descending thoracic aorta is usually possible for type IIIa with or without coverage of the left subclavian artery (LSA). In our experience, a primary entry of ruptured acute type IIIa is commonly located at a great curvature of distal aortic arch close to LSA as well as a primary entry of type IIIb. When using commercially available stent grafts as of 2011, there are cases in which LSA has to be sacrificed and covered by a stent graft in order to close a primary entry and to achieve a stable positioning of placed stent graft. Our current policy of TEVAR for aortic dissection is that a proximal

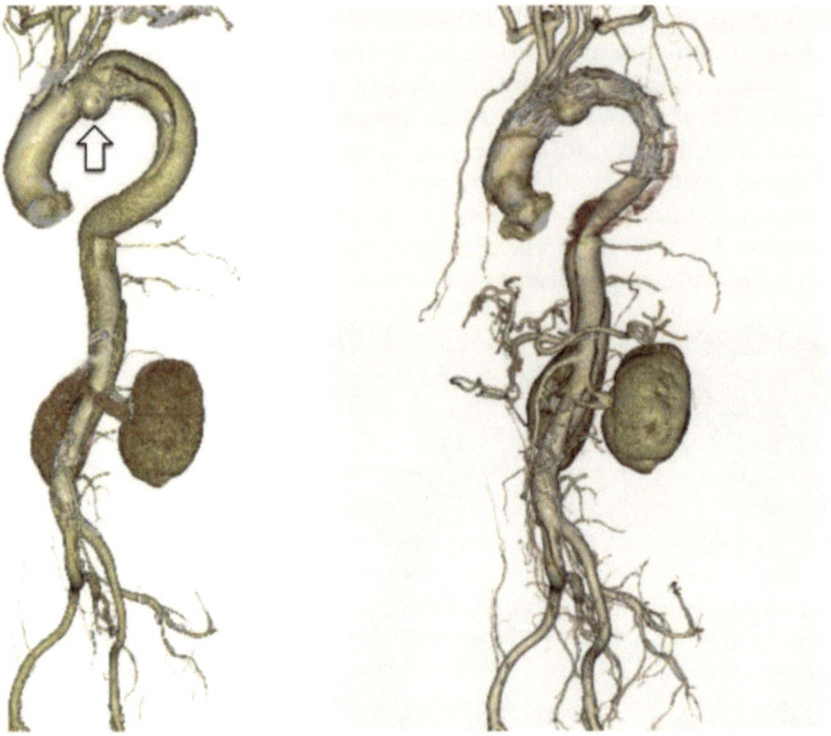

A 75-year-old man was transferred complaining left leg pain suddenly occurred 10 days after an initial onset of acute type B aortic dissection. VR-CT revealed small distal aortic arch aneurysm (White arrow in left) as well as acute aortic dissection. VR images were useful as a preoperative image study when a patient's condition allows reconstruction of original CT data. The hand-made fenestrated stent graft was placed from zone 0 with a simple coverage of the left subclavian artery preserving the brachiocephalic and left carotid arteries. Although type Ia endoleak into distal aortic arch aneurysm through a fenestration for the left carotid artery was observed, left leg ischemia was immediately improved just after TEVAR.

Fig. 2. Volume rendering (VR) computed tomographic (CT) images of left leg ischemia due to acute type B aortic dissection.

landing zone should be non-dissected aorta, generally, which is the aortic arch in cases of acute type B aortic dissection. Based on our study, there is a risk of complication around 5 % if LSA is simply covered by a stent graft (Kurimoto Y, et al., 2008a, 2009). In addition of cerebral complication, a simple coverage of LSA possibly increases a risk of spinal cord ischemia as postoperative complication. Although 10 % incident rate of spinal cord ischemia (Schoder M, et al., 2006) might be negligible considering a critical situation of ruptured acute type B aortic dissection, LSA should be reconstructed as much as possible if patient's general condition allows. Hybrid TEVAR combined with great-vessel, such as the brachiocephalic, the left common carotid and LSA, bypass-grafting, so called "debranching technique" (Schoder M, et al., 2006), has been commonly performed for cases in which a stent graft has to be placed from zone 0-2 (Fig. 5). In our hospital, we has chosen a hand-made fenestrated stent graft (Fig. 6) which enables preservation of great-vessels branched from the aortic arch without additional bypass-grafting in most cases of complicated acute type B aortic dissection.

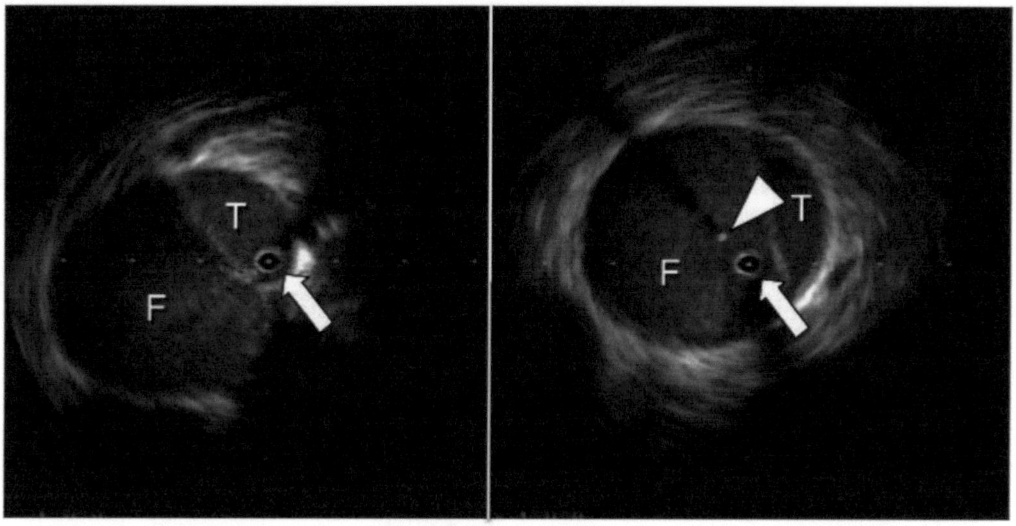

IVUS is useful to confirm a lumen of dissected aorta in which a guide wire is running. Stent-graft system should be advanced on a guide wire (White arrow) running in a true lumen from the iliac artery to the aortic arch (Left). In an elective case, a bailout guide wire in a false lumen (White arrow and arrow head) might be helpful just in a case of visceral organ ischemia secondary to malperfusion of false-lumen-branched organ following an entry closure by a stent graft (Right). T; true lumen, F; false lumen.

Fig. 3. Intra-vascular ultra-sound (IVUS) images during TEVAR for aortic dissection.

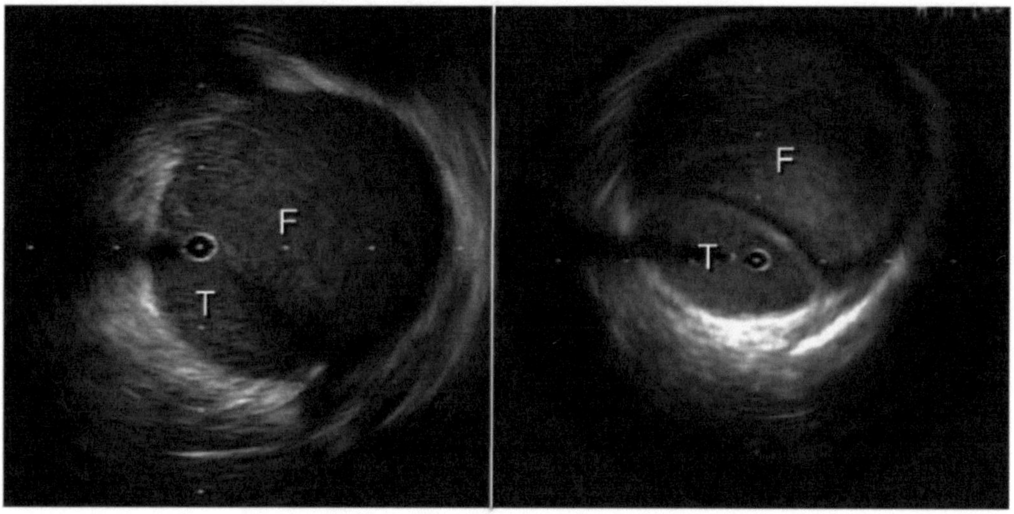

Smoke-like echo image, we call it "moya-moya echo", generally guarantees a thrombo-occlusion of a false lumen in the descending thoracic aorta (Right). In an elective case of chronic aortic dissection with a dilated false lumen, additional distal stent graft might be considered when "moya-moya echo" is not observed in IVUS after placement a 1st proximal stent graft (Left). T; true lumen, F; false lumen.

Fig. 4. Intra-vascular ultrasound (IVUS) images during TEVAR for aortic dissection.

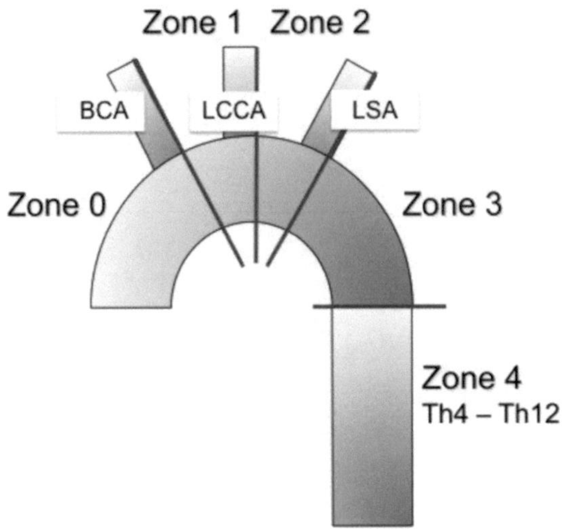

BCA; bracheocephalic artery, LCCA; left common carotid artery, LSA; left subclavian artery.

Fig. 5. Zone classification of proximal position of a stent graft in thoracic endovascular aortic repair (Mitchell RS, et al., 2002).

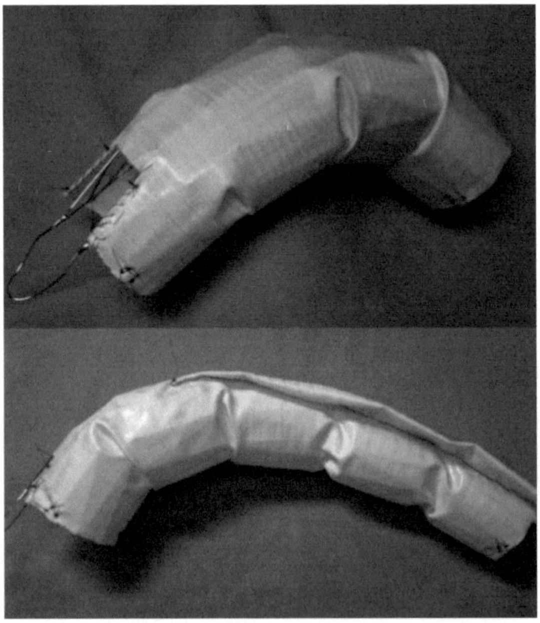

A proximal roof of a stent graft is fenestrated to preserve great vessels from the aortic arch (Upper). A stent graft is tapered in a case in which a diameter of a distal aortic neck is smaller more than 10 mm compared with one of a proximal aortic neck (Lower).

Fig. 6. Hand-made stent grafts in our facility.

2.1 Ruptured acute DeBakey type IIIa aortic dissection (Localized type)

Incidence of acute type IIIa aortic dissection is supposed to be rare compared with type IIIb. However, ruptured acute type B aortic dissection is likely to be more often experienced in type IIIa in a clinical setting (Steuer J, et al., 2011). This is very same in acute type A aortic dissection. Clinically, incident of acute DeBakey type II (localized type) is rare compared with type I (extended type). A high incidence of rupture in the localized type is probably due to lack of distal re-entry. However, once patients with ruptured acute type IIIa aortic dissection can be placed on the operating table as candidates of TEVAR, satisfactory early and long-term results can be expected if appropriate proximal and distal landing zones can be achieved (Fig. 7).

There is a possibility that emergency TEAVR can be almost a definitive treatment for ruptured acute type IIIa aortic dissection. As long as our 10-year experience of ruptured type IIIa, all 5 patients have been doing well with complete resolution of a false lumen without any dilatation of the descending thoracic aorta including proximal and distal landing zones (Fig. 8). Because of small number of patients and limited period of follow-up, we would like to wait for other reports regarding results of emergency TEVAR for ruptured type IIIa aortic dissection.

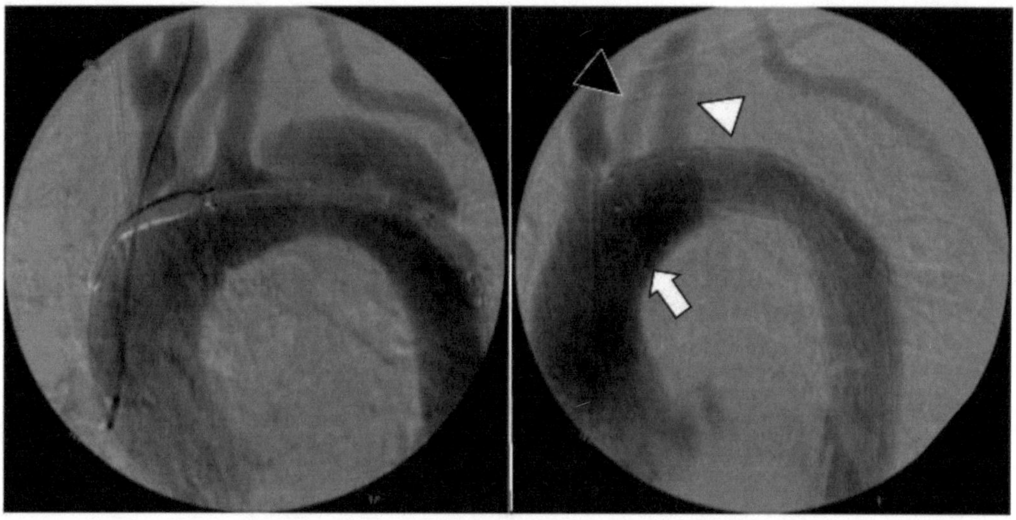

We think that a proximal landing zone for acute type B aortic dissection should be non-dissected aorta, which means that a stent graft is generally placed from the aortic arch. The left common carotid artery (LCCA) is always preserved and the left subclavian artery (LSA) is also preserved when a proximal entry is located more than 15 mm distally from LSA (Left), using a fenestrated stent graft without any debranching technique (Right). White arrow shows a proximal end of the stent graft with a fenestration to preserve LCCA (Black arrowhead) and LSA (White arrowhead)(Right).

Fig. 7. Digital subtracted angiographic (DSA) images of emergency TEVAR for ruptured acute type IIIa aortic dissection.

2.2 Ruptured acute DeBakey type IIIb aortic dissection (Extended type)

Ruptured acute type IIIb aortic dissection is rare, but a lethal complication. Although exact data is not unknown, most patients with ruptured acute type IIIb aortic dissection probably die before admission to hospitals. Based on reported thrombo-occlusion rate of more than 90%

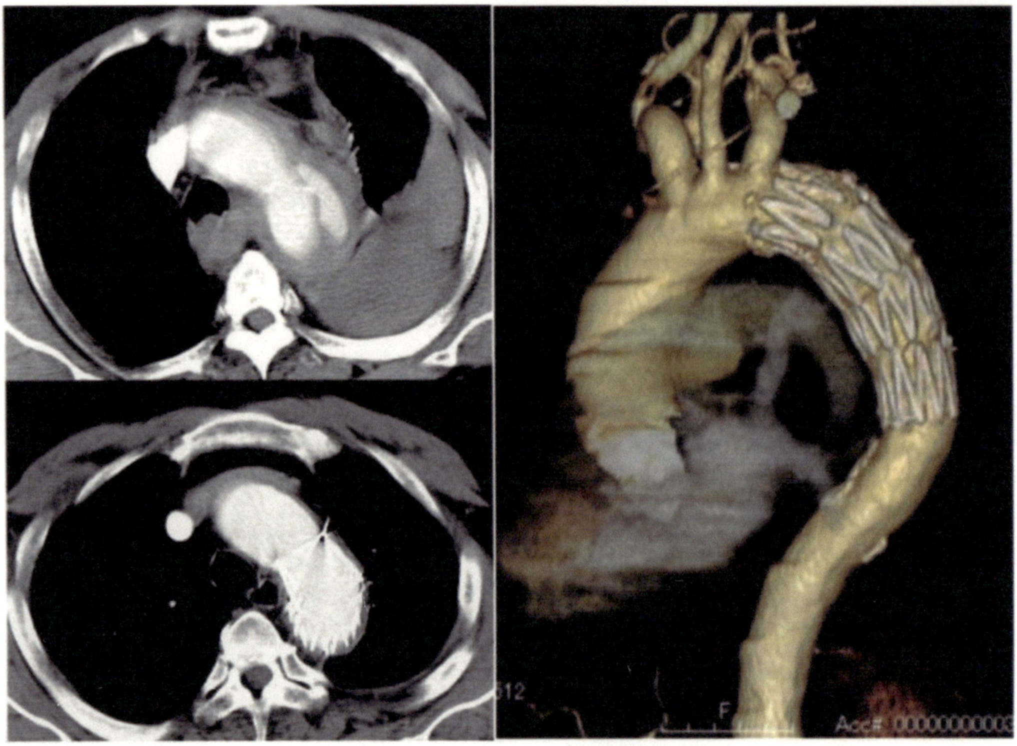

A 57-year-old man was transferred in a hemorrhagic shock due to mediastinal hematoma and left hemothorax (Left upper) and underwent emergency TEVAR. CT images at 2 months after TEVAR showed complete resolution of a ruptured false lumen (Left lower). 3D-CT image at 7 years after emergency TEVAR showed no problematic change in the descending thoracic aorta (Right).

Fig. 8. Computed tomographic (CT) images of ruptured acute type IIIa aortic dissection.

in a false lumen following elective TEVAR for acute aortic dissection, it makes emergency TEVAR to be a promising less-invasive treatment of choice for ruptured acute type B aortic dissection. A big concern is how much impact a retrograde blood flow via distal re-entries has for a ruptured false lumen following primary entry closure using a stent graft, which is totally different from a localized type IIIa wih rupture.

Based on our experience of early mortality rate 50% (2/4), there is no advantage in TEVAR for ruptured acute type IIIb compared with conventional open repair. However, emergency TEVAR is still thought to be a treatment of choice even for ruptured acute type IIIb (Fig. 9a,b) because of short operation time and feasibility of repeated TEVAR or open conversion as an urgent not emergent. Further experience will be necessary to conclude whether TEVAR is effective for ruptured acute type IIIb aortic dissection.

We experienced a difficult treatment in one case of ruptured type IIIb aortic dissection (chronic dissection, not acute). A 58-year-old man with 12-year history of hemodialysis and malignant rheumatic arthritis was transferred to our hospital by helicopter because of ruptured chronic type IIIb aortic dissection (Fig. 10a). Primary entry closure by placing a hand-made fenestrated stent graft from zone 1 to the level of Th 9 was effective to manage rupture into the mediastinum, but follow-up CT images revealed enlargement of the false lumen of ruptured descending thoracic aorta. To thrombo-occlude a false lumen of the entire aorta, 2nd and 3rd stent grafts were necessary to be placed from the aortic arch to the common iliac artery. The celiac and supra-mesenteric arteries were preserved using a hand-made fenestrated stent graft. Finally, the false lumen was completely thrombo-occluded and a diameter of the descending thoracic aorta was reduced (Fig. 10b). Considering a clinical course of this case and high early mortality rates of our experience, there is a risk that proximal entry closure does not work for ruptured type IIIb aortic dissection. To improve these high mortality rates, Sfyroeras GS, et al. mentioned in their report regarding malperfusion in acute type B aortic dissection that stent grafts should be placed in whole descending thoracic aorta from LSA to the celiac artery in cases associated with rupture accepting a possible increase of incident rate of spinal cord ischemia (Sfyroeras GS, et al., 2011).

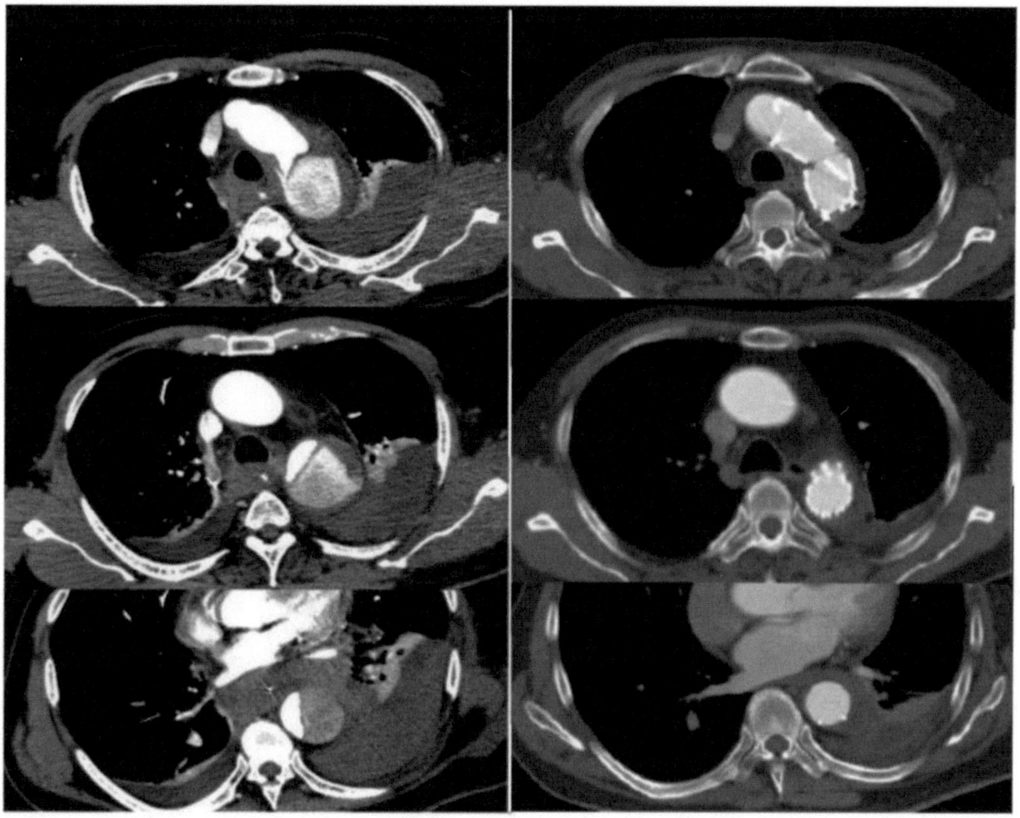

A 62-year-old man was transferred complaining severe back pain in a hemorrhagic shock. CT revealed acute type IIIb aortic dissection ruptured into mediastinum and bilateral pleural cavities (Left). Emergency TEVAR was chosen as an initial treatment because of deteriorated patient's general condition. CT at 2 months after emergency TEVAR showed complete resolution of a false lumen of the descending thoracic aorta (Right).

Fig. 9a. Computed tomographic (CT) images of emergency TEVAR for ruptured acute type IIIb aortic dissection.

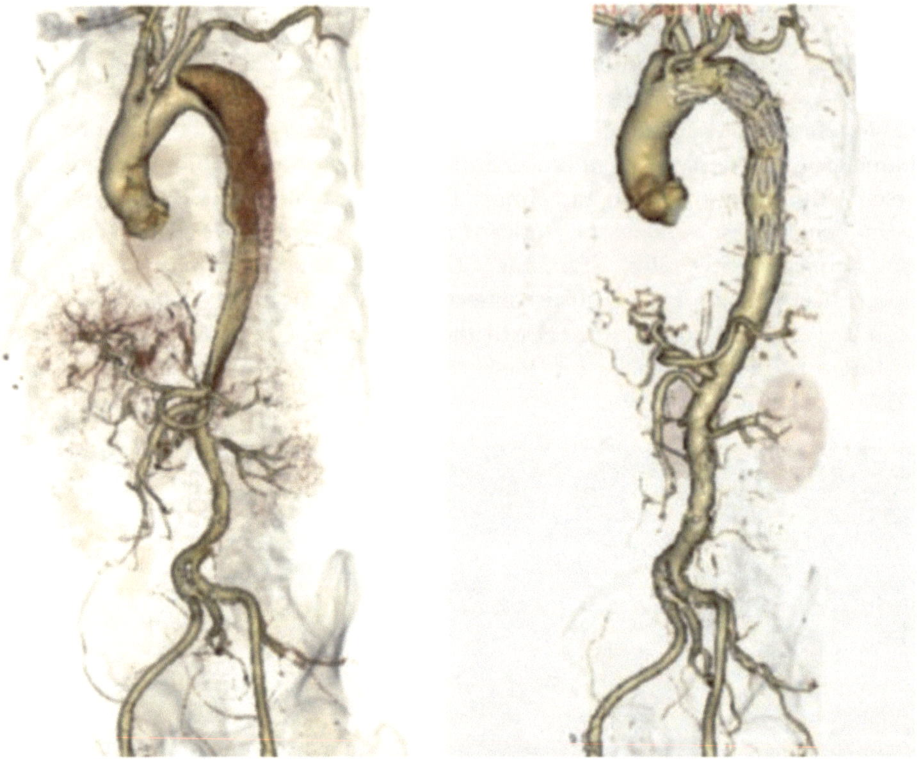

Preoperative VR-CT showed that all visceral main arteries were branched from a true lumen (Left). VR-CT at 2 months after emergency TEVAR showed full expansion of a true lumen of the entire aorta (Right).

Fig. 9b. Volume rendering (VR) computed tomographic (CT) images of ruptured acute type IIIb aortic dissection.

3. Visceral ischemia including leg ischemia secondary to acute type B aortic dissection

Malperfusion, especially mesenteric ischemia, secondary to acute aortic dissection is one of typical lethal complications as well as rupture above mentioned. Proximal aortic repair including excision of a primary entry seems to be too time-consuming to salvage visceral ischemia. Since before the era of a stent graft, a usefulness of percutaneous endovascular treatment has been reported as a creation of intimal fenestration for compressed and collapsed aortic true lumen or a bare stenting for dissected or occluded aortic branches. Theoretically, a creation of intimal fenestration can restore a blood flow in a collapsed true lumen of the aorta, but can not be a treatment of dissected aorta itself. Reported clinical results of catheter fenestartion is difficult to be understand because these reports include type A aortic dissection treated by open surgery following percutaneous catheter intervention. However, early mortality rate of 31 % and no dilatation of dissected aorta during mid-term follow-up (Midulla M, et al., 2011) might have been acceptable at least untill before an emergence of TEVAR.

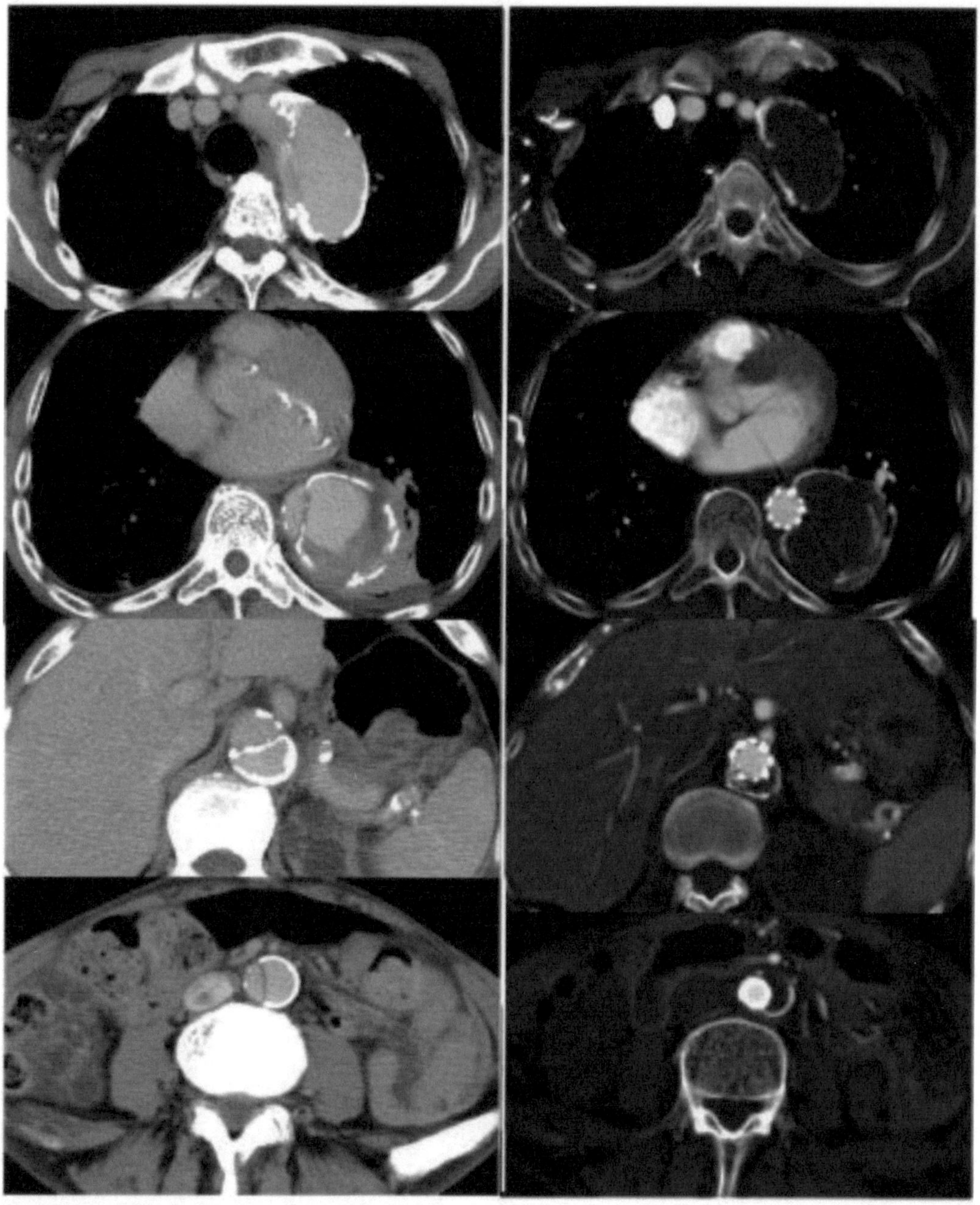

A 58-year-old man with a 12-year history of hemodialysis and malignant rheumatoid arthritis was transferred due to chronic type IIIb aortic dissection ruptured into the mediastinum (Left). Emergency TEVAR to close the primary entry was not able to thrombo-occlude a false lumen of the descending thoracic aorta. Additional EVAR and stent-grafting for thoracoabdominal aorta were necessary to thrombo-occlude a false lumen and to reduce a size of ruptured dissected aorta (Right).

Fig. 10a. Computed tomographic (CT) images before and after TEVARs and abdominal endovascular aortic repair (EVAR) for ruptured chronic type IIIb aortic dissection.

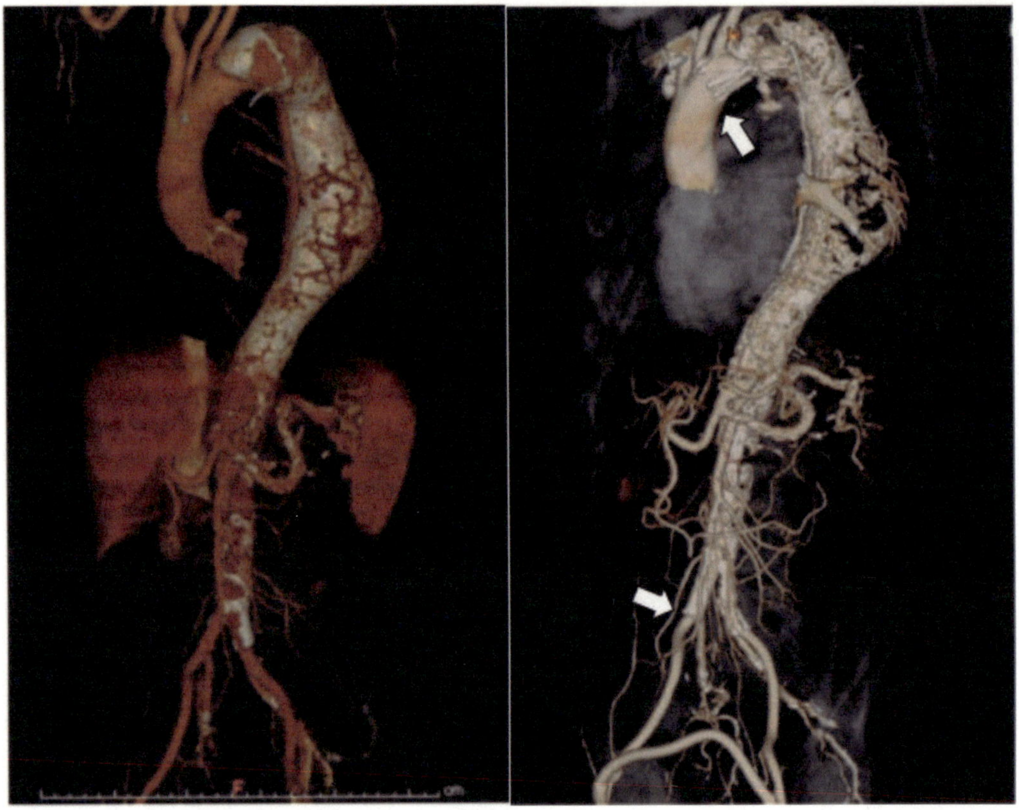

Preoperative VR-CT showed severely calcified false lumen of the entire aorta (Left). Because of insufficient thrombo-occlusion of a false lumen, Excluder (GoreTex, Japan) was placed in an aorto-uni-iliac fashion to close re-entries below a level of the supra-mesenteric artery (SMA) and a hand-made fenestrated stent graft to close re-entries around the thoracoabdominal aortic area was placed preserving the celiac and SMA without any debranching technique. As a result, 4 stent grafts were placed from zone 1 (White arrow) to the right common iliac artery (White arrow) and thrombo-occlusion of an entire false lumen was achieved (Right).

Fig. 10b. Volume rendering (VR) computed tomographic (CT) images of aortic stent-grafting for ruptured chronic type IIIb aortic dissection.

In cases of visceral ischemia due to malperfusion, emergency TEVAR can be applied based on a mechanism of malperfusion. In a case that dissected aortic branch itself is causing organ ischemia, conventional percutaneous catheter intervention using a bare stent should be chosen. In a case that thrombo-occluded aortic branch is causing malperfusion, direct bypass-grafting to ischemic organ usually has to be chosen. A catheter thrombectomy might be effective for limited cases of malperfusion. A primary entry closure by a stent graft is very effective for malperfusion caused by a collapsed true lumen compressed by an enlarged false lumen in the thoraco-abdominal aorta. This mechanism is called "dynamic obstruction" which is different from "static obstruction" above mentioned. Generally, it is not necessary to thrombo-occlude a false lumen in the descending thoracic aorta at least as an initial treatment for malperfusion. A minimum goal of emergency TEVAR for malperfusion is to reduce a blood flow in a false lumen and to re-expand a true lumen (Fig.

11). Therefore, emergency TEVAR is technically not demanding (Fig. 12) and should be more commonly considered as an initial management following accurate diagnosis of malperfusion mechanism. White RA et al. reported that early mortality rate following emergency TEVAR for malperfusion was 8.6 % (5/58). In our 7 cases of malperfusion, emergency TEVAR was effective for all cases except for one case associated with ruptured type IIIb aortic dissection which died due to re-rupture one day after TEVAR.

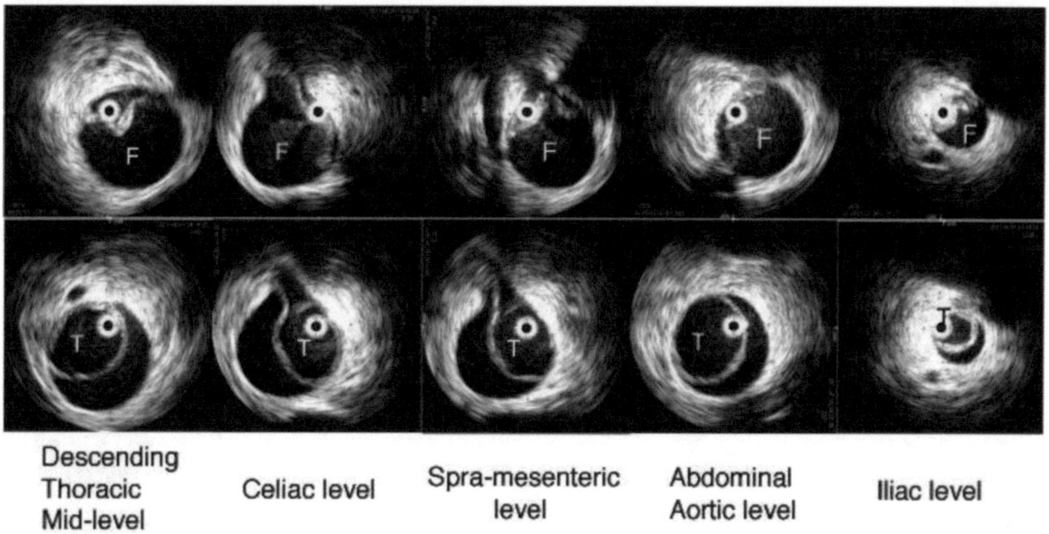

Preoperatively, a true lumen of the entire dissected aorta was critically compressed by an enlarged false lumen (Upper). Following emergency TEVAR to close a primary large entry at the distal aortic arch, a true lumen in each level was re-expanded (Lower). F; false lumen, T; true lumen.

Fig. 11. Intra-vascular ultrasound (IVUS) images during emergency TEVAR for malperfusion secondary to acute type B aortic dissection.

Procedure of emergency TEVAR for malperfusion secondary to acute type B aortic dissection is almost same as one for rupture already mentioned. In a case of ischemic leg, a stent-graft system should be approached via the side of ischemic leg because non-pulsatile femoral artery is usually perfused via a collapsed true lumen. In addition to confirmation of guide wire in a true lumen, IVUS is useful to determine a necessity of additional distal stent graft which can be placed until the level of the celiac artery with a little increasing risk of spinal cord ischemia. In our hospital, distal extension using a 2nd stent graft has not been employed when LSA is sacrificed to close a primary entry next to LSA because of a possible spinal cord ischemia. The facility where stent grafts have been placed on 87% of the descending thoracic aorta and LSA-reconstruction rate was 14%, reported that an incident rate of spinal cord ischemia following TEVAR for complicated type B aortic dissection was 15% (5/33) (Feezor RJ, et al., 2009). On the contrary, we have not experienced a spinal cord ischemia following 21 emergency TEVARs for complicated acute type B aortic dissection. Shu C, et al. also reported 0% of paraplegia following 45 emergency TEVAR for complicated type B aortic dissection (Shu C, et al., 2011). Our policy for acute aortic dissection is as same as ruptured aortic dissection. Proximal landing zone should be achieved at non-dissected

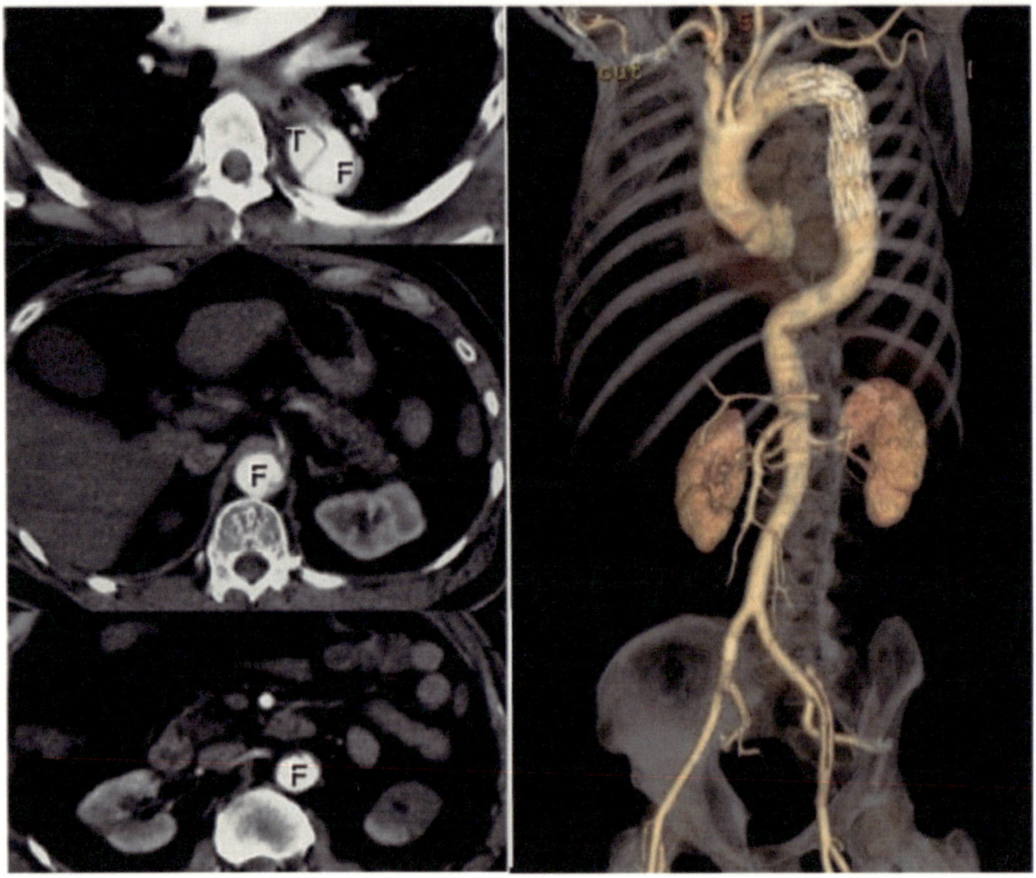

A 58-year-old man was transferred due to renal and right leg ischemia secondary to acute aortic dissection (Left). Emergency TEVAR was effective without any additional intervention. Volume rendering CT at 6 years after TEVAR showed a satisfactory remodelling of the entire aorta (Right). F; false lumen.

Fig. 12. Computed tomographic (CT) images of malperfusion secondary to acute aortic dissection.

aorta, usually the aortic arch, and great-vessels including LSA are preserved using a hand-made fenestrated stent graft as much as possible. Placement of stent graft from dissected aorta as a proximal landing zone has a risk of creation of a new entry (Fig. 13). Additional distal stent graft should be placed only for a case of ruptured acute type IIIb aortic dissection when necessary. A stent graft with proximal bare stent is not applied for acute aortic dissection when a hand-made fenestrated stent graft is available. A clinical impact regarding stent grafts with or without proximal bare stent for acute aortic dissection will be partially understood by the currently going clinical trials using Variant Captivia (Medtronic Vascular, CA, USA) and Gore cTAG (WL Gore & Associates Inc, AZ, USA). Although we currently have no experience of Relay NBS (no bare stent)(Bolton Medical SL, Spain), it might be suitable as a commercial device for acute aortic dissection instead of a hand-made stent graft (Zipfel B, et al., 2011).

Since TEVAR became available as a treatment for malperfusion secondary to acute type B aortic dissection, an early diagnosis of malperfusion has become more important. Most difficult and clinically important malperfusion is mesenteric ischemia. Since we reported a usefulness of a diameter of supra-mesenteric vein and increased level of arterial lactate (Kurimoto Y, et al., 2004, 2008b), we have never experienced massive mesenteric resection caused by delayed diagnosis of mesenteric ischemia. There is another reason why an early diagnosis is the key of success for re-canalization of ischemiac organ by TEVAR. Emergency TEVAR can re-expand collapsed true lumen of dissected aorta even more than several hours after onset, but obstructed aortic branches sometimes become thrombo-occluded, so called "static obstruction", and can not be re-canalized by a simple TEVAR (Fig. 14a,b,c). Further studies are necessary to determine what situation of malperfusion should be managed by direct open surgery including bypass-grafting to ischemic organ skipping primary TEVAR.

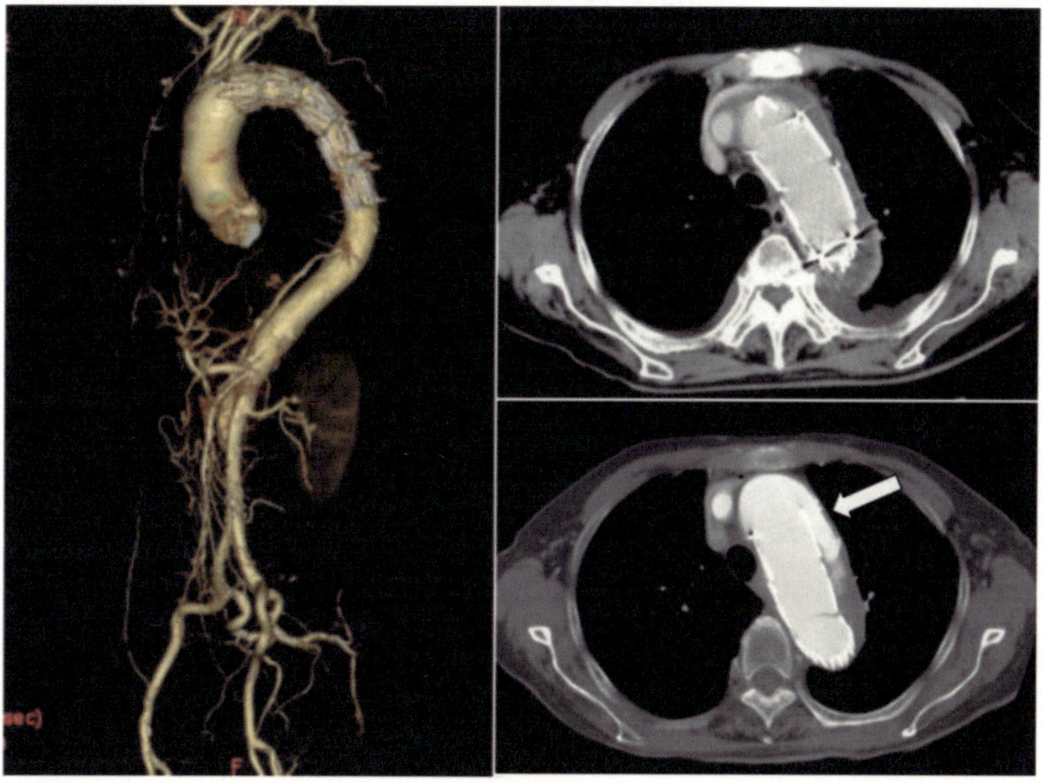

An 82-year-old woman was transferred due to bilateral leg ischemia secondary to acute type A aortic dissection with the thrombo-occluded false lumen of the ascending aorta and the primary entry at the proximal descending thoracic aorta. Although postoperative CT was satisfactory (Left and Right upper), follow-up CT at 18 months after emergency TEVAR revealed a new entry (White arrow) at the proximal end of placed stent graft in the aortic arch (Right lower).

Fig. 13. Computed tomographic (CT) images of malperfusion secondary to acute type IIIbR aortic dissection with a thrombosed false lumen of the ascending aorta.

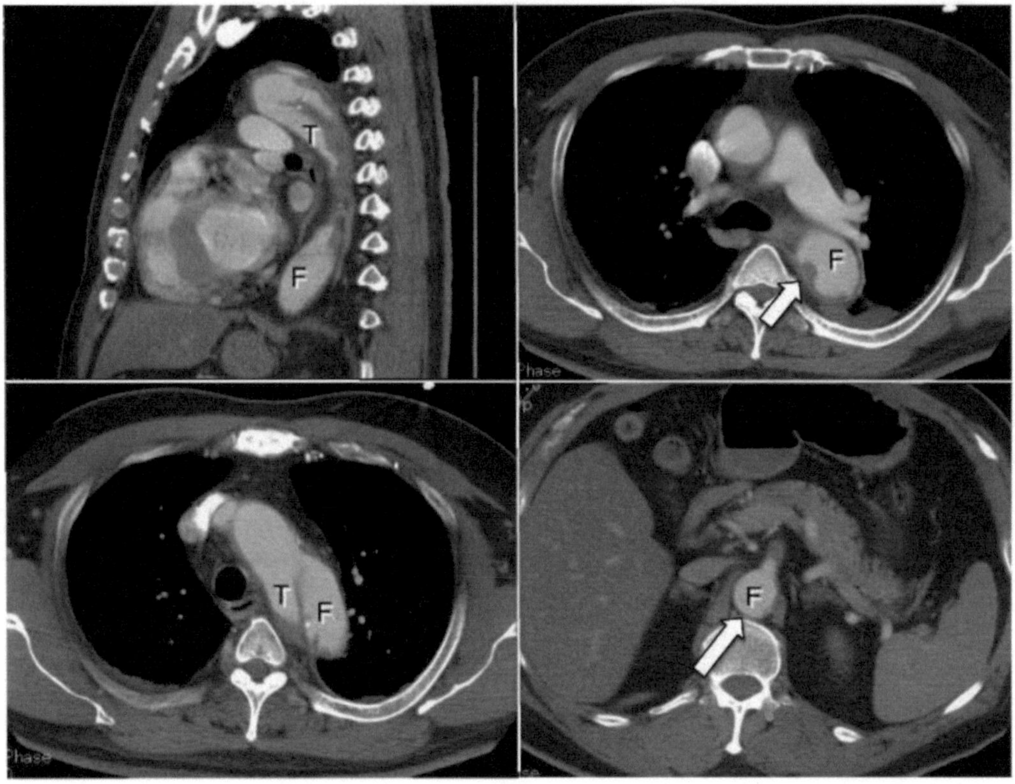

A 51-year-old man was transferred due to complicated acute type B aortic dissection 8 hours after onset. Preoperative CT including multiplanar reconstruction revealed a primary large entry at the distal aortic arch (Left) and completely collapsed true lumen (White arrow) of the descending thoracic aorta (Right). F; false lumen, T; true lumen.

Fig. 14a. Computed tomographic (CT) images of renal and left leg ischemia due to malperfusion secondary to acute type B aortic dissection.

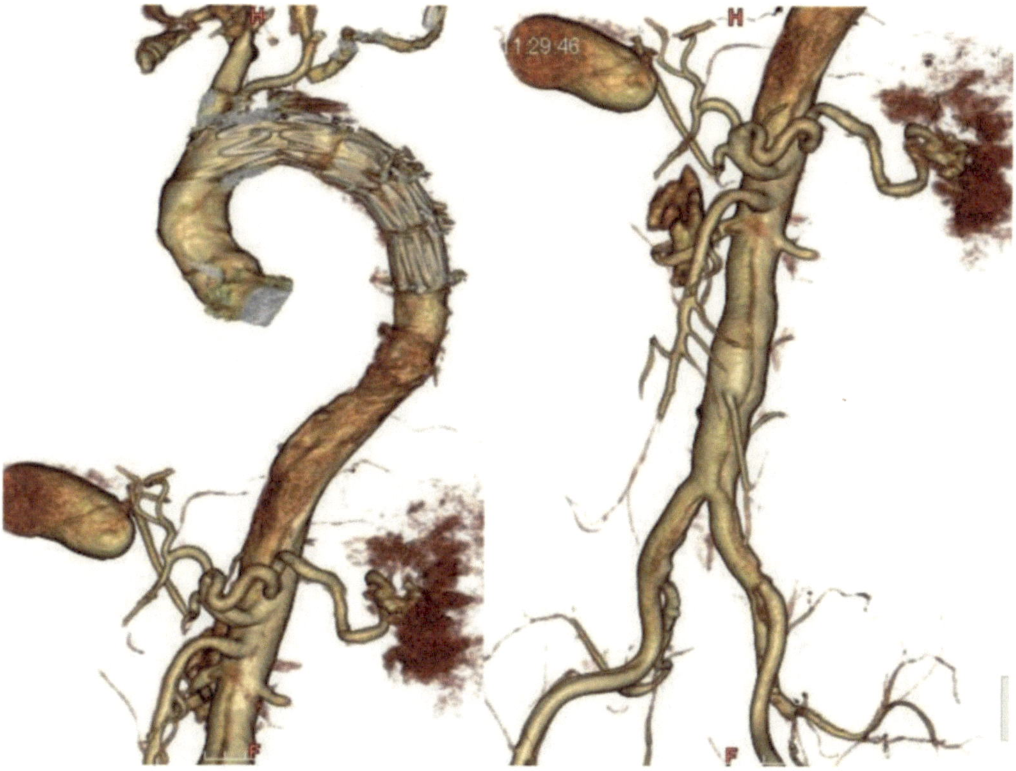

The hand-made fenestrated stent graft was placed from zone 0 with a simple coverage of the left subclavian artery 10 hours after onset of complication secondary to acute aortic dissection (Left). Although the true lumen was well re-expanded by a primary entry closure, bilateral renal arteries were already thrombo-occluded and re-canalization was not achieved (Right).

Fig. 14b. Postoperative volume rendering computed tomographic images of malperfuison secondary to acute type B aortic dissection.

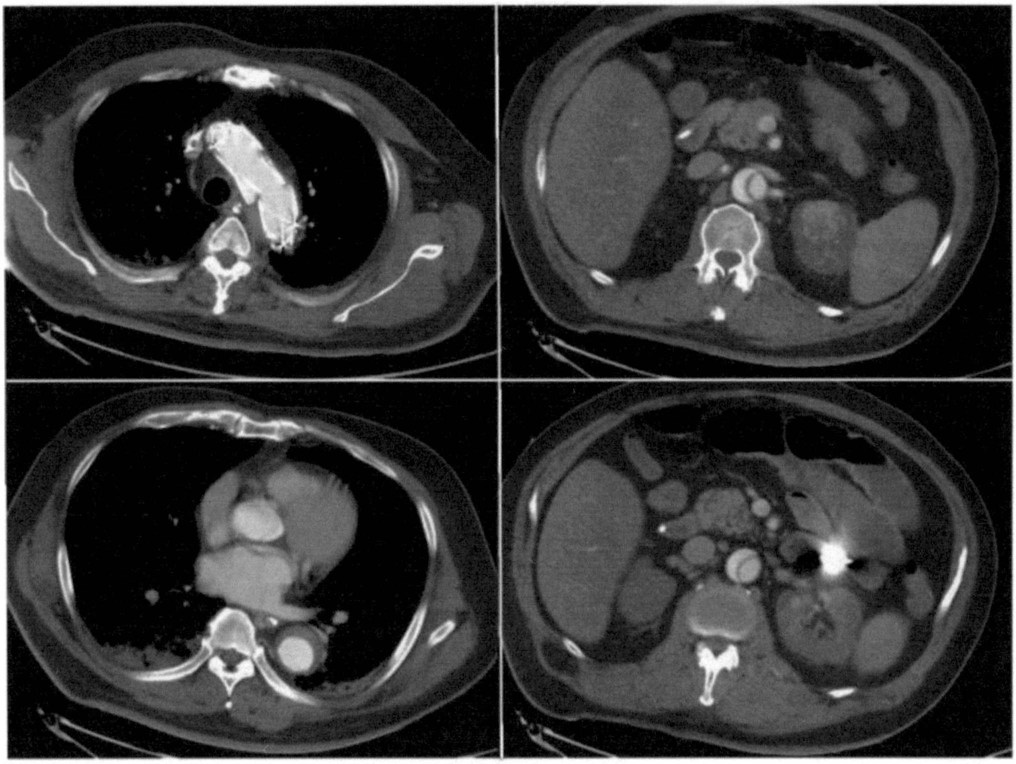

CT showed the successfully placed stent graft (Left upper) and satisfactory re-expanded true lumen with thrombo-occluded false lumen in the descending thoracic aorta (Left lower). Although the renal artery was enhanced, no flow in bilateral kidney was confirmed possibly due to long elapsed time from the onset (Right lower)

Fig. 14c. Postoperative computed tomographic (CT) images of malperfuison secondary to acute type B aortic dissection.

4. Conclusion

Emergency indication of TEVAR for acute aortic dissection is obviously expanding. Ruptured acute DeBakey type IIIa aotic dissection can be managed by emergency TEVAR with satisfactory early and long-term results. Although there are still points to evaluate about an efficacy of TEVAR for ruptured acute DeBakey type IIIb aortic dissection, currently reported results are relatively acceptable as an initial treatment for deteriorated patients. Malperfusion secondary to acute type B aortic dissection can be managed well by TEVAR when exact early diagnsis and mechanism of malperfusion are made. To reduce TEVAR-related complication rates, appropriate commercial device for acute aortic dissection should be developed based on clinical experiences.

5. References

Dake MD, Kato N, Mitchell RS, et al. (1999). Endovascular stent-graft placement for the treatment of acute aortic dissection. *N Engl J Med.* 340:1546-1552.

Fattori R, Tsai TT, Myrmel T, et al. (2008). Complicated acute type B dissection; is surgery still the best option? A report from the International Registry of Acute Aortic Dissection. JACC Cardiovasc Interv. 14:395-402.

Feezor RJ, Martin TD, Hess Jr PH, et al. (2009). Early outcomes after endovascular management of acute, complicated type B aortic dissection. *J Vasc Surg.* 49:561-567.

Kurimoto Y, Morishita K, Fukada J, et al. (2004). A simple but useful method of screening for mesenteric ischemia secondary to acute aortic dissection. *Surgery.* 136(1):42-46.

Kurimoto Y, Ito T, Harada R, et al. (2008a). Management of left subclavian artery in endovascular stent-grafting for distal aortic arch disease. Circ J. 72(3):449-453.

Kurimoto Y, Kawaharada N, Ito T, et al. (2008b). An experimental evaluation of lactate concentration following mesenteric ischemia. Surg Today. 38(10):926-930.

Kurimoto Y, Kawaharada N, Ito T, et al. (2009). Less-invasive management of left subclavian artery in stent-grafting for distal aortic arch disease. Interact Cardiovasc Thorac Surg. 8(5):548-552.

Mitchell RS, Ishimaru S, Ehrlich MP, et al. (2002). First international summit on thoracic aortic endografting: roundtable on thoracic aortic dissection as an indication for endografting. J Endovasc Ther. 9(Suppl 2):II98-II105.

Midulla M, Renaud A, Martinelli T, et al. (2011). Endovascular fenestration in aortic dissection with acute malperfusion syndrome: Immediate and late follow-up. *J Thorac Cardiovasc Surg.* 142:66-72.

Nienaber CA, Rousseau H, Eggebrecht H, et al. (2009). Randomised comparison of strategies for type B aortic dissection: the INvestigation of STEnt Grafts in Aortic Dissection (INSTEAD) trial. *Circulation.* 120:2519-2528.

Sachs T, Pomposelli F, Hagberg R, et al. (2010). Open and endovascular repair of the type B aortic dissection in the nationwide inpatient sample. *J Vasc Surg.* 52(4):860-866.

Sfyroeras GS, Rubio V, Pagan P, et al. (2011). Endovascular management of malperfusion in acute type B aortic dissections. *J Endovasc Ther.* 18:78-86.

Shu C, He H, Li QM, et al. (2011). Endovascular repair of complicated acute type-B aortic dissection with stentgraft: Early and mid-term results. *Eur J Vasc Endovasc Surg.* (in press).

Schoder M, Grabenwoger M, Holzenbein T, et al. (2006). Endovascular repair of thoracic aorta necessitating anchoring of the stent graft across the arch vessels. *J Thorac Cardiovasc Surg.* 131:380-387.

Steuer J, Eriksson MO, Nyman R, Bjorck M, Wanhainen A. (2011). Early and long-term outcome after thoracic endovascular aortic repair (TEVAR) for acute complicated type B aortic dissection. *Eur J Vasc Endovasc Surg.* 41(3):318-323.

Svensson LG, Kouchoukos NT, Miller DC, et al. (2008). Expert concensus document on the treatment of descending thoracic aortic disease using endovascular stent-grafts. *Ann Thorac Surg.* 85:S1-41.

White RA, Miller DC, Criado FJ, et al. (2011). Report on the results of thoracic endovascular aortic repair for acute, complicated, type B aortic dissection at 30 days and 1 year from a multidisciplinary subcommittee of the Society for Vascular Surgery Outcomes Committee. *J Vasc Surg.* 53:1082-1090.

Zeeshan A, Woo EY, Babaria JE, et al. (2010). Thoracic endovascular aortic repair for acute complicated type B aortic dissection: superiority relative to conventional open surgical and medical therapy. *J Thorac Cardiovasc Surg.* 140(6 Suppl):S109-115.

Zipfel B, Czerny M, Funovics M, et al. (2011). Endovascular treatment of patients with types A and B thoracic aortic dissection using Relay thoracic stent-grafts: Results from RESTORE patient registry. *J Endovasc Ther.* 18:131-143.

7

Endovenous Laser Treatment of Incompetent Superficial and Perforator Veins

Suat Doganci and Ufuk Demirkilic
Gulhane Military Academy of Medicine, Department of Cardiovascular Surgery
Turkey

1. Introduction

Varicose veins are a common disorder and occur in about 40% of men and 32% of women. However the prevalence of the varicose veins has variability according to the age, gender, duration of reflux, and localization (superficial and/or deep veins). According to the Bonn Vein Study according to the duration of reflux (>500 ms) prevalence of the varicose veins in all veins was 35.3% (superficial veins: 21.0%, deep veins: 20.0%). The effect of venous insufficiency on patients' quality of life is comparable with other common chronic diseases such as arthritis, diabetes and cardiovascular disease. (1, 2)

Traditional treatment of great saphenous vein (GSV) varicosities includes ligation of the sapheno-femoral junction (SFJ) combined with GSV stripping (complete/partial). (3) For the small saphenous vein (SSV) and the perforator veins, situation is a little more complicated. Due to their anatomic challenges and variations, surgery for the SSV and the incompetent perforator veins is sometimes very difficult and may cause adverse events and complications.

Conventional surgery for SSV incompetence presents a high incidence of recurrence (up to 52% at 3 years) and is frequently associated with neurovascular injury. (4) In many instances this is the result of inaccurate ligation of saphenopopliteal junction (SPJ). Even in experienced hands saphenopopliteal ligation is not always technically successful. This is mainly due to the diverse anatomic anomalies of the SPJ and its proximity to the tibial and sural nerves. (5) Unlike the saphenofemoral junction of GSV which is almost constant, the SPJ is variable in terms of level, site of implantation into the popliteal vein, as well as termination and tributaries. (6) Rashid et al. (7) have shown that ligation of the SPJ is not achieved in 30% of the cases, even if the junction is marked pre-operatively under ultrasound guidance. The incision made in the popliteal fossa is associated with wound healing problems and infection in 19-23% of cases. (5)

Incompetent perforator veins (IPVs) are also a significant source of venous hypertension and it is important to treat IPVs. (8) Traditional methods such as Linton procedure and the modifications have a relatively high incidence of wound complications ranging from 20% to 40%. (9) These procedures require general or regional anesthesia and involve a hospital stay of 3-5 days. Postoperative pain significant and may require narcotics. Subfacial endoscopic perforator surgery (SEPS) overcomes some of Linton's limitations but have some of its own. (10) Percutaneous ablation of IPVs by using laser energy is a relatively new technique and has been performed very recently.

Associated morbidity and patient dissatisfaction associated with the traditional surgical treatment have led to the development of alternative techniques. (3) Endovenous treatment modalities (laser ablation, radiofrequency ablation, steam, and foam sclerotherapy) have been readily accepted by both patients and doctors.

2. Historical background

Endovenous laser ablation (EVLA) of the GSV was first described by Puglisi (11) in 1989 in the International Union of Phlebology and the first successful results were reported by Navarro (12) in 2001. Although no multicenter clinical trials of the safety and efficacy of this procedure in humans have been published, many case series and some analysis of pathophysiological effects have been published subsequently.

Endovenous laser treatment of GSV was approved by FDA in 2002 and SSV was approved in 2003. (13, 14) However, percutanous laser treatment of IPVs is a very new procedure. Proebstle (15) published early results of this procedure in 2007.

3. Technological issues

Lots of manufacturers produce laser generators, all of which seems to be effective in the thermal ablation of the incompetent varicose veins.

Semiconductor (diode) lasers have been the main laser type employed for this treatment although some reports have mentioned the neodymium: yttrium-aluminium-garnet (Nd:YAG) laser. Laser wavelengths reported include 810nm, 940nm, 980nm, 1064nm, 1320 nm and 1470 nm. (3, 16)

Clinical trial experience with diode lasers has produced extremely low rates of deep vein thrombosis (DVT) and paraesthesia, a low risk of skin burns, and no documented cases of pulmonary embolism; both paraesthesia and skin burns have been associated with 1064 nm laser treatment. The most common side effects seen with all laser types are bruising, localised pain, induration and discomfort along the treated vein, and superficial phlebitis. (17) Longer wavelengths (>1000nm) show greater water absorption but are overall less strongly absorbed in blood than shorter wavelengths and may have some advantages for endovenous laser ablation. (18-20) The 1470 nm diode laser operates at a relatively new wavelength for this treatment and has been in use since 2006. (16)

There has also been progress in the field of laser fibers (Figure 1). Recently, new fibre tips (jacket-tip fibres, glass, metal, ceramic, diffusion, radial, and tulip) were developed. There are promising results with radial laser fibers. (21) These new generation fibers also more echogenic than the old bare-tip fibers and can easily be seen on Doppler ultrasound.

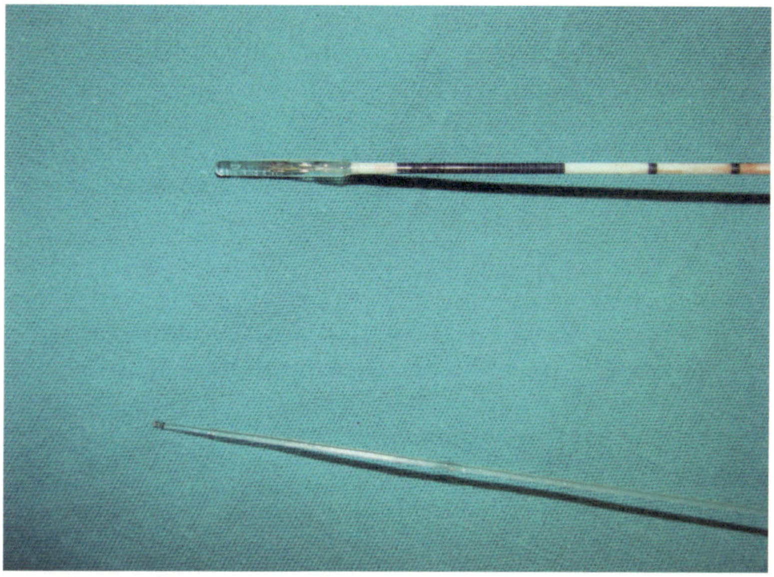

Fig. 1. Picture of bare-tip and radial laser fibers.

With the evolving technology, nowadays it is very difficult to follow technologic advances in the field of endovenous treatment modalities. However, we believe that in the near future technologic advances will overcome all the limitations of these procedures and endovenous procedures will definitely take the place of traditional surgical methods in the treatment of venous insufficiency.

4. Patient selection

Inclusion criteria consist of symptoms and signs of venous insuffiency. Any patient that has the indication for treatment of varicose veins can be treated by endovenous laser ablation method.

In our clinical experience, we perform EVLA for patients other than absolute contrindications (22) (arteriovenous malformation, deep vein thrombosis and restricted immobility). Although there are some relative contraindications (22) documented in the literature such as deep vein reflux, previous treatment, large-vein diameter, anticoagulant therapy, hormone replacement therapy, tortuos vein, and aneurysmal vein segments, in our clinical practice we perform EVLA to all these patients with our increasing clinical experience. In our clinical experience deep vein reflux (less than 6 seconds) without extremity diameter increase (more than 3 cm) is not a contraindication for EVLA.

EVLA may also be performed in patients not really suitable for surgical therapies. Such patients are patients taking anticoagulant therapy for various reasons (i.e. atrial fibrillation, mechanical valve prosthesis etc.). Those patients can be treated with EVLA without cessation of anticoagulation. In a study, Theivacumar et al. (23) evaluated the effects of Coumadin usage on surgical outcomes and recanalization rates. They reported no major complication and a slight difference in recanalization rate in Coumadin group.

Presence of very tortuous or dilated veins does not prevent endovenous laser ablation. Besides the new laser fibers (such as radial fibers) and the longer wavelengths (1320 nm and

1470 nm), tumescent anesthesia and Trendelenburg position during the ablation procedures make endovenous laser ablation procedure possible for even the most dilated veins by shrinkage and circumferential ablation of the vein. It is sometimes difficult to advance the laser fiber in very tortuous veins. Skin stretching and positioning the vein sometimes help to advance the laser fiber. However, a second vein puncture may be necessary to complete the whole segment ablation of the diseased vein. By help of these techniques, we can simply say that almost every vein can be treated by EVLA.

Another problematic issue is the veins that are located very subdermally. Laser ablation of this vein is not a problem. However at the postoperative period patients may feel the presence of these ablated veins as a palpable cord just under the skin and may also feel stretching. Sometimes those veins may cause hyperpigmentation in the long-term period. In order to prevent these negative effects such subdermal veins may be ablated until the end of the deeper part and the superficial subdermal part may be removed surgically.

5. Procedure and technique

Endovenous laser ablation of the varicose veins may be divided into four sections:

1. Anesthesia regimen
2. Vein puncture and positioning the laser fiber
3. Ablation procedure
4. Postoperative care

5.1 Anesthesia regimen

It is possible to perform EVLA under any kind of anesthesia; however it is contrary to the nature of this minimal invasive procedure to perform under general or spinal anesthesia. Tumescent local anesthesia is sufficient for this procedure. If concomitant phlebectomies are performed, additional local anesthesia is applied to the area of varicosities. Tumescent local anesthesia should be applied under ultrasound control into the interfascial space around the saphenous vein. If correctly applied, tumescent anesthia forms a heat shield around the vein and protects the perivascular tissues (i.e. nerves) and the skin from the high temperatures caused by the laser energy. The temperature at the tip of the laser fibre may reach 720 °C and although tumescent anaesthesia reduces heat transfer to adjacent tissue irreversible nerve injury may occur at temperatures above 45 °C. In a previous study measurements adjacent to the GSV have confirmed that following adequate infiltration of tumescent anaesthesia the perivenous temperature reaches a median of 34.5 °C and thus nerve injury should be avoided. (24) This is particularly important when treating SSVs which is very close to the diffent nerves (posterior femoral nevre, tibial nerve, common peroneal nerve and sural nerve) due to its anatomic course. The authors recently published their experience for the importance of puncture site selection in the prevention of postoperative nerve injuries following SSV EVLA. (24) Different mixtures of solutions have been reported for tumescent anesthia. Either lidocaine or prilocaine are suitable in concentrations between 0.05 and 0.2%. In our clinical experience we prefer to use the following mixture: 1000 ml saline 0.9%, 50 ml lidocaine 2%, 1 ml Epinenephrine 1:1000,10 mEq $NaHCO_3$. A total volume of 100-500 cc is given according to length of the vein is reported in the literature. We use a simple formula for the amount of tumescent anesthesia and give an amout of 10 ml/treated vein centimeter. There are different techniques for administering tumescent anesthesia. But according to authors' experience, injection of the solution by the help of a motor pump is an easy method. However, if this is not avaliable then the solution can be injected via syringes under the ultrasound guidance.

5.2 Vein puncture and positioning the laser fiber

For a successful vein puncture there are some important rules. There should be a comfortable temperature in the surgical suit. Cold environment may cause vein spasm especially in sensitive patients. Patient also should be positioned in the reverse Trendelenburg position in order to fill the vein. Then the patient is cleaned. The ultrasound probe covered sterile and taken into the operating field. To preserve the minimal invasive nature of the procedure vein should be punctured percutaneously under ultrasound guidance. In the experienced hands it very easy to cannulate the vein percutaneously. Until gaining experience in the percutaneous cannulation, biopsy apparatus of Doppler probes may help to ease your cannulation. However if this is not possible, vein access can be done via stab incision and hooking of the saphenous vein.

After gaining access to the vein, a guide-wire inserted (Figure 2) through the needle and 5 or 6-F introducer sheath was placed over the guide-wire into the GSV. If a radial laser fiber is

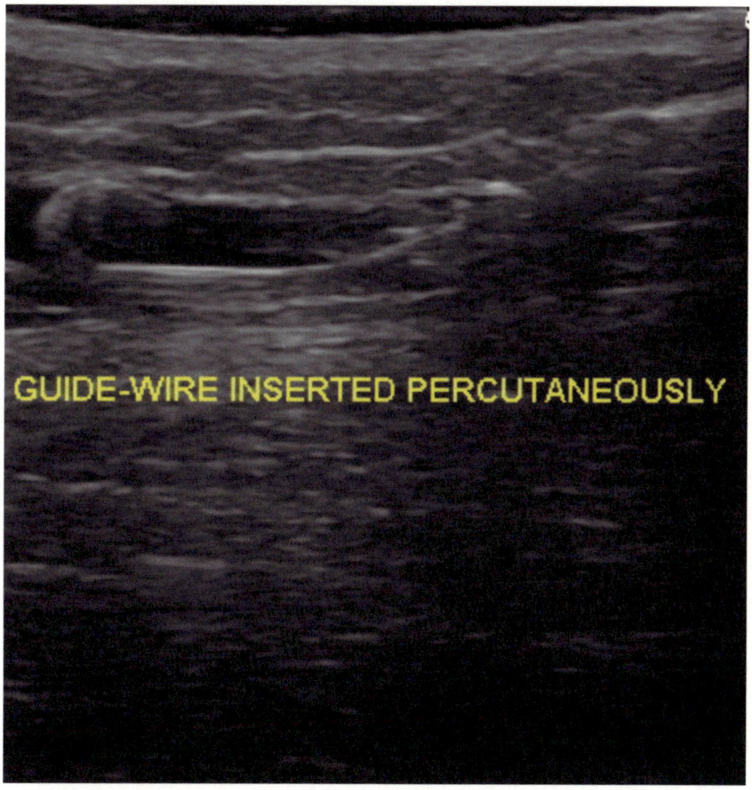

Fig. 2. Guide-wire in the sapheonus vein.

used a short guide-wire and short introducer is enough to advance the fiber in GSV. However if it is preferred to use a bare-tip fiber, long guide-wires and sheaths must be used. Regardless the type of the used laser fiber, fiber is advanced till a safe distance from the saphenofemoral junction (SFJ) under the ultrasound guidance. This distance is changing in the published literature between 1-2 cm and 3-4 cm. In our experience, with 980 nm and bare-tip laser fiber we keep the distance 1-2 cm below SFJ. However we can go up till 0.5-1 cm below the SFJ with 1470 nm and radial laser fiber (Figure 3). For SSV ablation the distance from the saphenopopliteal junction should be decided according to the connection place and type of the SSV with popliteal vein. According to classification by Kosinski and Creton, SSV connects to the popliteal vein in very different types. (6) And incidence of nerve injury increase as the saphenopopliteal junction goes up to the popliteal crease. Usually as a simple rule at least a 2 cm distance should be kept between saphenopopliteal junction and the fiber for positioning.

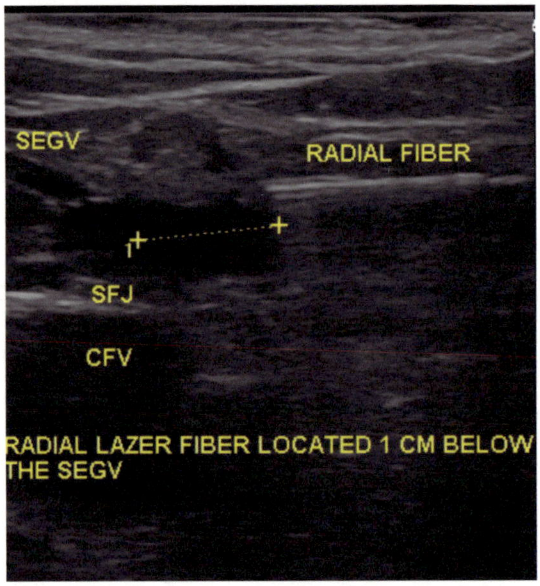

Fig. 3. Radial fiber in the saphenofemoral junction.

Sometimes it is difficult to advance the fiber in tortuous veins. Usually straightening of the leg or guiding the fiber by external manipulation and compression may solve the problem. If these maneuvers do not solve the problem a second puncture of the above the impeded vein segment is necessary to achieve a complete ablation.

The correct positioning of the fiber (just inferior to the entrance of the superficial epigastric vein into the GSV for GSV treatment and just inferior to the deep penetration of the SSV) is a very important step which must be done very cautiously to prevent any adverse event related with the procedure. The position must also be confirmed after injection of tumescent anesthesia, just before the beginning of the ablation (Figure 4). Since the echogenity of the bare-tip fibers is not so good, it needs good ultrasound skills and experience. Especially after the injection of tumescent solution, it is sometimes difficult to see the fiber due to the confounding effect of the solution. The radial fiber is more Doppler friendly and can also be seen easily after tumescent solution. (Figure 5)

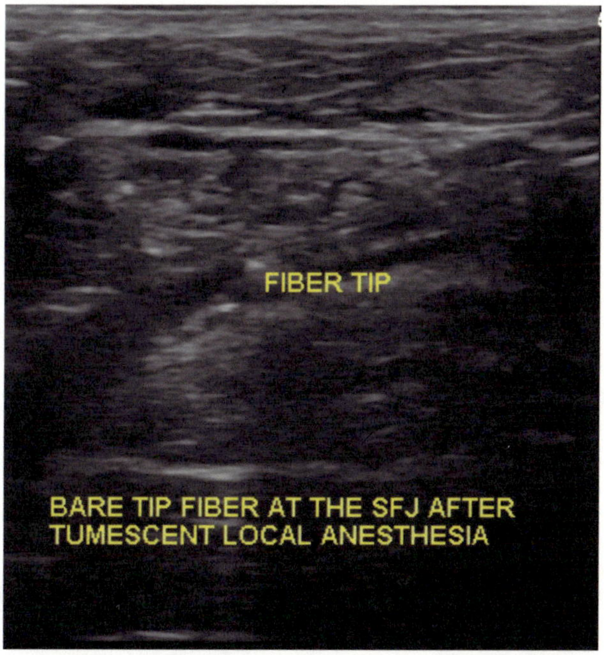

Fig. 4. Control of the position of laser fiber at the saphenofemoral junction.

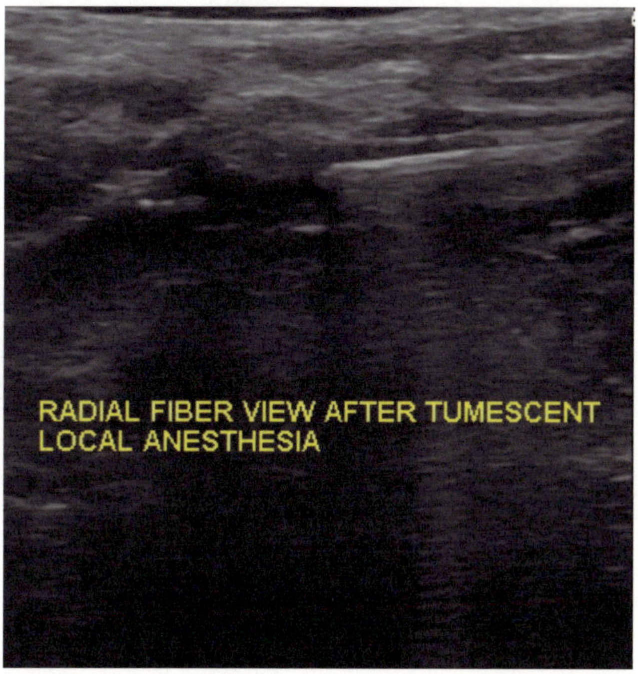

Fig. 5. View of radial fiber after tumescent local anesthesic solution.

5.3 Ablation procedure

After confirming the correct position of the fiber, patient is placed in Trendelenburg position to further empty the vein. This is especially important in treating the dilated veins.

Ablation procedure may be performed in a pulsed or continuous fashion. In our experience we prefer continuous method. (Figure 6, 7) The fiber and/or sheath are withdrawn at a speed of 1-3 mm per second. This speed is determined by the given energy to treated vein centimeter. This is called as Linear Endovenous Energy Density (LEED). Generally 60-100 J/cm LEED is delivered to the vein wall according to the diameter of the treated vein. Withdrawal speed should be a little slower at the proximal part than the distal part. During the withdrawal of the fiber, external hand compression over the ablated vein segment may help ever further narrowing the vein wall for increasing the vein wall laser energy interaction. Our goal is to achieve successful ablation while minimizing the rate of adverse events such as pain and bruising.

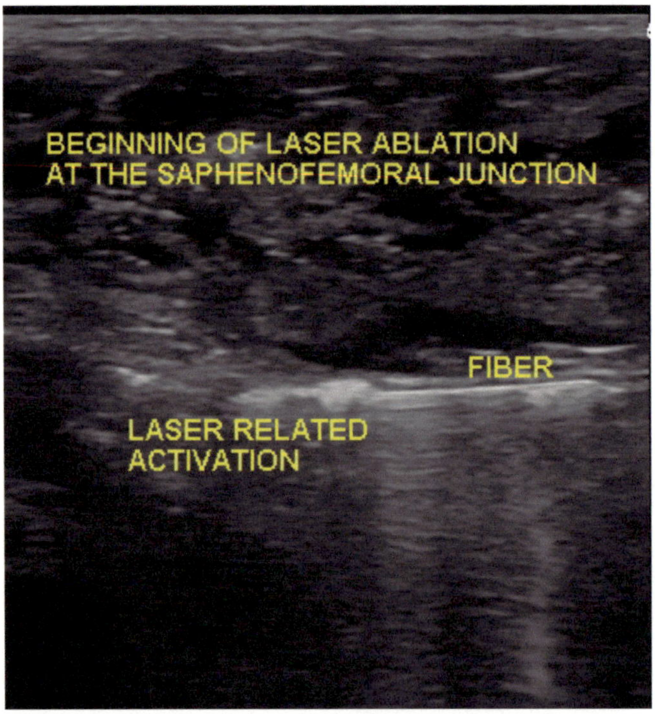

Fig. 6. Beginning of the laser ablation at the safenofemoral junction.

On the conclusion of the ablation procedure immediate Doppler confirmation is crucial. (Figure 8) Patencies of the deep veins (femoral vein, popliteal vein) as well as occlusion of the treated saphenous veins are recorded.

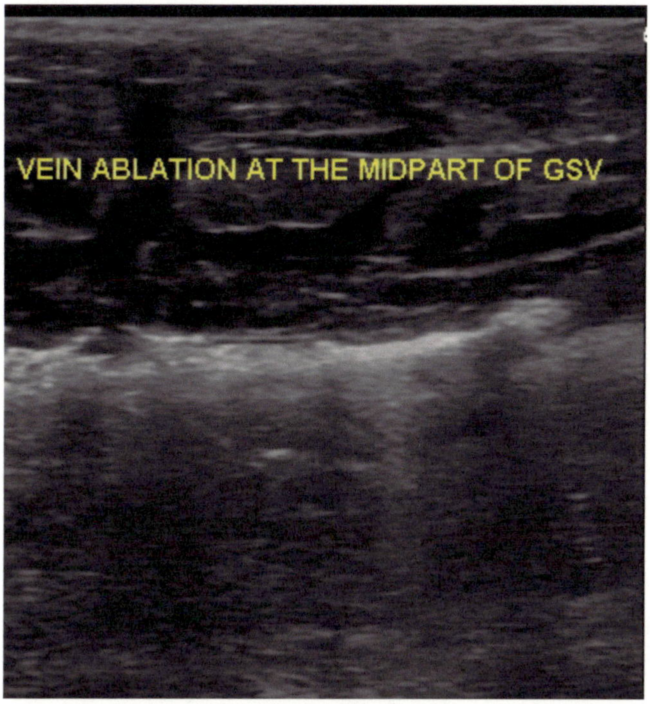

Fig. 7. Ablation at the midpart of great saphenous vein.

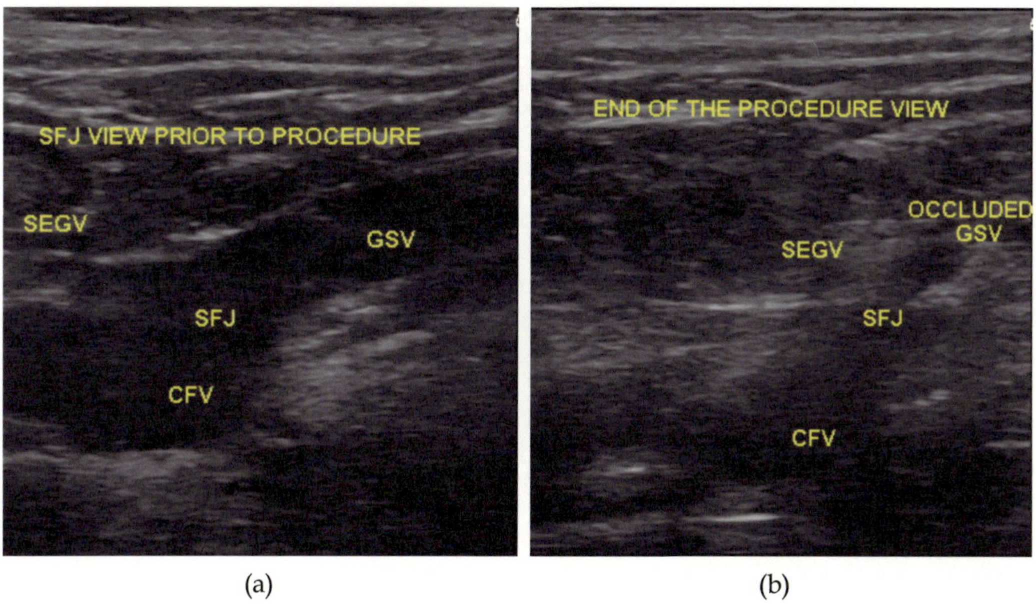

Fig. 8. Picture showing the saphenofemoral junction preoperative (a) and immediate (b) after the procedure.

EVLA for incompetent perforator veins (IPVs) is a more demanding procedure when compared to GSV and SSV ablation. The key point in the EVLA of perforator vein is the vein access. Patient is placed in a reverse Trendelenburg position and a direct puncture is made under ultrasound guidance with a 21 Gauge micropuncture needle or 16 Gauge angiocatheteter. There is no specific catheter or fiber system for treating perforator veins. However, 400µm, 600 µm fibers can be used. Recently, Biolitec Company introduced a 200 µm slim radial fiber for the treatment of IPVs. After gaining access, confirmation is performed by aspiration of the blood. Then the laser fiber should be positioned at the fascia level. Following the confirmation of the correct position, tumescent local anesthesia is administered around the vein. Then energy is applied to the vein. External compression with ultrasound probe may help to increase vein wall the contact. In our clinical experience, while treating IPVs we do not use continuous pull back, rather we prefer pulsed mode. Since there are conflicting results and high recanalization rates in the literature, we prefer to ablate every vein segment twice and to treat the possible longest vein segment. (8) After completion of laser ablation a compression should be applied over the vein for several minutes. Following the compression, confirmation of the occlusion of the vein is made with ultrasound and recorded.

5.4 Postoperative care

After the completion of the ablation procedure, patients should be placed on compression therapy. There are different compression therapy protocols in the literature. In our clinical experience, we have two different policies which are determined by the applied procedure. In the patient that we performed concomitant extensive phlebectomies, we use the external compression bandages (short-stretch) for the following 24 hours and then we use 23-32 mmHg compression stockings (thigh high) for the following 4 weeks. If we do not perform concomitant phlebectomies, we directly use compression stockings for the following 4 weeks. There are different conflicting recommendations about the duration and the need for the postoperative compression therapy. In a preliminary study by Berland et al., (26) it was reported that no detrimental effect was shown with the absence of post-procedural compression therapy.

In the earlier studies low molecular weight heparin was recommended for the 8days following the procedure. In the beginning of our experience we also used this protocol. However after gaining experience, we do not use low molecular weight heparin in our patients excluding patients with obesity and older age. We use non steroid antiinflamatory drugs (i.e. diclofenac potassium, 75 mg, bid, p.o.), if necessary. Patients are advised to walk regularly during recovery from treatment.

6. Follow-up

Since there is the possibility of recanalization and/or incomplete ablation, patients should be controlled at appropriate intervals with physical examination and color-flow Doppler ultrasound. In the physical examination, any recurrent and/or new refluxing tributaries are recorded. Any signs or symptoms related with chronic venous insufficiency are also recorded. With the color-flow Doppler ultrasound occlusion of the ablated vein is examined. In our clinical protocol patients are seen at 1st week, 1st month, 3rd month, 6th month, 1st year and yearly thereafter. (Figure 9)

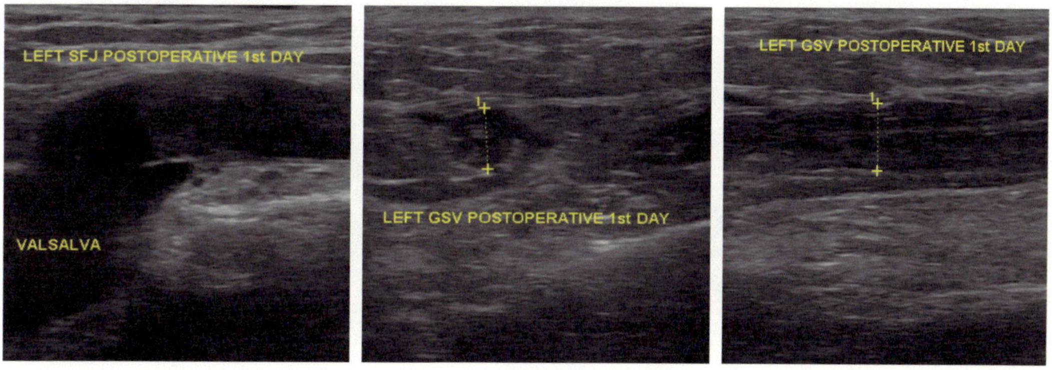
LEFT SFJ POSTOPERATIVE 1st DAY
VALSALVA
LEFT GSV POSTOPERATIVE 1st DAY
LEFT GSV POSTOPERATIVE 1st DAY

(a)

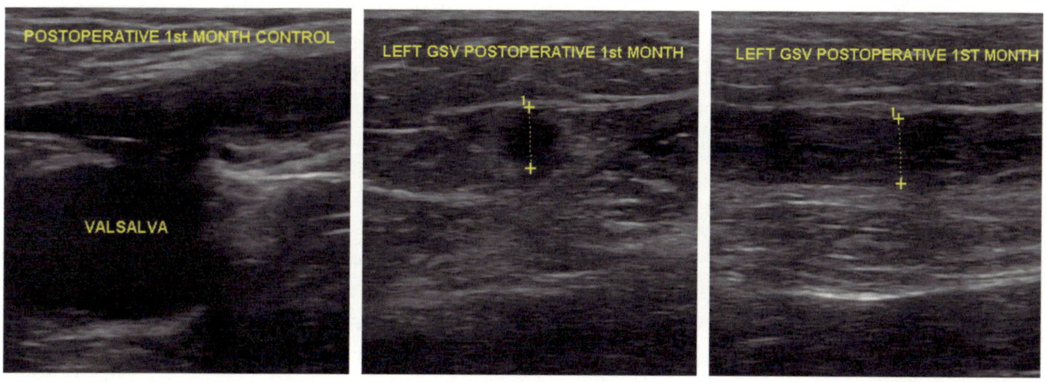
POSTOPERATIVE 1st MONTH CONTROL
VALSALVA
LEFT GSV POSTOPERATIVE 1st MONTH
LEFT GSV POSTOPERATIVE 1ST MONTH

(b)

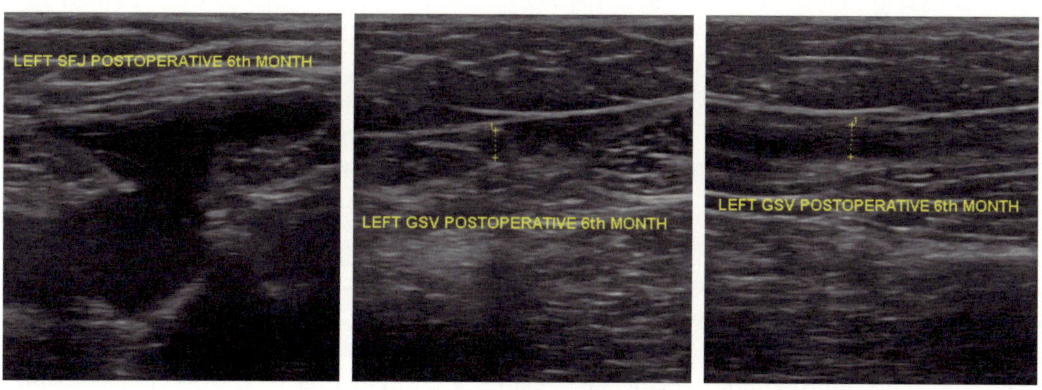
LEFT SFJ POSTOPERATIVE 6th MONTH
LEFT GSV POSTOPERATIVE 6th MONTH
LEFT GSV POSTOPERATIVE 6th MONTH

(c)

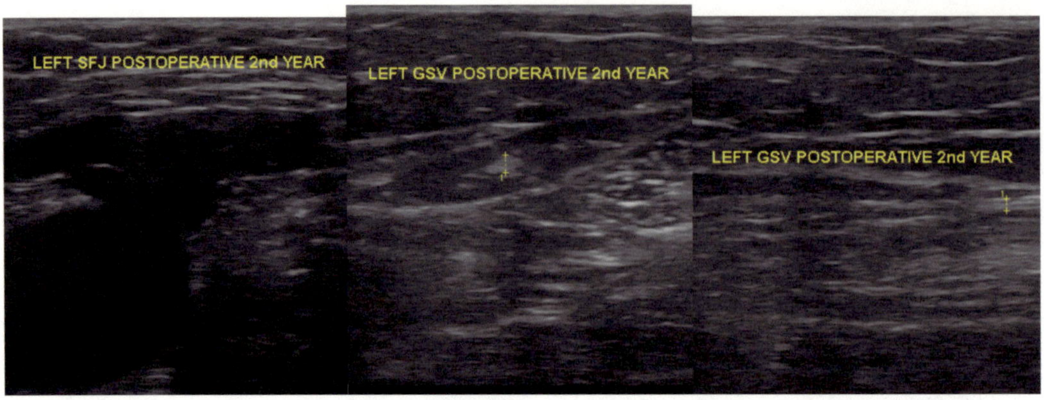

(d)

Fig. 9. Postoperative follow-up doppler images of the same patients postoperative 1st day (a), postoperative 1st month (b) 6th month (c), 2nd year (d)

7. Complications

Complications of EVLA may be divided as procedure related and post-procedural events. Procedure related complications are generally related with technical difficulties. These are vein access and fiber advancement problems. As mentioned above warm and comfortable operating rooms may solve the problems related with venospasm. Also determining the most suitable place for puncture by Doppler ultrasound is important. A straight and appropriate size vein segment usually solves the problem.

Postoperative bruising, pain, paresthesia, and induration are the most common adverse events. However, there are also other adverse events such as superficial thrombophlebitis, skin burn, deep vein thrombosis, infection, arteriovenous fistula and skin burn. Although these later adverse events are literally possible, they are uncommon. (16)

Bruising is generally minimal and self-limiting and usually lasts less than two weeks period. (Figure 10) There are different rates of bruising in the literature (between 11-100%). (26) Bruising rates are higher with wavelengths that use hemoglobin as cromophore such as 810 nm and 980 nm. However, Laser systems with emission wavelengths of 1320 nm and 1470 nm have their main absorption in water. There are reduced postoperative pain and bruising with 1320 nm when compared to shorter wavelengths. In our previous randomized study, we compared 1470 nm with 980 nm for early postoperative adverse events and found that 1470 nm wavelength was superior with reduced postoperative pain, bruising, and paresthesia. Furthermore patient satisfaction was also higher with 1470 nm. (27)

Incidence of postoperative paresthesia is reported between 7 and 9.5%. Paresthesia is also mild and usually resolves average an 8 week period. It is mainly seen following the full length ablation of the GSV. However the situation is different for SSV which has very close relationship with nerves along with its anatomic course. In some studies temporary paraesthesia is reported as frequently as in 40% of limbs following the EVLA for the SSV. (25) In our clinical experience, incidence of paresthesia following EVLA for GSV with 1470 nm is very low (1/54 limbs). The incidence may be reduced with partial (over the knee)

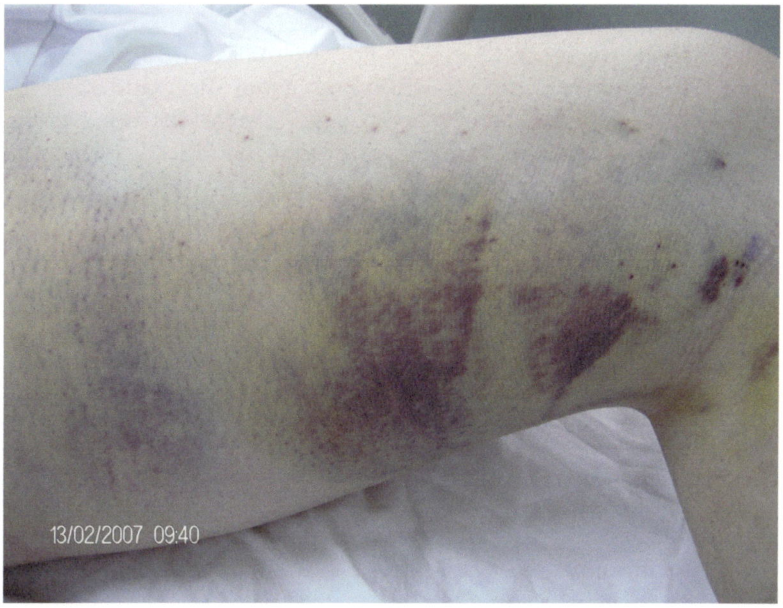

Fig. 10. Postoperative bruising. (980 nm and bare-tip fibre)

ablation and accurate administered perivenous tumescent local anesthesia. In another study, we compared the postoperative nerve injury following SSV EVLA. Puncture site from the midcalf level was shown to decrease the paresthesia. (25).

Indurations happen along the treated veins after EVLA that resembles either a palpable cord or the feeling of a shortened muscle at the medial part of the thigh. According to our study induration is more common with bare tip fibers, shorter wavelengths (i.e. 810nm, 980 nm), and higher LEED levels. Since they ablated the vein only the places that they contact the vein wall, bare tip fibers especially at the higher LEEDs may perforate the vein and extravasation of the leukocytes cause pain and the induration. Nowadays with use of radial fibers, longer wavelengths (such as 1470 nm), and lower LEED levels, the incidence of induration decreased dramatically. (28)

Skin burn is vey rare complication. In the literature excluding the study by Chang et al. (29) in which no tumescent anesthesia was used, only nine cases of burns have been reported; two occured when no local anesthetic was used and two during treatment of tributaries. This situation emphasizes the importance of tumescent local anesthesia, especially in the very superficial veins. In our experience, we have never seen skin burns.

Infection is very rare complication. However, there is a case report of septic thrombophlebitis following EVLA. (30) With adequate sterile technique infection is avoided. Skin burn is also a rare complication. This can be avoided by scrupulous technique plus injection of correct and adequate amount of tumescent local anesthesia. We have never seen infection and skin burn related with the EVLA procedure so far.

Although it is rare, deep vein thrombosis is the most severe complication. In our experience no deep vein thrombosis was recorded so far. Endotermal Heat Induced Thrombosis (EHIT) (Regardless of the energy, either laser or radiofrequency) is now used for the propagation of thrombus in to the deep system as a new terminology. (Table 1) EHIT II is considered to be significant, since it is a precursor to deep vein thrombosis. In a study by Sadek et al. incidence of EHIT II in patients treated with endovenous laser and radiofrequency was evaluated. They concluded that there was no significant difference between laser and radiofrequency for the incidence of EHIT II, and upon identification it should be treated using anticoagulation. (31)

Hyperpigmentation along the ablated vein occurs in up to 12% patients, although most authors report a much lower incidence. It usually improves in time. (27)

I	Thrombosis to the level of the saphenofemoral (SF) junction
II	Extension into the deep venous system, cross-sectional area ≤50%
III	Extension into the deep venous system, cross-sectional area ≥50%
IV	Occlusion of the femoral vein

Table 1. Endotermal Heat Induced Thrombosis (EHIT) classes (30)

Complications related with the laser ablation of the incompetent perforator veins are also similar with great/small saphenous veins such as skin injury, nerve injury and deep vessel injury. However there is no clear data about the prevalence of these complications due to the limited number of studies with limited patient volumes. In one study, redness, numbness or blistering was reported as complication. (8)

8. Outcomes

Since the first publication of Navarro et al. in 2001, (12) many authors reported their experience on different wavelengths, fibers and veins. Also Van den Bos et al. (3) published the first review of endovenous therapies of lower extremity varicosities in 2009. There are almost similar results with successful ablation and low adverse events rates. Some of the studies and their results are summarized in Table 2.

In some studies EVLA was compared to surgical stripping. Especially in the randomized trials, it was suggested that abolition of GSV reflux, improvements in quality of life, patient satisfaction and cosmetics are similar for both treatment modality. Although pain levels appear similar in both techniques, return to normal activity or work was reported earlier after EVLA. (3)

Importance of wavelength is also matter of question. There is not so much data regarding the effects of wavelengths that can be used for a decision-making tool for the treatment of varicose veins. Proebstle et al. (19) compared 1320 nm Nd:YAG laser with 940 nm diode laser and concluded that endovenous laser treatment using a 1320 nm Nd:YAG laser causes fewer side effects compared with 940 nm diode laser. In our randomized clinical study we compared the 1470 nm diode laser with commonly used 980 nm diode laser for the adverse event and the varicose venous clinical severity scores (VCSS). At early postoperative period 1470 nm diode laser was superior in both adverse events and VCSSs. (28)

There is now also experience in patients with recurrent varicosities. Theivacumar et al. (32) reported their experience on 104 limbs of 95 patients with recurrent varicose veins. They successfully ablated these varicosities and concluded that EVLA was a safe and effective

Author	Number of limbs	Occlusion Rate (%)	Follow-up Period
GSV			
810 nm	499	93	2 year
Min, 2003	1076	97	3 years
Agus, 2006			
940 nm			
Ravi, 2006	990	97	3 years
Proebstle, 2003	41	95	6 months
980 nm			
Gibson, 2007	210	96	4 months
Pannier, 2008	67	88.1	2.2 years
1470 nm			
Pannier, 2009	128	100	1 year
Doganci, 2010	54	100	6 months
SSV			
810 nm			
Huisman	169	98	3 months
980 nm			
Desmyttere, 2009	147	97	1 years
Park, 2008	55	100	3 years
1470 nm			
Doganci, 2011	68	100	6 months

Table 2. Outcomes following endovenous laver ablation

option for the treatment of recurrent varicose veins. In our clinical experience between February 2010 and February 2011, we treated 46 limbs of 39 patients with recurrent varicose veins. Our results are also similar to Theivacumar's results. Treatment of recurrent varicosities especially in patients with previous surgical stripping is very easy and safe. As a simple rule it can be said that "if you cannulate, you can treat any vein" with indication of treatment.

Due to its anatomic localization treatment of incompetent SSV with endovenous laser ablation is superior to surgical stripping. Rashid et al. (7) have shown that ligation of the saphenopopliteal junction (SPJ) is not achieved in 30% of the cases, even if the junction is marked pre-operatively under ultrasound guidance. In the endovenous laser ablation, there is not a problem like that. If there is anatomic SPJ, you can treat the incompetent SSV without having any surgical difficulties. As it is summarized in Table 2 the results are very promising so far.

In the review by Van Den Bos et al. (3) success rate of EVLA after a five year period was 95.4%. Although there are articles with very promising results, there is still a need for randomized controlled studies with long term results.

In our clinical experience (not published yet), we treat 717 patients (1066 limbs) with 1470 nm diode laser and radial laser fiber between September 2009 and March 2011. There was no recanalization so far in this cohort of patients during the follow-up period.

Results for endovenous treatment of IPVs are not so much as it is in GSVs. Kabnick et al. (33) presented data using a 980 nm wavelength. Twenty-five IPVs with an average size of

4.4 mm were treated. Closure rate was 85% at a 4 month period. In another study Murphy et al. (34) reported 100% closure rate at a 6 months period.

9. Discussion

Traditional surgical methods to treat varicose veins are associated with significant complications, high recurrence rates and some patient dissatisfaction. In a randomized trial of SFJ ligation methods for primary saphenous incompetence, the two year clinical recurrence rate was 33% and Doppler ultrasound (DUS) proven recurrence was up to 22%. However, the clinical benefits and cost-effectiveness of surgery are well established. (35)

Minimally invasive techniques such as EVLA are a popular choice for patients and doctors because of the low risk of complications, short ''downtime,'' and excellent cosmetic results. When applied properly, these techniques also seem to be effective and safe. For efficacy and safety, it is essential that professionals well trained in phlebology and ultrasound examination perform these complex procedures, but pain and ecchymoses seem to be inherent to all (minimally invasive) procedures of varicose veins including EVLA. (17)

In recently published studies, high success rates after EVLA have been reported. These have been based mainly on duplex US assessment of the treated veins.

Three recent systematic reviews, two with meta-analysis, have attempted to analyse all of the relevant literature comparing surgical outcomes to UGFS, RFA and EVLA, and another has compared safety and efficacy of EVLA and surgery. The largest meta-analysis examined 64 eligible studies, which included over twelve thousand limbs, with DUS findings as outcome. Average follow-up was 32 months and estimated pooled success rates at 3 years were highest for EVLA with 94%, followed by RFA (84%), surgery (78%) and foam sclerotherapy (77%). EVLA was significantly superior to all other methods to abolish saphenous incompetence. (3, 35) RFA and UGFS were equally effective as surgery. This analysis has had some criticism, as most studies reviewed had not used survival analysis, so the success rates are probably inflated. In a separate meta-analysis, the improved effectiveness of EVLA is confirmed over surgery, with better post-operative outcomes. However venous clinical severity scores (VCSS) were equivalent between EVLA and surgery at end of followup. Another systematic review compared safety and efficacy of all treatments, new and old, where articles reported comparisons between at least two treatments. This review demonstrated better safety records for both EVLA and RFA compared to surgery, although major surgical complications were rare. Surgery consistently caused more post-operative bruising overall and more post-operative pain than both EVLA and RFA. Paraesthesia was the most common serious adverse event associated with surgery occurring at a median rate of 11.7% (4.1-30.3%) reported among 517 limbs and ten studies. (35)

In the EVVERT study comparing laser and radiofrequency, 810 nm laser and bare-tip laser fibers compared with VNUS ClosureFast catheter. As it is expected in the result part, pain scores was lower in the radiofrequency group, and bruising was greater in the laser group. (36) However, it is comparison is not well balanced. Simply saying, in this study the authors compared the brand new catheter of VNUS (ClosureFast) with the oldest laser technology. There is now new generation laser and fiber system commercially in use from a very long time. And the conclusion should not be laser generates greater perioperative bruising and pain than radiofrequency. Instead, it should be as 810 nm laser and the bare-tip fiber generates greater bruising and pain than radiofrequency. Thus, this study should be designed to compare the new generation laser systems (i.e. 1470 nm diode or 1320 Nd:YAG lasers and radial laser fibers). In our previous study, 1470 nm diode laser and radial laser fibers were compared with 980 nm and bare-tip fibers in randomized controlled groups. We found that side effects such as pain, induration (14 vs 3 (radial)), ecchymosis (13 vs 2 (radial)) and paraesthesia (9 vs 1(radial)) were significantly reduced with the 1470 nm laser and radial catheter system compared to the 980 mm bare-tip laser fibre.

In the review by Van den Bos et al., (3) besides anatomic success rates, patient-reported outcomes such as health related quality of life (HRQOL), treatment satisfaction, symptom relief, and side effects were analyzed. Compared with surgery, EVLA-treated patients appreciated EVLA more than surgery because they reported fewer side effects and their HRQOL improved better and faster.

In our study, patient satisfaction and patient preference were questioned. Most of the patients in 1470 nm and radial laser-fiber group replied as "very satisfied-satisfied" and "definitely-probably yes". The difference was statistically significant ($p<0.05$). Venous Clinical Severity Scores also evaluated. VCSSs in the fisrt month were also favorably lower in 1470 nm and radial laser fiber group.

In another study which is similar to ours, Gerard JL et al. (37) questioned "Is bare-tip fiber out-dated?" in their study. They used 1470 nm diode laser and compared bare-tip fiber with radial fiber. As a conclusion they declared that protected fibers should be recommended as bare-tip fibers have proved to be out-dated.

Laser fibers are evolving with the technological advances. Nowadays after learning the importance of fibers, many fibers come-out. Direct vein wall contact of the tip of the fiber cause carbonization of the wall. This can induce perforations leading to bruising and pain related to white blood cell extravasation. (28) For avoiding direct wall contact of the fiber many manufacturers produced alternative fibers such tulip, jacket-tip and radial fibers.

Another point is the amount of delivered energy. There are many different formulas to calculate the amount of energy per centimeter which is known as LEED. As a simple rule a minimum of 10 J/cm/diameter is an effective amount. In our experience we generally use this formula.

In our clinical experience, after gaining experience and seeing results of our patients; we gradually decreased our watt and LEED levels. At the beginning of our 1470 nm and radial fiber experience, we begin with 15 Watts and 90 J/cm LEED level. There was no recanalization, and minimal postoperative morbidity. Then we gradually decreased our watt level to 12 W and LEED level to 70 J/cm. These parameters are very effective. They do not affect the recanalizastion rates. Furthermore our adverse event rate is nearly approach to minimum. With these improvements we are now gradually decreasing the amount of tumescent local anesthesia.

These improvements increase the office-based nature of the endovenous laser treatment modality. Patients tolerate this procedure well.

However there is still a need for the long-term results and strong evidences, especially in the area of HRQOL and follow-up protocols. There is still an ongoing competition between the endovenous treatment modalities. Recently steam ablation and the mechanochemical ablation devices (ClariVein) added to this competition area. The results of these new modalities are also beginning to come.

Evolving Doppler ultrasound technology will also help the physicians to increase their success in endovascular techniques by providing excellent diagnostics and perioperative imaging options.

In our opinion next decade will witness the outcome of some other new techniques. Long-term result of the treatment modalities will be available and by these results strong evidences will also be available.

According to the American Venous Forum Guidelines (4.10.0) recommendation endovenous laser therapy of GSV is safe and effective and has a grade 1A recommendation level. Recommendation for the IPV (4.21.0) has a lower evidence level and is grade 2C. (8, 22)

10. Summary

Endovenous laser ablation is a safe and effective treatment modality in the treatment of incompetent great and small saphenous veins. With an obsessive approach to all technical steps and patient selection criterion, incidence of adverse events and complication is very low. Although we still need long-term result and strong evidences longer wavelengths and new generation laser fibers seem superior to the shorter wavelengths and bare-tip fibers. Multicenter randomized controlled trials with larger patient volume and standard long-term follow-up protocols are still needed to answer our questions.

However, with the available results and patient/physician preferences it can be said that conventional high ligation plus stripping of the incompetent saphenous veins is no longer the gold standard treatment choise.

In the very near future, reticular veins, incompetent tributary veins, perforator veins beside main trunk varicosities will be treated by endovenous modalities and the patiens will have the opportunity to have these procedures in best cosmetic and the least invasive ways without having stab incisions.

11. References

[1] Maurins U, Hoffman BH, Lösch C, Jöckel KH, Rabe E, Pannier F. Distribution and prevalence of reflux in the superficial and deep venous system in the general population--results from the Bonn Vein Study, Germany. J Vasc Surg. 2008 Sep;48(3):680-7.

[2] Evans CJ, Fowkes FGR, Ruckley CV, Lee AJ. Prevalence of varicose veins and chronic venous insufficiency in men and women in the general population: Edinburgh vein Study. J Epidemiol Community Health 1999;53:149-53.

[3] Van den Bos R, Arends L, Kockaert M, Neumann M, Nijsten T. Endovenous therapies of lower extremity varicosities: a metaanalysis. J Vasc Surg 2009 Jan;49(1):230-9.

[4] van Rij AM, Jiang P, Solomon C, Christie RA, Hill GB. Recurrence after varicose vein surgery: a prospective long-term clinical study with duplex ultrasound scanning and air plethysmography. J Vasc Surg 2003;38:935-43.

[5] Huisman LC, Bruins RM, van den Berg M, Hissink RJ. Endovenous laser ablation of the small saphenous vein: prospective analysis of 150 patients, a cohort study. Eur J Vasc Endovasc Surg 2009; 38:199-202.

[6] Gerard JL. Small saphenous vein ablation: particularities and precautions. In: Becquemin JP, Alimi YS, Gerard JL, editors. Controversies and updates in vascular surgery 2009. Torino:Edizioni Panminerva Medica; 2009. p. 450-4.

[7] Rashid HI, Ajeel A, Tyrrell MR. Persistent popliteal fossa reflux following saphenopopliteal disconnection. Br J Surg 2002;89:748-51.

[8] Elias S. Percutaneous ablation of perforating veins. In: Gloviczki P, editors. Handbook of venous disorders. London:Hodder Arnold; 2009. P. 536-44.

[9] Sato DT, Goff CD, Gregory RT. Subfascial perforator vein ablation: comparison versus endoscopic techniques. J Endovasc Surg 1999;6:147-54

[10] Nezlen D. Prospective study of safety, patient satisfaction and leg ulcer healing following saphenous and subfascial endoscopic perforator surgery. Br J Surg 2008; 87:86-91.

[11] Puglisi B, Tacconi A, San Filippo F. L'application du laser ND-YAG dans le traitement du syndrome variquex. [Application of theND-YAG laser in the treatment of varicose syndrome]. In: Davey A, Stemmer R, editors. Phlebology' 89. London: J Libby Eurotext; 1989. p. 39-842.

[12] Navarro L, Min RJ, Bone C. Endovenous laser: a new minimally invasive method of treatment for varicose veins: preliminary observations using an 810 nm diode laser. Dermatol Surg 2001; 27:117-22.

[13] Forrestal MD, Min RJ, Zimmet SE, Isaacs MN, Moeller MR. Endovenous laser treatment (EVLTTM) for varicose veins—A review. In: Todays Ther Trends. Princeton Junction, NJ: Communications Media for Education. 2002. 20(4): 299–310.

[14] Proebstle TM, Gül D, Kargl A, Knop J. Endovenous laser treatment of the lesser saphenous vein with a 940 nm diode laser—Early results, Dermatol Surg. 2003. 29: 357–361.

[15] Proebstle TM, Herdeman S. Feasibility of incompetent perforator vein ablation by endovenous laser treatment. In: Presented at the German Phlebologic Society Annual Meeting, September 2005

[16] Pannier F, Rabe E, Maurins U. First results with a new 1470-nm diode laser for endovenous ablation of incompetent saphenous veins. Phlebology 2009;24:26-30.

[17] Van Den Bos RR, Neumann M, De Roos KP, Nijsten T. Endovenous laser ablation-induced complications: review of the literature and new cases. Dermatol Surg 2009 Aug;35(8):1206-14.

[18] Van den Bos RR, Kockaert MA, Neumann HA, Nijsten T. Technical review of endovenous laser therapy for varicose veins. Eur J Vasc Endovasc Surg 2008;35:88-95.

[19] Proebstle TM, Moehler T, Gul D, Herdemann S. Endovenous treatment of the great saphenous vein using a 1320 nm Nd:YAG laser causes fewer side effects than using a 940 nm diode laser. Dermatol Surg 2005;31:1678-83.

[20] Almeida J, Mackay E, Javier J, Mauriello J, Raines J. Saphenous laser ablation at 1470 nm targets the vein wall, not blood. Vasc Endovascular Surg; 2009 Jul 23.

[21] Kabnick LS, Caruso JA. No-wall touch laser fiber vs bare-tip laser fiber for endothermal venous ablation of great saphenous vein: are the results the same? In: Gerard JL, editor. Controversies and updates in vascular surgery. 1st ed. Torino: Edizioni Panminerva Medica; 2008. p. 401-2.

[22] Morrison N. Laser treatment of the incompetent saphenous vein. In: Gloviczki P, editor. Handbook of venous disorders. London:Hodder Arnold; 2009. P. 418-28.
[23] Theivacumar NS, Gough MJ. Influence of warfarin on the success of endovenous laser ablation (EVLA) of the great saphenous vein (GSV). Eur J Vasc Endovasc Surg. 2009 Oct;38(4):506-10
[24] Theivacumar NS, Beale RJ, Mavor AI, Gough MJ. Initial experience in endovenous laser ablation (EVLA) of varicose veins due to small saphenous vein reflux. Eur J Vasc Endovasc Surg 2007; 33:614-8.
[25] Doganci S, Yildirim V, Demirkilic U. Does puncture site affect the rate of nerve injuries following endovenous laser ablation of the small saphenous veins? Eur J Vasc Endovasc Surg. 2011 Mar;41(3):400-5.
[26] Berland T, Kabnick L, Rudarakanchana N, Chasin C, Sadeck M, Rockman C, Maldonado T, Cayne N, Jacabowitz G, Lamparllo P, Mussa F, Adelman M. Compression vs. no compression after endovenous ablation of the great saphenous vein. In: Jean-Pierre Becquemin, editor. Contoversies and Updates in Vascular Surgery 2011. Torino (Italy): Edizioni Minerva Medica; 2011.p. 622-26.
[27] Darwood RJ, Gough MJ. Endovenous laser treatment for uncomplicated varicose veins. Phlebology. 2009;24 Suppl 1:50-61.
[28] Doganci S, Demirkilic U. Comparison of 980 nm laser and bare-tip fibre with 1470 nm laser and radial fibre in the treatment of great saphenous vein varicosities: a prospective randomised clinical trial. Eur J Vasc Endovasc Surg. 2010 Aug;40(2):254-9
[29] Chang CJ, Chua JJ. Endovenous laser photocoagulation (EVLP) for varicose veins. Lasers Surg Med 2002;31: 257–62
[30] Dunts K, Huemer G, Wayant W, Shamiyeh A. Diffuse phlegmonos phlebitis after endovenous laser treatment of the greater saphenous vein. J Vasc Surg 2006; 43:1056-8.
[31] Sadek M, Kabnick L, Berlant T, Chasin C, Rudarakanchana N, Rockman C, Maldonado T, Cayne N, Jacobowitz G, Lamparllo P, Musa F, Adelman M. Vein thrombosis induced by laser or radiofrequency: the winner is… In: Jean-Pierre Becquemin, editor. Controversies and Updates in Vascular Surgery 2011. Torino (Italy): Edizioni Minerva Medica; 2011.p. 653-57.
[32] Theivacumar NS, Gough MJ. Endovenous laser ablation (EVLA) to treat recurrent varicose veins. Eur J Vasc Endovasc Surg. 2011 May;41(5):691-6.
[33] Kabnick L. Perforator vein treatment. In: Presented at the Vein Meeting, Uncasville CT, June 2006.
[34] Murphy R. Comparison of radiofrequency and laser for perforator treatment. American College of Phlebology, Poster Session, November, 2006.
[35] McBride KD. Changing to endovenous treatment for varicose veins: how much more evidence is needed? Surgeon. 2011 Jun;9(3):150-9.
[36] Nordon IM, Loftus IM. EVVERT comparing laser and radiofrequency: An update on endovenous treatment options. In: Greenhalgh RM, editor. Vascular and Endovascular consensus update. London. BIBA Publishing; 2011.p.381-88.
[37] Gerard JL, Daoud M. Is bare-tip fiber out-dated? … In: Jean-Pierre Becquemin, editor. Controversies and Updates in Vascular Surgery 2011. Torino (Italy): Edizioni Minerva Medica; 2011.p. 648-52.

8

Iatrogenic Complications Following Laser Ablation of Varicose Veins

Carolina Vaz et al.*
Department of Angiology and Vascular Surgery, Hospital de Santo António,
Centro Hospitalar do Porto,
Portugal

1. Introduction

During the past decade, Endovenous Laser Ablation (EVLA) has been introduced as a minimally invasive alternative to high ligation and open surgical stripping of the incompetent Great Saphenous Vein (GSV) or Short Saphenous Vein (SSV). There is great variability in EVLA protocols and at the present time there is data from more than 60 publications with more than 15000 EVLA treatments reporting good clinical results but also undesired side effects. Post-operative pain in the operated area is rated from slight to moderate by most patients (81, 5%),post-operative induration of the truncal vein can be expected in 78, 1% of patients and perivenous ecchymosis and hematoma are observed in an average of 52% of patients. Further complications such as persistent dysesthesia after nerve lesions (0, 8%) and burns on the skin (0, 2%) are reported in a minority of cases. Great care must be taken to ensure adequate tumescent anesthesia and light dosimetry in order to avoid post-operative paresthesia.

Thrombus propagation to the deep venous system (0, 2%) or pulmonary embolism (0, 02%) are seldom observed. Careful sonografic examination of the sapheno-femoral or sapheno - popliteal junctions is required during the procedure. Inappropriate energy densities can lead to side effects such as transmural ablations, perforations and alteration in perivenous tissue. So far it has not been possible to establish general valid recommendations for appropriate energy density nevertheless it seems clear that the use of laser systems with longer wavelengths will lead to a reduction of undesired tissue side effects.

2. Endovenous laser therapy

The first application of endoluminal laser was described by Bone in 1999 (Bone, 1999). EVLA received Food and Drug Administration approval in January 2002 and acts through a mechanism of nontrombotic venous occlusion of the target vein through the delivery of laser energy into the vein lumen via a laser fiber. Laser (light amplification by stimulated emission of radiation) creates high-energy bundled light that is monochromatic (of an unique wavelength) and releases direct thermal energy that heats both the blood and

---

* Arlindo Matos, Maria do Sameiro C. Pereira, Clara Nogueira, Tiago Loureiro,
Luís Loureiro, Diogo Silveira and Rui de Almeida

adjacent vein wall (Van den Bos et al. 2008).The tip fiber reaches temperatures in the region of 800°C. This results in destruction of the intima, collagen denaturation of the media and eventually fibrotic occlusion of the vein. Lasers with wavelengths of 810, 940, 980 (haemoglobin specific) and 1319, 1320 and 1470 nm (water specific) have been successfully used. The light of these wavelengths are not visible to the human eye and for orientation purposes, visible light is additionally emitted as a pilot beam. In the last ten years EVLA has evolved into an accepted option for the treatment of underlying truncal vein reflux causing varicose veins.

2.1 Preoperative duplex imaging

Duplex ultrasound has become the reference standard in assessing the morphology and hemodynamics of the lower limb veins. Preoperative duplex planning for EVLA is extremely important in order to avoid potential complications. Almost all modern ultrasound scanners used for imaging peripheral venous disease should be suitable for preoperative imaging and for guiding endovenous procedures. Typically linear array transducers with a frequency in the range of 5-12 MHz are suitable. During this examination it is important to evaluate the anatomy and the physiology of both the superficial and deep venous systems. EVLA is a good treatment option for eliminating reflux in a straight superficial venous segment. Indications for ablation include reflux in a truncal vein of a duration greater than 0, 5 seconds, that is responsible for patient symptoms or skin changes. Measurement of the vein diameter should be carried out during the course of pre-operative ultrasound for the calculation of the appropriate energy density. The duplex ultrasound inclusion criteria for this treatment are: veins with a 2mm or more diameter but preferably with 3mm or more and a treatable length of at least 10-12 cm. The course of the saphenous vein, from the saphenofemoral or saphenopopliteal junction to the insertion site is mapped by ultrasound. An indelible marking pen is used to mark incompetent sources of venous reflux under duplex ultrasound guidance before the procedure (figure 1).

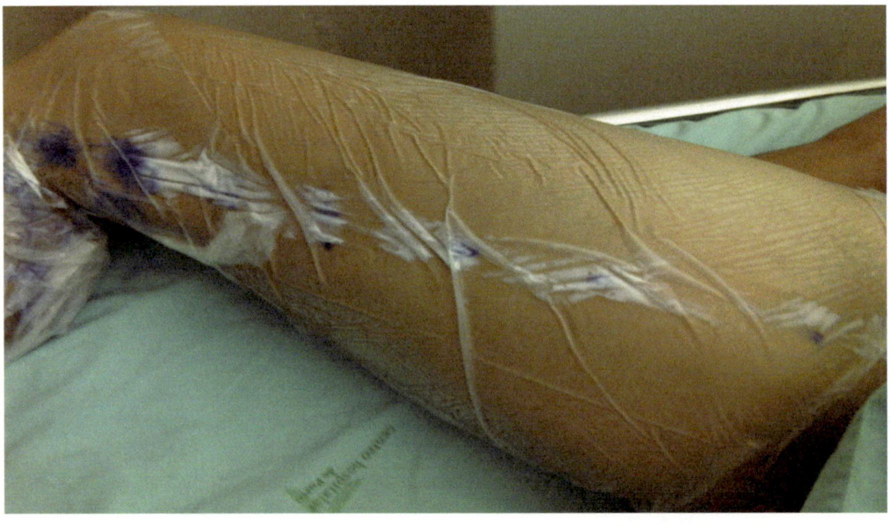

Fig. 1. Pre-operative marking of the vein, topic anesthesic on the length of the vein being treated

Veins with acute thrombophebitis or partially obstructed saphenous vein on the duplex examination are exclusion criteria for this kind of treatment. Patients with ropy varicose veins located immediately under the skin or those with aneurismal dilations of the sapheno-femoral junction are probably better served with conventional surgery(Gloviczki et al 2011).The use of EVLA to close incompetent perforating veins has been described. At this point, the indications and contraindications, as well as the success rates and safety of this approach have only recently begun to be evaluated (Proebstle et al 2009). The use of EVLA to directly close surface varicose veins is not encouraged. These veins are usually too tourtous for current generation devices to pass through. Also these veins are very superficial; EVLA of these veins carries a high risk of thermal skin injury.

2.2 The procedure

EVLA begins with ultrasound evaluation and disinfection of the skin. The area to be operated on is covered with sterile dressings. The groin area has to be accessible as a sonographic examination of the sapheno-femoral junction is required. In addition, an intra-operative switch to conventional open surgery with high ligation and stripping must be possible if necessary. The patient is placed in the reverse Trendelenburg position and an insertion site is chosen to maximize the treatment length. For GSV, this is around the knee level where the vein is usually superficial, the portion below the knee beeing in close proximity to the saphenous nerve carrying an increased risk of parestesia from the puncture or thermal nerve injury by the laser energy delivered.

After infiltration with local anesthetic at the insertion site, an introducer needle is inserted into the vein or a small incision is made and the vein is elevated with a phlebotomy hook. Although efficient this second approach is not preferred because of the increased risk of trauma or venospasm. A microguidewire is inserted into the vein, followed by the placement of a 4F microsheath. With the help of a floopy guidewire, the sheath is exchanged for a 5F sheath. The wire is advanced so it that runs across the SFJ, always with ultrasound guidance. It is not uncommon for the wire to loop, especially in dilated areas of the vein. The laser fiber is then introduced through the sheath into the GSV or SSV and advanced proximally to the SFJ or SPJ. The fiber tip extends proximaly 1-2 cm beyond the end of the sheath, and its position should be marked. This is important since the fiber tip can be heated up to several hundred degrees Celsius during the procedure and if there is no sufficient distance between them, this can lead to the melting of the sheath material. To treat reflux of the GSV beginning at the SFJ, the device is generally positioned just below the junction of a competent *epigastric vein.* Theoretically this preservers flow at the junction and prevents thrombus from extending upwards. For SSV ablation, the tip of the device is positioned just beyond the take-off point of a gastrocnemius vein. If this vein is not identified by ultrasound evaluation, ablation generally begins at the cephalic end of the intrafascial SSV before it passes below the muscular fascia.

Once the device is appropriately placed for ablation, the patient is placed in Trendelenburg position to facilitate vein emptying and perivenous tumescent anesthesia is then delivered. Optimal delivery of this fluid into the saphenous space is accomplished with real time duplex ultrasound examination. The tumescence has four main goals; firstly it provides cooling and offers some perivascular tissue protection against heating or burns. Secondly it provides pain relief. Thirdly, the vein tends to collapse, removing blood and improving surface contact between the laser and the vein wall and finally it will ensure that there is at least 1 cm between the vein and the skin surface to avoid skin burns. Once the vein is surrounded by tumescence, the position of the laser tip must be rechecked to ensure it has not been accidentally displaced. The thermal energy is then delivery using protocols inherent to each device (Table 1). Currently 50 to 80 J/cm is the average treatment energy most often used for EVLA procedures.

Laser Generators	Wavelength	Recommended Pullback
Diomed	810 nm	1 cm every 3-5 seconds
Varilaser	810 nm	50-70 J/cm
Dornier	940 nm	1 cm every 3-5 seconds
AngioDynamics	980 nm	50-80 J/cm
Sciton	1319 nm	Unknown
Cool Touch	1320 nm	Automated fiber pullback device at 1 mm/second
Biolitec	1470 nm	UnKnown

Table 1. Endolaser Ablation Devices

The goal is to achieve successful ablation while at the same time minimizing the incidence of postoperative pain and bruising.

Ultrasound should be used to follow the catheter pullback, the energy supplied to the laser tip also heats the surrounding blood and this can be clearly seen as echogenic areas.

At the end of the procedure, ultrasound can then be used to ensure the patency of the common femoral vein, and to confirm successful obliteration of the saphenous vein. Its lumen is usually reduced and filled with strongly echoing thrombus material.

If a patent segment is identified, re-treatment is advisible.

Ancillary ambulatory phlebectomy or sclerotherapy may be performed immediately after the EVLA procedure or several weeks later to treat any residual branch varicose veins (figure 2).

2.3 Post-procedural care

The entry site is covered with a SteryStrip bandage as well as the phlebectomy sites, if performed. Graduated compression stockings with an ankle pressure of 30-40 mmHg or an elastic wrap is placed on the limb at the end of the procedure and should be kept at least one week after the procedure. (Figure 3)

Immediately following EVLA, patients are instructed to ambulate regularly to promote the vessel occlusion process and decrease the incidence of deep venous thrombosis (DVT). But vigorous exercise is generally discouraged for the first week.

There is no convincing data to support the routine use of anticoagulants with EVLA. Selected patients with a history of thrombophlebitis, DVT, or obesity are candidates for thrombosis prophylaxis (Geerts et al 2008). In Europe the use of a short course of post procedural prophylactic dose of low molecular weight heparin is common (Proebstle 2003). The complication rate following its use does not seem substantially increased.

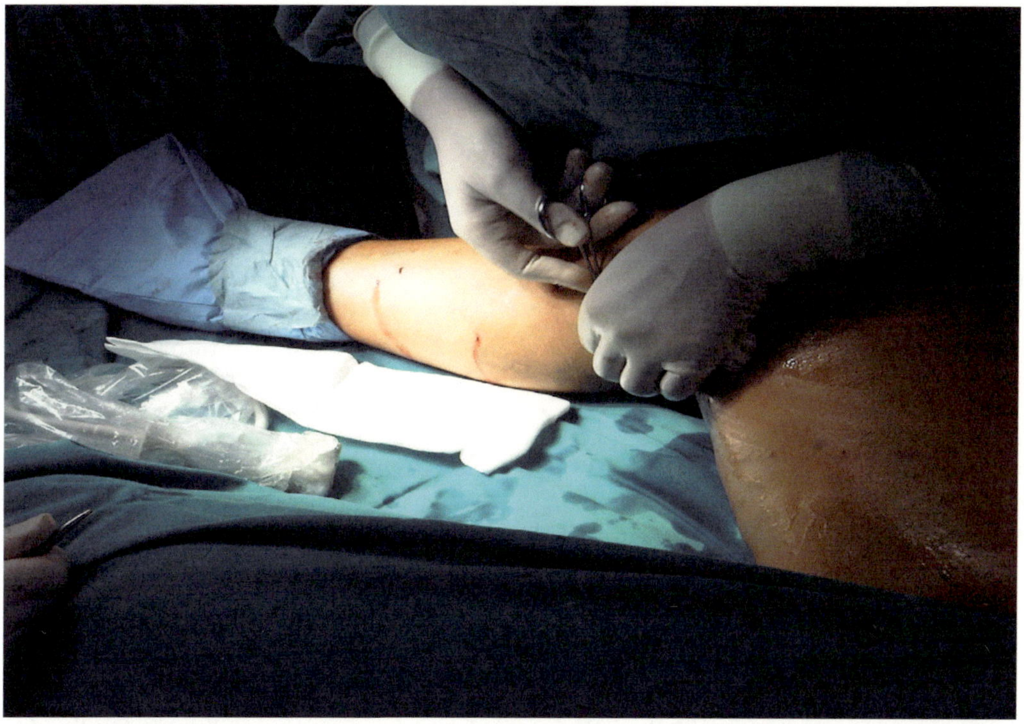

Fig. 2. Ancillary ambulatory phlebectomy performed immediately after the EVLA procedure

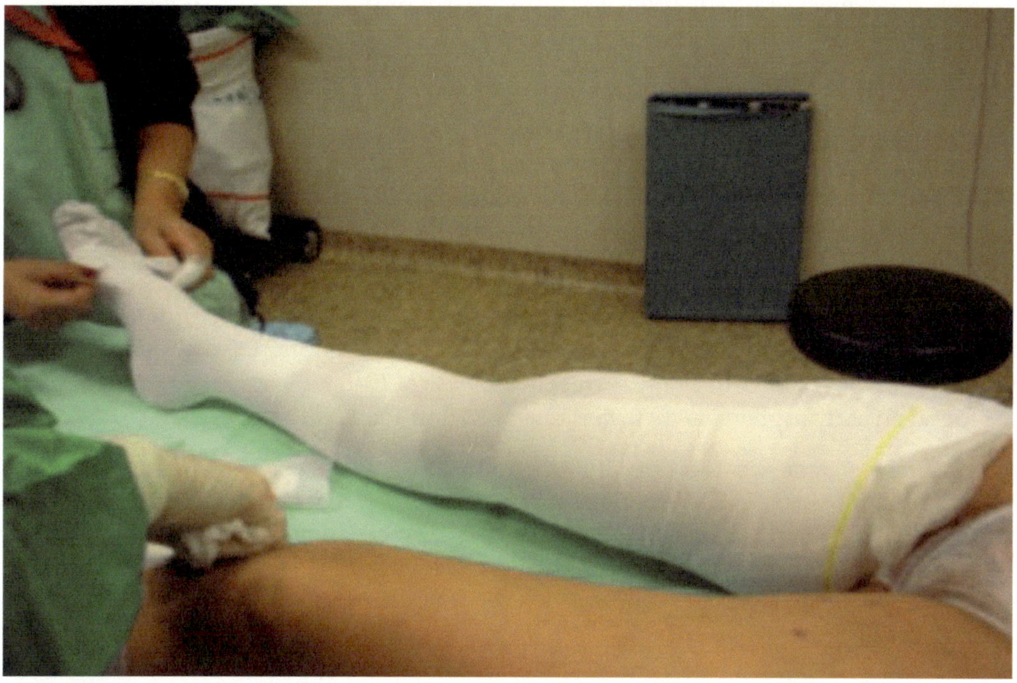

Fig. 3. Graduated compression stockings placed at the end of the procedure

Some patients will experience mild discomfort over the treated vein, beginning a few hours after the procedure that usually resolves in 24 to 48 hours and a nonsteroidal anti-inflammatory drug may be taken daily as needed.

2.4 Follow - up

Clinical success after EVLA is defined as permanent occlusion of the treated vein segments with improvement in clinical syntomatology. Patients should return for periodic clinical and duplex ultrasound evaluation to confirm vein closure and exclude early complications. At minimum, patients should be examined at 1 week, 6 months and one year following laser ablation of the saphenous vein. But if a physician is trying to identify thrombus extension across the SPJ or SFJ, duplex ultrasound in the first 72 hours after EVLA should be performed.

The natural history of a successfully treated truncal vein includes acute vein wall thickening without significant intraluminal thrombus in the first weeks after treatment followed over the next months by progressive vein shrinkage and eventual disappearance on ultrasound examination (Min et al 2003). This venous contraction, produces a delayed (4 to 6 weeks after the procedure) sensation described by the patient as "pulling". This pain is most likely secondary to venous fibrosis as the treated vein undergoes permanent closure. Follow up duplex will no longer be needed when the treated vein is no longer visible.

Additional periodic follow up may be necessary to evaluate the aetiology of any new tributary varicosities to determine whether they are related to a recurrence of reflux in the treated vein segment or progression of the disease in a different venous pathway.

3. Clinical outcomes

Sucess rates with EVLA of the GSV have generally been reported between 72% and 100%, and the follow up for these evaluations varies from 3 months to 4 years. Currently there is data from more than 60 publications with altogether more than 15000 EVLA treatments available. With the appropriate selection of patients, EVLA treatment can technically be carried out in more than 99 % of the patients. (Elmore, 2008)

In a large single center, Myers and Jolley treated 509 limbs with an 810 nm laser during a 5 year period. The rate of primary occlusion at 4 years was 76% and the secondary occlusion rate was 97%.(Myers et al 2009). A systematic review of EVLA for varicose veins by Mundy et al found an early saphenous occlusion rate of 88% to 100%. (Mundy et al 2005).

There is fewer data for the SSV but the published results are qualitatively similar. Proebstle et al observed a 100% occlusion rate at 6 months by using 940 nm diode laser to treat SSV in 41 patients. (Proebstle et al 2008). In a prospective cohort study, Huisman et al treated the SSV in 169 limbs with an 810 nm diode laser. The treated length averaged 23 cm (range 6 - 53 cm). Occlusion of the SSV after 3 months was achieved in 98%. (Huisman et al 2009)

It has been reported that most incompletely ablated veins will develop reflux recurrence in the first few months following treatment.

Most EVLA recanalizations occur in the first 6 months, and all occurred in the first 12 months. This has been interpreted as suggesting that recanalization may be related to insufficient thermal energy delivered to the segment of the vein being treated.

On the majority of the cases the 1-2 cm proximal segment of the vein below the SFJ or the SPJ remains patent. Inferior success rates of closure of this proximal vein segment may be related to an increased likelihood of insufficient thermal transfer to this portion that is usually of larger caliber that the remaining vein, more difficult to empty, and less likely to develop spasm during tumescent anaesthetic administration. As a result, it is difficult to obtain device and vein wall apposition in this segment.

There is a correlation between the amount of thermal energy delivered and the occlusion rate. Energy deposition has been described as the amount of energy delivered per centimetre of vein length (J/cm). Durable vein occlusion was demonstrated as more likely when the energy applied was a mean of 80 J/cm. (Sadick et al 2004).

As previously said successfully treated veins have been demonstrated to occlude and shrink with time. The average mean duration for a treated GSV to shrink to a fibrous cord of less than 2,5 mm diameter is 6 months.(Yang Ch 2006).

Late clinical recurrence is extremely unlikely in an occluded vein that has shrunken to a non compressible cord. Based on this and on surgical data that demonstrates that the pathologic events that lead to recurrence usually take place within 2 years, later clinical recurrences are more likely related to development of incompetence in untreated veins. It seems that late clinical success after EVLA is predicted by the natural history of the venous insufficiency and the ability of the physician to identify and eliminate all incompetent pathways.

Comparing two wavelengths of delivered laser energy (940 nm and 1320 nm) in a retrospective analysis, showed equivalent occlusion rates, when used at similar rates of energy deposition. (Proebstle 2005)

Several studies have documented significant and durable improvements in validated assessments of Quality of Life (QOL) following EVLA. Some studies demonstrated significant improvements in the Aberdeen Varicose Veins Questionnaire (AVVQ) as long as 6 months following laser ablation. (Mekako et al 2006); (Rasmussen et al 2007)

Ulcer healing has been reported after EVLA. One report documented an 84% success in ulcer healing with a combination of EVLA and microphlebectomy , with 77% of these healings occurring within 2 weeks after the procedure (Ravi et al 2006).

Several studies have reported that EVLA is more effective than venous stripping and other endovenous procedures in terms of obliteration and lower recurrence rates in the range of 1 to 5%. (Bos et al 2009) It is also important to mention that cosmetic results are in the majority of the cases very good when compared with high ligation and stripping.

As with as other treatment options for superficial venous insufficiency, EVLA treatments and indications are in constant evolution. Neglen et al, demonstrated good outcomes combining laser ablation with deep vein stenting for superficial venous insufficiency and concomitant deep vein obstruction. (Neglen et al 2006)

As above indicated EVLA for the treatment of venous superficial reflux is an efficient treatment option.

4. Complications

Complications after EVLA may be divided into early and late complications (Table 2 and 3). The most serious potential complication involves misidentification of the anatomy with duplex ultrasound leading to the placement of the tip in a wrong position or even in a deep vein.

Complications	
Early Complications	Vessel Perforation
	Vein Spasm
	Vein Trombosis
	Excessive Pain
	Skin Burns
	Hematoma
	Hemorrhage
	Irrradiation of Nontarget tissue
	Thromboplhebitis
	Deep vein Thrombosis
	Pulmonary Embolism
	Arteriovenous fistula

Table 2. Early complications of EVLA Procedure

Complications	
Late Complications	Recanalization of the Vein
	Skin Necrosis
	Paresthesia
	Infection

Table 3. Late complications of EVLA Procedure

In an international endovascular working group registry that included 3696 procedures, bruising after EVLA was observed in 75% of the cases, paresthesia in 3%, thrombophlebitis in 1,87%, skin burns in 0,46% and DVT in 0,27% and there is a single report of pulmonary embolism (Kabnick et al 2006). But in majority of the series reported in the literature the complication rates are variable (Table 4).

Study	Number of veins treated	Complication Rate
Navarro et al	40	Any
Proebstle et al	41	6% thrombophlebitis
Chang and Chua	252	1,6% thrombophlebitis 36,5% paresthesia 4,8% skin burn
Timperman et al	111	1% deep vein thrombosis 1% skin burn
Huang et al	230	1% skin burn 7% paresthesia
Vuylsteke et al	118	4% skin burn 14% paresthesia
Almeida and Raines	819	0,2% deep vein thrombosis 0,2% paresthesia 2% thrombophlebitis
Min et al	121	Any
Meyers et al	404	0,2% severe pain

Table 4. Complications after EVLA reported in the literature

Ecchymosis (Figure 4) over the treated segment frequently occurs and normally can last approximately ten days. The mechanism of the EVLA procedure that causes ecchymosis remains unclear, although some experts speculate that these complications are due to perforation of the vein wall by laser energy.

Superficial phlebitis is another uncommon side effect that is reported in approximately 5% of procedures (Min 2003). The major complications more frequently reported are neurologic injuries, skin burns and DVT. But the overall rate of these complications has been shown to be higher in low volume hospitals compared with high - volume hospitals. The nerves at highest risk include the saphenous nerve, adjacent to the GSV below the Knee and the Sural nerve adjacent to the SSV, but both of these nerves have only sensory components, and the most common manifestation of nerve injury is paresthesia or dysthesia, which is often transient (Rutherford 2010). The nerve injury can occur with sheath and catheter introduction, during the delivery of tumescent anaesthesia, or by direct thermal injury. The rates of permanent paresthesias typically reported for laser are approximately 0-10% for GSV treatment. Only a few series look at the SSV nerve injuries and the reported rates of temporary paresthesia following SSV EVLA are 0-10% in some series. It is reported that the rate of paresthesia is inversely related to the operator experience with perivenous ultrasound -guided anesthesia(Morrison et al 2011). It has also been suggested that greater volumes of tumescence may be required during ablation of the SSV to prevent any thermal injury to the sural nerve which is in close proximity to the vein.

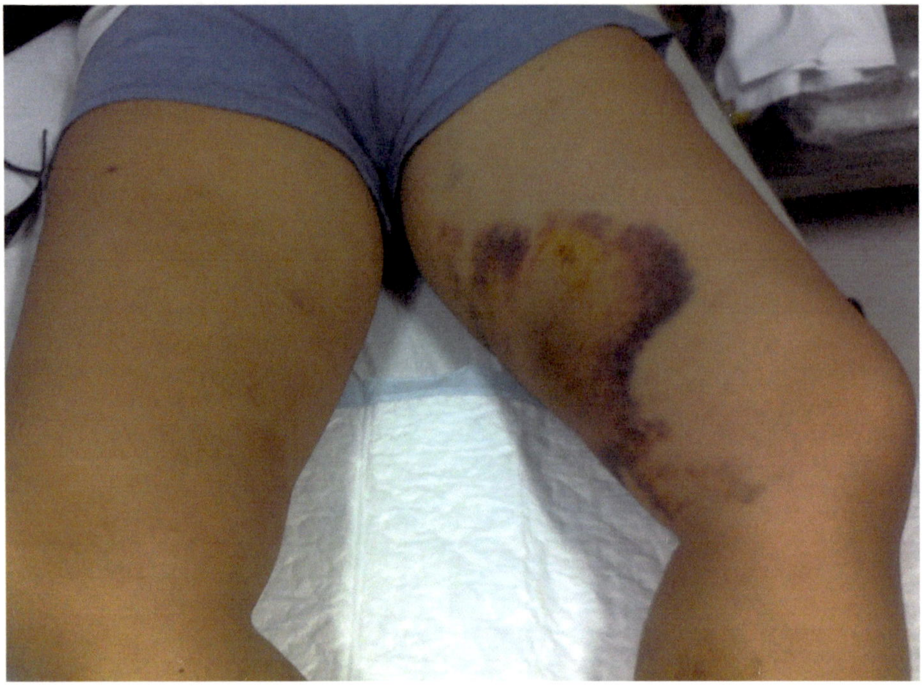

Fig. 4. Ecchymosis on the left lower limb after a bilateral EVLA procedure

Skin burns following EVLA have been reported but are relatively rare and seem avoidable with adequate tumescent anesthesia.

DVT following EVLA is unusual and can occur as an extension of thrombus formation from the treated truncal vein across the junctional connection into the deep vein or in the calf or femoral popliteal veins. The reported rates of junctional thrombosis following GSV EVLA are variable. This variability may relate to the ultrasound duplex timing after the EVLA procedure. Most series using early duplex ultrasound document a proximal thrombus extension of approximately 1% and those performing the ultrasound duplex later (after 72 hours) identify a lower rate. But it is also possible that this different thrombus propagation rates are variable because the ultrasound is performed by different operators. Data from different series suggests that the incidence of DVT is approximately of 0,3% after laser ablation. But this type of DVT is almost universally asymptomatic. The significance of this type of thrombus extension into the femoral vein seems to be different from the native deep vein thrombosis (Kabniick et al 2006). But treatment should be started immediately usually in an outpatient basis with compression, ambulation, anti - inflammatory medication and anticoagulation. A close follow up evaluation with ultrasound should be performed. Reports in the literature based on careful follow up evaluation of these thrombo extensions concluded that they retract over the course of 7-10 days and none produced clinical symptoms suggestive of pulmonary embolus. (Morrison et al 2011). The incidence of junctional extension of thrombus after SSV ablation has been described to be inferior to 6 %(Ravi et al 2006). In a particular study the rate of popliteal extension of SSV thrombus after EVLA was thought to be related to the anatomy of the SPJ (sapheno-popliteal junction) (Gibson et al 2007). The incidence of DVT in other peripheral deep veins after EVLA has not been well evaluated.

There are some case reports in the literature of an arteriovenous fistula between a small popliteal artery branch and the SSV (Vaz et al 2008). Although thought to be related to a heat induced injury caused by thermal energy from the laser device, an a arteriovenous fistula could be caused by a needle injury during tumescent anaesthetic administration. To minimize the risk of these arteriovenous fistulas is necessary a careful advancement of the intravascular devices, atraumatic delivery of the tumescent fluid, the use of adequate amounts of tumescent fluid and the subfascial portion of the SSV where the popliteal artery branches exist, should be avoided. (figure 5).

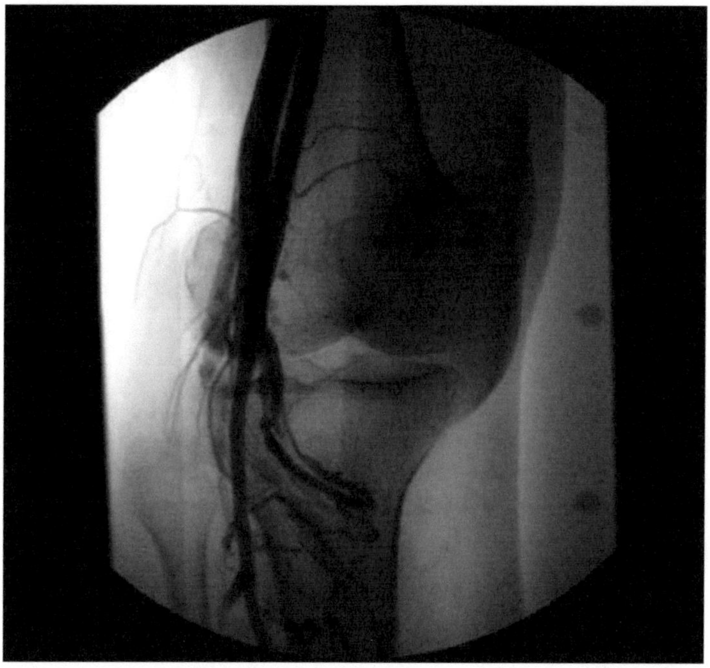

Fig. 5. Popliteal stage arteriography depicting an AV fistula between branches of the popliteal artery and a genicular vein after an EVLA procedure.

If there is evidence of a perivenous structure (artery or nerve) that is impossible to isolate from the vein by the tumescent anesthesia, probably skipping this venous segment and use a combination of concomitant therapies would be a more prudent choice(Perrin et al 2007).

During the procedure, adverse patient events may occur, which are rarely reported. A transient vagal reaction is often described secondary to the patient's anxiety, there are some reports of dysrhytmia and transient pain due to inadequate anesthetic infiltration.

Infection is extremely rare, but there is one case report of septic thrombophlebitis following an EVLA procedure requiring surgical intervention (Dunst et al 2006).

Neovascularization has been reported only in one case on the literature three years after the EVLA procedure (Morrison et al 2011). The endovenous laser ablation procedure deliberately leaves the superficial epigastric vein intact, which, it is believed, has contributed to the lack of neovascularisation reported so far. More case reports are necessary to establish a mechanism of this type of neovascularisation after an EVLA procedure.

Laser fracture or retained venous access sheaths have been reported on the literature (Ravi et al 2007).Caution in handling the laser should help to minimize these situations, and the possibility of a laser fracture should always be considered with the removal of the device. Care to deliver thermal energy only beyond the introducer is essential to avoid damage of some segments of these catheters.

Some evidence suggests that higher wavelength lasers produce less pain and bruising as well as minimize other types of complications; however a large scale study evaluating all wavelengths available is needed to confirm these initial findings.

A new adaptation of the laser fibbers has emerged,that appears to have some beneficial effect on the vein wall perforation, the jacket tipped fibers. This newly advance constitutes on a stainless steel or a ceramic jacket that completely covers the tip of the fiber, with the end of the tip being recessed within the jacket, thus preventing the tip contact with the vein wall. One study has been described on the literature comparing the efficacy and the complications of jacket tipped fibers versus bare tipped fibers. At 72 hours after the procedure, both groups demonstrated 100% success treatment and in the jacket tipped group pain and ecchymoses scores appeared to be lower.

5. Discussion

Endovascular techniques have been introduced as minimally invasive alternatives to high ligation and open surgical stripping of the incompetent GSV or SSV. The Endovenous laser therapy has established itself in the last few years among the range of endovascular therapy options for the treatment of truncal vein insufficiency. Nevertheless the significance of this reflux in itself still remains a matter of debate. A duplex ultrasound detected reflux should not be in itself an indication for treatment. We think that EVLA, as well as other treatment modalities, is only indicated in patients with clear symptoms and clinical signs of chronic venous insufficiency (varicose veins, skin changes or ulcer).

Studies looking specifically at the success and complication rates associated with laser ablation are extensively being reported. But the effects of laser on tissue, and therefore on clinical results, are clearly very variable because of the use of different wavelengths, different pull back protocols and different energy densities and so EVLA can hardly be standardized. Mechanisms to determine the accurate energy density to be used in EVLA are lacking. This makes the appropriate dosage of light for the sufficient thermal alteration of tissue harder to achieve. In addition to transmural damage, wall perforation is being reported with great variability in most of the series.

In order to eliminate these disadvantages and create endothermal occlusion more effectively and in a more reproducible fashion, EVLA continues to find itself in a dynamic process of development. Treatment planning, technical details and postprocedural care is of paramount importance to this procedure and to the operator. Every patient undergoing endovenous procedures should do an early post-operative duplex scan to rule out major complications (Perrin et al 2007). The learning curve in EVLA treatment of the SSV is still going up, and further experience and research with this modality will better delineate its risks, complications and long term efficacy.

6. Conclusion

The Endovascular technology has transformed the evaluation and treatment of venous disease during the past decade. As with any new technique, there is a learning curve in terms of patient selection and the different steps of the procedure itself. Once mastered it seems that EVLA can safely eradicate GSV and SSV reflux with a low rate of minor complications and a lower rate of major complications.

7. References

Almeida J, RainesJ et al (2006) *Radiofrequency ablation and laser ablation in the treatment of varicose veins,* Ann Vasc Surgery, 20 :547-52

Bone, C. (1999).*Tratamiento endoluminal de las varices con laser de Diodo. Estudio preliminary,* Review Patology vascular, 5, 35-46

Bos, RVD, Arends L et al (2009) *Endovenous therapies of lower extermity varicosities are at least as effective as surgical stripping or foam sclerotherapy : meta – analysis and meta – regression of case series and randomized clinical trails,* Journal of vascular Surgery, 49 :230-239

Chang CJ, Chua JJ et al, (2002) *Endovenous laser photocoagulation (EVLP) for varicose veins. Laser Surg Med 31 :257-62*

Dunst K, Huemer G et al.*(2006) Diffuse phlegmonous phlebitis after endovenous laser treatment of the greater saphenous vein. J Vasc Surg 43 : 1056-8*

Elmore FA, Lackey D,(2008) Effectiveness of endovenous laser treatment in eliminating superficial venous reflux, Phlebology 23 :21-31

Gibson Kd, Ferris Bl et al, *(2007), Endovenous laser treatment of the short saphenous vein : efficacy and complications, J Vasc Surg 45 :795-801*

Geerts, Wh, Bergqvist D, et al,(2008) *Prevenction of venous Thromboembolism : American College of Chest Physicians Evidence – based Clinical Practice Guidelines. Chest ; 133 :381-453s*

Gloviczki et al (2011), *The care of patients with varicose veins and associated chronic venous diseases : Clinical pratice guidelines of the society for vascular Surgery and the American venous Forum, Journal of Vascular Surgery, 53 :16s 2-27*

Huang Y, Jiang M et al.*(2005) Endovenous laser treatment combined with a surgical startegy for treatment of venous insufficiency in lower extremity : a report of 208 cases, J Vasc Surg 42 :494-501*

Huisman LC, Bruins Rm et al (2009), *Endovenous laser ablation of the small saphenous vein : prospective analysis of 150 patients, a cohort study. Euro J vasc Endovasc Surg 38 : 199-202*

Kabnick LS, Ombrellino M et al, *(2006) Endovenous heat induced thrombus (EHIT) at the superficial deep venous junction : a new post-treatment clinical entity, classification and patient treatment strategies.* Presented at the American Venous Forum 18 th Annual Meeting February 23

Kabnick LS. (2006) Complications of endovenous therapies : statistics and treatment. Vascular, 14 (suppl1) : S31-2

Mekako AI, HattieldJ, et al (2006), *A nonrandomized controlled trial of endovenous laser therapy and surgery in the treatment of varicose veins, Annals of Vascular Surgery* ;20 :451-457

Min Rj, Khilnani NM et al (2003), *Duplex ultrasound evaluation of lower extremity venous insuffinciency, Journal of Vascular Intervetion Radiology, 14 :1233 – 1241*

Min Rj, Khilnani NM et al (2003*), Endovenous laser treatment of saphenous vein reflux : Long term results* J Vasc Interv Radiology, 14 : 991-6

Myers K, Fris R et al (2006) *Treatment of Varicose veins by endovenous laser therapy : assessment of results by ultrasound surveillance,* Med J Aust 85 :199-202

Myers KA, Jolley D. (2009) *Outcome of endovenous laser Therapy for saphenous reflux and varicose veins : medium – term results assessed by ultrasound surveillance*, Eur J Vasc Endovasc Surg 37 :239-45

Mundy L, Merlin TL et al (2005), Systematic review of endovenous laser treatment for varicose veins, Br J Surg 92 : 1189-94

Navarro L, Min R, et al.*(2001) Endovenous laser : a new minimally invasive method of treatment for varicose veins – preliminary observations using an 810 nm diode laser. Dermatology Surgery27 :118-22*

Neglén P, Hollis K et al,(2006) *Combined saphenous ablation and iliac sten placement for complex severe chronic venous disease, J Vasc Surg 44 :828-33*

M.Perrin (2007) *Traitement Chirurgical endovasculaire des varices des membrers infériurs. Techniques et resultants.* EMC, Techniques chirurgicales - Chirurgie vasculaire, 43-161

Proebstle TM, Gul D et al, (2003),*Endovenous laser treatment of the lesser saphenous vein with a 940 – nm diode laser :early results. Dermatology Surgery29 :357-61*

Proebstle TM, Gul D et al, (2003), *Infrequent early recanalization of greater saphenous vein after endovenous laser Treatment, Journal of vascular surgery,* 38 :511-516

Proebstle TM, Moehler T et al (2005),*Endovenous treatment of the great saphenous vein using a 1,320nm Nd : yag laser causes fewer side effects than using a 940 nm diode laser, Dermatology Surgery,* 31 :1678-1683

Proebstle TM, Vago B et al (2008),*Threatment of the incompetent great saphenous vein by endovenous radiofrequency powered segmental thermal ablation : first clinical experience, J Vasc Surg, 47 :151-6*

Proebstle, Thomas M. (2009),*Handbook of venous Disorders, Guidelines of the American Venous Forum,* pp-390-398, Hodder Arnold(Ed)

Ravi R, Rodriguez – Lopez JA et al (2006) *Endovenous Ablation of incompetent saphenous veins : a large single center experience. J Endovascular Therapy* 13 : 244-248

Ravi R,Bhutani A et al(2007) *No sheath left behind, J Endovasc Ther, 14 :265-267*

Rasmussen LH, Bjoern L, Lawaetz et al, (2007), *Randomized trial comparing endovenous laser ablation of the great saphenous vein with high ligation and stripping in patients with varicose veins : short term results, Journal of Vascular Surgery ; 46 :308-315*

Rutherford (2010). *Rutherford´s Vascular Surgery,* Sauders Elsevier, ISBN 871-888, Philadelphia, USA

Sadick Ns, Waser S. (2004) *Combined endovascular laser with ambulatory phelebectomy for threatment of superficial venous incompetence : a 2 – Year perspective. J Cosmet Laser Therapy, 24 :149-153*

Timperman P, Sichlau M et al(2004) *Greater energy delivery improves treatment sucess of endovenous laser treatment of incompetent saphenous veins.* J Vasc Interv Radiol 15 :1061-3

Van den Bos R, Kockaert M, Neumann H et al (2008) *Technical review of endovenous laser Therapy for varicose veins.* European Journal of vascular and Endovascular Surgery 35 : 88-95

Vaz C, Matos A. et al (2009), *Iatrogenic arteriovenous Fistula following endovenous laser therapy of the short saphenous vein, Annals of Vascular Surgery,412*

Vuylsteke M, Van den Bussche D et al (2006) *Endovenous Laser obliteration for the treatment of primary varicose veins.* Phlebology 21 : 80-7

Yang CH, Chou HS et al (2006) *Incompetent great saphenous Veins treated with endovenous 1,320 nm laser: results for 71 legs and morphologic evolvement study. Dermatology Surgery; 32:1453 - 1457*

Part 3

Preoperative Care, Complications and Others

9

Preoperative Care, Anesthesia and Early Postoperative Care of Vascular Patients

Zsófia Verzár[1], Endre Arató[2], Attila Cziráki[3] and Sándor Szabados[3]
[1]*University of Pécs, Faculty of Medicine, Institute of Anesthesiology and Intensive Care,*
[2]*University of Pécs, Faculty of Medicine, Department of Vascular Surgery,*
[3]*University of Pécs, Faculty of Medicine Heart Institute,*
Hungary

1. Introduction

The changes in the operation technic in the last twenty years may reduce morbidity and mortality of traditionally high - risk vascular surgical procedures. (White CJ&Gray WA, 2007) The indrease of median age, the number of elderly patients will also elevate the number of vascular procedures. Careful preoperative evaluation of patients undergoing vascular surgical intervention holds great significance since this group of patients has almost the highest percentage of accompanying diseases with poor outcome. It is well-known that vascular disease - irrespectively of its manifestation - is a generalized disorder, the majority of patients with vascular disease smoke and have chronic pulmonary disease, also suffers from diabetes and hypertension. Hypertension and diabetes are often associated with coronary artery disease which determines the short and long-term survival of vascular procedures. Coronary artery disease is one of the most frequent cause of the perioperative mortality and morbidity (1-5%). Goldman et al.(drew the attention to the frequency of cardiac complication of vascular operations as far back as 1977 and aimed to establish a multi-factorial score index. Based on detailed surveys which covered a large patient population the perioperative incidence of myocardial infarction among patient undergoing vascular surgical procedures is 2, 1 - 8, 0 %, whilst the mortality is 0, 6 - 5, 4 %. These examinations did not consider the type of operations - open or endovascular. Beside Goldman's classic risk index numerous task forces have established their own score system for the assessment of perioperative cardiac risk. All of these highlight the significance of the fact that after being aware of the clinical risk, consultation and mutual decision making of cardiologists, anesthetists and vascular surgeons in evaluation the long-term efficiency and risk ratio is essential. The most important weak point of all score system is the utilization of data derived from patients underwent elective operations. Kertai et al. developed a simplified risk index, which is suitable for the assessment of perioperative mortality of either acute or elective patients undergoing vascular surgical operations. The American College of Cardiologist and the American Heart Association has developed a guideline (2007) for the assessment of Cardiovascular risk among patients with different diseases who are undergoing non-cardiac surgery. This guideline includes the risk assessment for the patient undergoing vascular surgery. Three categories of cardiac risk have been classified in the guideline, high, intermediate and low. High cardiac risk involves the history of acute coronary syndrome, congestive heart failure, significant arrhythmias and severe heart valve diseases. Among non-cardiac surgeries associated with higher cardiac risk, the acute operations, surgery on extremely old patient, operations of the aorta, prolonged operations, operations with excessive fluid or blood loss are considered to be high-risk while carotid endarterectomy should be considered within the intermediate-risk category. The most simple clinical determining factors of cardiac risk are the age, body weight, known diabetes, congestive heart failure, angina pectoris, history of myocardial infarction and previous coronary revascularization.

2. Preoperative evaluation

Preoperative examination should include the assessment of patient's functional capacity. In the presence of lower extremity peripheral vascular disease performing exercise stress test may be difficult, thus pharmacological stress test or specific upper body exercise test should be carried out. Severely impaired functional capacity further increases the cardiac risk. Diseases of the aorta are frequently associated with severe coronary artery disease.The incidence and severity of coronary artery disease are remarkably higher at the diseases of the aorta.

Preoperative examination should include the following:

Assessment of cardiac risk using different noninvasive examinations. Noninvasive stress testing are the following: dipyridamole myocardial perfusion scintigraphy, radionuclide ventriculography, Holter ECG monitoring, dobutamine stress echocardiography. Several authors (Eagle and collegues, Lee and coworkers) have examined the sensitivity and specificity of these methods, and have found the dobutamine stress echocardiography to be the most appropriate test to assess this group of patients. This examination not only assesses the left ventricular dysfunction but also provides other valuable information on the ground of echocardiography. However, choosing the most appropriate type of test is undoubtedly influenced by local availabilities and cost effectiveness, as well.

After assessing the cardiac risk, what therapeutic options are available to decrease it?

Beta-blocker therapy at high-risk vascular patient has been proven to improve not only the perioperative but also the long term survival. **Manago et al**. carried out a study, which covered a large number of patients on the effect of bisoprolol and atenolol on mortality and cardiovascular morbidity after non cardiac surgery. Treatment of hypertension: blood pressure fluctuation at high-risk vascular patients further increases the cardiac risk. Previous anti-hypertensive therapy should be broadened by administration of beta-blockers and the directly acting, alpha-2 agonist,clonidine. In the last few years, the **American College of Cardiology Foundation/American Heart Association** focused on beta-blocker therapy. Based on this update beta-blockers should be continued in patients , who are receiving them for treatment of conditions with ACCT/AHA indications (Class I)

Perioperative ACE-inhibitors therapy may cause intraoperative hypotension, thus administration of them are not recommended.

What further medical therapy is available to decrease the perioperative risk?

Poldermans and colleagues evaluated the effectiveness of statin therapy, and they found that the perioperative statin therapy is associated with lower postoperative mortality.

Of smoking among patients with vascular risk factors are also important, so increased the perioperative complications between the role of pulmonary complications. Chronic obstructive pulmonary disease and chronic bronchitis, which often encounter. The kidney complications should be considered. First, the generalized vessel disease associated with hypertension, the renin-angiotensin system leads to damage, and the second associated with diabetes to nephropathy.

3. For each type of vascular surgery

3.1 Aortic reconstruction - lesions affecting the abdominal aorta

Growing the progressive aortic aneurysm rupture in the final output. In ruptured cases, the deaths of over 50% indicate a value and this value has not changed significantly over the past 40 years, developments in technology and the introduction of the endovascular technique does not like routine. If known and expanding aortic aneurysm is detected, and reconstruction is the surgical mortality rate is between 0.4 to 2.3%.

The technique of anesthesia during general anesthesia supplemented with epidural anesthesia benefits. We must work towards the introduction of anesthesia, the hemodynamic stability, to eliminate changes caused by intubation. Cross-clamping of the aorta, causes a sudden increse in the afterload. This growth, provoke arrhythmias and myocardial ischemia and left ventricular failure.

3.2 If a patient with acute surgery

Aortic aneurysm rupture due to a significant amount of blood in the abdomen, in any event be deemed hypovolemic. The abdominal muscle tone affects the capacity for intraabdominal blood vessels, this relaxation is terminated and the formation of the blood

pressure to fall, then a further decrease in blood pressure by opening the abdominal cavity should be expected. So close to the team's work comes to the fore the importance of continued vigilance isolation inhalating 100% oxygen, and then rapidly after induction

opening the stomach , fast and high aortic cross clamp immediately save the patient's life. This type of surgery with surgical mortality of 50% is over, and over the past 4 decades has not changed.

3.3 Thoracic-thoraco abdominalis aneurysm

The anesthesia and surgical technique despite the development of the aorta during surgery thoracoabdominalis section of the complications and mortality has not changed significantly over the past 20 years. High-traffic, high number of sick institutions in 5-14% mortality rates reported.The paraplegia, paraparetikus complication rate of 50-40% of the shares are known.

The percentage of complications depends on which section of the aorta, the exclusion should be carried out. The neurological complications after pulmonary complications to be expected. The monitoring of the thoracic aneurysm surgery should be extended. Close cooperation is required between the vascular surgeon and anesthesiologist, the surgical plan must be designed carefully crafted after (follow the protocol), the every aspect of the monitoring and the distal aortic perfusion technique. Important aspects of the arteries of the spinal cord and the renal arteries perfusion ensure and the adequate oxygenation. If the exclusion (cross clamping) is happening, a retrograde perfusion provides security for patients. In surgery for thoracic aortic aneurysm general anesthesia of suitable technology The most important is protection of the spinal cord, 20-30 minute cross clamping time is safe for the patient . The hypothermia is one of the most suitable method for neuroprotection.

4. Preoperative management

The patient who has been diagnosed with significant coronary artery disease during preoperative examination and is a candidate for high-risk vascular surgery is the most challenging. In elective patients coronary revascularization should be carried out.

If the vascular procedure is not urgent, CABG operation is preferable over PCI. Elective non-cardiac surgery is not recommended within 6 weeks of coronary revascularization with PCI and stent implantation. In these cases careful risk assessment and effectiveness evaluation is necessary. Among patients with vascular disease tobacco smoking is a significant risk factor, thus perioperative pulmonary complications are frequent. Chronic obstructive pulmonary disease and chronic bronchitis are the most common ones. Perioperative blood gas analysis can be useful in assessing the risk. If the arterial carbon dioxide partial pressure is higher than 45 mmHg, the risk for postoperative pulmonary complication is increased. If a tobacco smoking patient is presented at the preoperative evaluation meeting 2-4 weeks prior to the operation, it is reasonable to try to persuade the patient to cease the cigarette smoking, although, cessation will increase the amount of bronchial discharge. Smoking cessation 2-3 days prior to the surgery only results in decrease of the blood carboxi-hemoglobin level. In case of history of COPD and asthma preoperative glucocorticoid therapy (40 mg of prednisolon for two days) can decrease the risk of pulmonary complications. Treating the bronchial spasm, mobilizing the bronchial discharge and performing chest physiotheraphy would improve the patients' condition. One to two days prior to surgery preoperative pulmonary function test should be performed. Decreased FEV1/FVC ratio suggests obstructive pulmonary disease. Performing regional anesthesia can lower the operative risk by eliminating the administration of the respiratory depressive opiates. On the other hand intraoperative blood CO2 pressure monitoring is important, since the probability of developing hypercapnia is high, as well as the postoperative CO2 level follow up, since the pain can lead to hypoventilation. Thus adequate pain management is strongly advisable.

Renal complications should also be taken into consideration, because of the pre-existing hypertension which is usually accompanied to generalized vascular disease and which can lead to impairment of the renin-angiotensin system. Preexisting diabetic nephropathy can also influence the development of perioperative renal complications. All the anesthetic and operative techniques and perioperative events that decrease blood pressure and cardiac output have the potential to alter renal function. The blood flow redistribution in the kidney can decreased the glomelural filtration.

5. Anaesthetic management

5.1 Infrarenal aortic aneurysm:

The final outcome of aneurysms that present progressive growth is the rupture. In case of aneurysm rupture the mortality reaches the 50 %, this ratio has not changed over the last 40 years, despite the technical development and the introduction and routine application of endovascular techniques. Postoperative mortality rate of reconstruction of previously known and growing aortic aneurysm varies from 0,4 to 2,3 percents.

Preparation for the operation includes setting up the following:

1. two 14 G peripheral venous line
2. central venous line
3. arterial line
4. ECG monitoring from 5 different points
5. pulsoxymetry
6. urinary catheter
7. gastric tube
8. body temperature monitoring
9. noninvasive blood pressure measurement (from the opposite side than the direct arterial pressure line)
10. In case of impaired ejection fraction (less than 30 %) or suprarenal aortic cross-clamping, routine monitoring should be completed by the use of PICCO or Swan-Ganz catheter. In case of patients with significant diastolic dysfunction continuous intraoprative TEE (trans-esophageal echocardiography) monitoring can help to evaluate the need of fluid or catecholamine therapy.

The anticoagulation maintained with use of heparin 100 unit/kg, additional heparin necessary if the clamping time prolonged. Heparin can be reversed by protamine (4mg/kg over 15 minutes) it may lead to anaphylaxis, pulmonary hypertension and myocardial depression.

At aortic operations it is recommended to prepare 4 - 6 units of red blood cell transfusion, if possible, autologous transfusion should be performed. The use of cell saver (intraoperative cell salvage machine) improves the efficacy of transfusion therapy, if it is not available normovolaemic hemodilution is required. Hemodilution does not increase the oxygen deficit of the myocardium. During fluid therapy close monitoring the 24-hour diuresis and warming the fluid infusions increases patients' safety.

During anesthesia, general anesthesia can be completed by the benefits of application epidural anesthesia. The thoracic epidurals decrease the stress response to surgical procedure. During induction of anesthesia care must be taken to maintain the patient's hemodynamic stability and to eliminate the hyperdynamic response caused by the intubation. In case of aortic operation close attention must be paid to physiologic changes during aortic cross-clamping. In case of abdominal aortic operation the level of cross-clamping is infrarenal, i.e. aorta is fully cross-clamped under the origin of renal arteries. Changes in patient's condition appear rapidly, thus taking prompt actions are necessary. Aortic cross-clamping causes sudden increase in systemic vascular resistance, i.e. in afterload. This increase can provoke myocardial ischemia, arrhythmia and left ventricular failure. The more proximal the cross-clamping is, the more severe the myocardial adverse consequences are. Administration of vasodilators and activation the epidural anesthesia before the cross-clamping can stabilize the patient's condition and have beneficial effect. During aortic cross-clamping the lower extremities and certain parts of large intestines receive minimal blood flow through collateral circulation, but the renal circulation are also impaired. As a result of these circulatory changes inflammatory mediators are released by leukocytes, platelets and endothelial cells.

Cessation of aortic cross-clamping causes sudden decrease in afterload, which is on the one side caused by the discontinuation of mechanical obstruction but the accumulated vasodilator mediators by getting back into the systemic circulation plays also an important role in this. Beside vasodilation, metabolic acidosis and increased capillary permeability aggravates the condition. Providing adequate circulatory volume and maintaining stable blood pressure is necessary before releasing the aortic cross-clamp. Administering mannitol and pressor drugs can be helpful to fulfill this. Every efforts must be made in order to reach as short hypoperfusion time as possible.

In the postoperative period the close monitoring should be continued and care must be taken of the adequate pain management. If the infrarenal cross-clamp time exceeds 60 minutes, the subsequent pressure rise in the renal arteries may cause systemic hypertension in the early postoperative period, which is usually transient.

Patients require monitoring after abdominal aortic aneurysm operation. The postoperative pain management is important, the early extubation, and the enteral nutrition. Appropriate thrombotic profilaxis and postoperative gastrointestinal ulcus profilaxis, the use of antacids.

5.2 Emergency AAA surgery

In case of acute operation of ruptured aortic aneurysm, the patient should be considered hypovolaemic under all circumstances due to the excessive amount of extravascular blood found in the abdominal cavity. Increased abdominal muscle tone has a pressor effect on the intraabdominal capacity vessels, which is ceased if muscle relaxants are administered during the anesthesia and this causes subsequent blood pressure drop. Hypotension is further aggravated by the opening of abdominal cavity. This fact underlines the importance of team work. Isolation and draping of the operative field is carried out while the patient is awake, under simultaneous 100 % of oxygen inhalation, followed by rapid induction, quick opening the abdominal cavity and immediate high aortic cross-clamp which actions can only save the patient's life. Heparinization is not required until the aorta is not cross clamped. After the aorta is cross clamped the fluid resuscitation can be instituted with colloids and blood. The dilutional coagulopathy is precnse, FFP and platelets ordered for the patient, and heparin is omissioned. Mortality rate of these operations exceeds the 50 percents and has not changed over the past four decades. The predictors of the survival are the patients age, the total blood loss, and the time of hypotension.

Preparation for the operation includes setting up the following:

1. two 14 G peripheral venous line
2. blood count, electrolytes coagulation screen
3. arterial line
4. ECG monitoring from 5 different points
5. pulsoxymetry
6. urinary catheter
7. gastric tube
8. body temperature monitoring

9. noninvasive blood pressure measurement (from the opposite side than the direct arterial pressure line)

Drugs and fluids:

6-10 units of cross matched blood, fresh frozen plasma and platelets

Crystalloids and colloids

Inotropes (ephedrine 3 mg/ml, adrenaline 1:100 000) and vasopressor agents (phenylephrine 100 mcg/ml, metaraminol 0.5 mg/ ml)

5.3 Thoracic – thoracoabdominal aneurysm

Operative complications and mortality rate of thoracoabdominal aneurysm surgeries has remained remarkably high despite the development of anesthetic and surgical techniques. High, 5-14 % of mortality rates have been reported by even specialized aneurysm centers which are dealing with a large number of patients. Paraplegia and paraparesis, as postoperative complications develop at 5 - 40 % of all cases. The incidence of complications is influenced by the site of the cross-clamp. The most commonly occurring neurological complications are followed by the pulmonary ones. At thoracic aneurysm operations more vital signs is required to be monitored. It also demands closer collaboration between the vascular surgeon and the anesthetist, because every step of the monitoring has to be set up after developing the operative plan. Particular attention must be paid to the perfusion technique of the distal aorta. Providing adequate perfusion of vertebral and renal arteries and application of satisfactory ventilation are also very important.

Preparation for the operation includes setting up the following:

1. High flow venous catheter, 2 peripheral venous line and 3-lumen central venous line
2. Radial arterial cannula, inserted in the right side if the cross-clamp is placed proximally to the left subclavian artery.
   Femoral arterial cannula, if the bypass is used to maintain the distal aortic flow.
   Radial + femoral , more information can be obtained about the circulation of the lower part of the body
3. Transesophageal echocardiography -intraoperative information: LVEDP, the myocardial function and the valves status
4. Preparation for unilateral ventilation
5. Positioning the double-lumen tube can be helped by bronchofiberoscopic intubation.
6. Ten units of red blood cell transfusion, FFP and platelet transfusion.
7. Monitoring of SSEPs (somatosensory evoked potentials)
8. Body temperature monitoring: core and peripheral temperature.

The Type A - when the ascending aorta is destroyed, need an urgent surgical procedure.

If cross-clamping is applied, significant pressure elevation proximally to the cross-clamping is common. Administration of nitrates and vasodilators is recommended, in case of patient with preserved myocardial systolic function administration of isofluran and desfluran is also suggested. Nitrates can optimize the preload and are able to decrease the left ventricular wall tension. If the operation is performed under the protection of cardiopulmonary bypass (CPB), patient safety is improved if retrograde aortic perfusion is used. In order to ensure appropriate therapy, direct arterial pressure monitoring is registered from two separate regions, above and under the cross-clamping.

In case of thoracic aortic aneurysm surgery balanced anesthesia is the appropriate technique of choice. Protection of the vertebral spine is the most important task, from 20 to 30 minutes of cross-clamping time is considered to be safety. Spinal blood pressure is equal to the difference of mean distal aortic pressure and the cerebrospinal fluid pressure. Cerebrospinal fluid pressure is approximately equal to the central venous pressure. The spinal perfusion autoregulation is similar to the cerebral, appropriate blood flow is maintained between 60-120 mmHg of perfusion pressure. Applying hypothermia is one of the best solution to ensure adequate neuroprotection, 32 - 34 degrees of Celsius of body temperature is recommended during the operation. Impairment of renal circulation can also lead to severe complications, administration of mannitol and loop-diuretics and applying hypothermia can prevent these adverse outcomes. During anesthesia strict attention must be paid to maintain the patient's body fluid and electrolyte balance. If the procedure is done with the patient in the left lateral thoracotomy the CPB is constructed through the femoral artery with venous drainage through right atrial, bicaval, or femoral venous cannulation. Systemic hypothermia is used , with a circulatory arrest. Surface cooling is used along with core cooling and rewarming through the CPB heat exchanger. The cooling of the head with ice during core cooling and kept cold until the period of arrest is important. The core temperature is monitored in the esophagus or tympanic membrane.

Drugs and fluids:

6-10 units of cross matched blood, fresh frozen plasma and platelets

Crystalloids and colloids

Inotropes (ephedrine 3 mg/ml, adrenaline 1:100 000) and vasopressor agents (phenylephrine 100 mcg/ml, metaraminol 0.5 mg/ ml).

It is very important during induction is to minimize the hypertensive response to laryngoscopy and intubation, which may lead to further spreading of the tear and result in rupture of an aneurysm or propagation of a dissection. Dispite the factthat we could make a long surgery, a large doses of pancuronium are generally avoided. This drug has a vagolytic and norepinephrine releasing effects, which produce hypertension and tachycardia. In patients with significant reduced myocardial function etomidate 0.2 to 0.3 mg/kg may provide the hemodynamic stability during induction. Anesthesia is maintained with inhalation agents, opiates and non-depolarizing muscle relaxants.

Airway management: lesions of the ascending and transverse aortic arch are managed with a single-lumen endotracheal tube. If the aortic lesions may cause tracheal or bronchial compression better to use a left-sided double-lumen tube (DLT). The tube should be placed with using fiberoptic bronchoscopy.

Bleeding and hematologic dysfunction: A thoracic aortic surgery involves using large amounts of blood. The amount of blood used for depends on the bypass time. The time of deep hypothermia has an effect on the clotting system.

Aneurysms of the descending thoracic and thoracoabdominal aorta

Aneurysm of descending thoracic aorta involves different part of the thoracic aorta and may extend to the abdominal aorta too. Several techniques can be used to control upper- and lower-body blood flow during the operation.

- Aortic cross-clamping, This is the method for resection in a short period of time. The problems are the organ ischemia because of arterial hypertension, and metabolic acidosis. The cross clamp duration and severity of complications is directly proportional. A cross-clamping time longer than 30 minutes increases the risk of spinal cord injury
- Passive shunts, the most commonly used shunt is the 9-mm heparin-coated conduit (Gott shunt), which does not require systemic anticoagulation.
- Centrifugal pump bypass flow, the left atriofemoral centrifugal pump bypass may be useful in patients with decreased left ventricular function, coronary artery disease, renal failere. and anticipated longer then 30 minutes aortic cross-clamping time.
- Partial Cardiopulmonary Bypass, it is used from the femoral vein to the femoral artery, or from the right atria to the femoral artery. This techique adds the use of oxigenator.
- Deep Hypothermic Circulatory Arrest has been used to protect vital organs and the spinal cord. Despite the detailed research work has not found the perfect way to protect the spinal cord. Containing a high number of patients in studies based on the present position is that hypothermic protection with CPB and DHCA may be the useful methods.

5.4 Endovascular procedures

Endovascular stent graft implantation is one of the most suitable alternatives to open aortic aneurysm surgery today. Aortic operations have remarkably changed since the introduction of endovascular techniques. Extremities of implantation technique have been reported in the scientific literature, from the stent-grafts implanted in the X-ray lab percutaneously toward the open stent-graft implantation procedures. Stent-graft implantation is less invasive, more tolerable for the patients, the length of surgery is shorter, less transfusion is required and the shorter ICU and hospital stay are also the advantages of this technique. Based on our experience stent-graft implantation is considered at those patients, who are referred to be high-risk due to the large number of severe accompanying diseases. In our institute we intend to perform epidural anesthesia at abdominal aortic aneurysm stent-graft repair operations and balanced anesthesia at thoracic cases. Standards of the monitoring technique are the same as that is described at the open procedures. Monitoring improves patient's safety.

Preparation for the procedure includes setting up the following:

1. two 14 G peripheral venous line
2. laboratory exams : blood count, electrolytes , coagulation screen
3. arterial line
4. ECG monitoring from 5 different points
5. pulseoxymetry
6. urinary catheter
7. body temperature monitoring - prolonged operations

8. noninvasive blood pressure measurement (from the opposite side than the direct arterial pressure line)

At the endovascular procedures hemodynamic changes caused by the cross-clamping are not presented. The postoperative period is better tolerated, the pain is milder and the cardiovascular status is more stable. Endovascular stent-graft repair of aortic aneurysms. At present, aortic stent-grafts are most frequently used to repair infrarenal aortic aneurysms. The hemodynamic consequences of infrarenal endovascular balloon inflation are minimal compared with those of suprarenal, supraceliac, or thoracic aortic occlusion. More significant hemodynamic changes are likely to be encountered during stent-graft repair of the descending thoracic aorta.

The high-risk patients undergoing endovascular stent-graft aortic repair appear to have greater hemodynamic stability compared with for the traditional open technique was. Despite this, hypotension and hemodynamic instability could detected, especially during manipulation with expended balloon. Causes of hypotension include hemorrhage and loss of blood into the aneurysm sac after graft implantation, release of endothelial vasoactive substances, and/or an autonomic reflex in response to endovascular balloon inflation.Along the course of the operation, theres is a significant advamtage with the change int he opersation technique, and that the clamping of the aorta is left out or restricted to only a few minutes. During the positioning of the graft , the measured systemic vascular resistence increases but the value (9,2 ±3%)compared to total aortic clamping (32,8 ± 7,6 %) is significantly lower. At this point , following clamping of the abdominal aorta, we experienced a decrease in stroke volume and cardiac output which reached 38% in the cross clamping patients. In patients with stent graft technique this value remained under 9% . The decrease in venous backflow is much lower and therefore the decrease in end diastolic pressure is also lower which influences the left ventricular filling pressure. In a series of 12 patients undergoing infrarenal aortic repair with an EVT endovascular graft under neuroaxial blockade (epidural or continuous spinal), 25% of patients had sudden severe bradycardia and hypotension necessitating immediate therapy. Accordingly, blood must be immediately available, and large-bore intravenous access must be obtained before the procedure. Because of the high incidence of CAD, careful monitoring and aggressive treatment of myocardial ischemia is essential. Conversion to open repair may be required in 2% to 20% of patients (average, 9%) due to technical difficulty with graft deployment or acute surgical complications such as aneurysm rupture or arterial injury. With increasing experience, the need for emergency conversion to open repair is decreasing to approximately 2% to 5% of cases but is still associated with increased morbidity and mortality in these high-risk surgical patients

In patients with significant coexisting atherosclerotic vascular disease of major organs (heart, brain, kidneys), induced hypertension should be avoided altogether or its duration minimized. A stent-graft that does not require hemodynamic manipulations for its deployment would be more desirable in such patients. The anesthetic technique may consist of general anesthesia, regional anesthesia (epidural, spinal, or continuous spinal), or local anesthesia plus sedation . The choice of technique is influenced by multiple factors, including local customs and the experience of the surgical and anesthetic teams. Consideration should be given to the potential for intraoperative hemodynamic instability and the possible need to react rapidly to surgical complications. The anesthetic goals include analgesia, sedation, anxiolysis, patient immobility, and maintenance of hemodynamic stability. General anesthesia was the most commonly used method during the initial experience with endovascular infrarenal aortic repairs because it provided the ability to rapidly convert to open surgical repair. With envolving experience, regional anaesthesia (epidural or spinal) and even local anesthesia with sedation and monitoring are being increasingly used for endovascular aortic repairs A variety of drugs have been used successfully for general anesthesia, including etomidate, propofol, potent synthetic opioids, volatile anesthetics, and muscle relaxants In patients with severely impaired left ventricular function, etomidate together with a potent opioid such as fentanyl or sufentanil provides adequate hemodynamic stability. Advantages of regional anesthesia include minimization of systemic drug use, continuation of pain relief into the postoperative period, and the improved ability to detect symptoms of myocardial ischemia in patients who can report the occurrence of chest pain. Central neuroaxial blockade was shown to reduce the postoperative hypercoagulable state, which may result in a decreased incidence of deep vein thrombosis and vascular graft occlusion . The infrarenal cross clamping acts on kidney function only bedside refle and hemodinamic changes. In our stent graft patients we did not experienced a decrease in the renal functions. The infrarenal aortic clamping convincingly increases renin release from the kidney. The increase in plasma renin and angiotensin levels causes a postoperative increase in blood pressure, compared to preoperative values. Because of the variable and unpredictable duration of these procedures, epidural anesthesia is the most commonly used technique because it has the flexibility of providing anesthesia of indefinite duration. Careful titration of the dermatomal level helps minimize the sympathectomy-related hypotension. Continuation of epidural blockade beyond the operating room is an excellent method of providing postoperative analgesia. A normal coagulation profile must be assured before catheter placement and removal. Continuous spinal anesthesia using an intrathecally placed epidural catheter provides a more rapid onset of a more dense neuroaxial block than does epidural anesthesia.

Endovascular aortic stent repair, especially of the infrarenal segment, has also been performed under monitored anesthesia care. **Drake** et al. used general anesthesia in 103 patients undergoing endovascular repair of the descending thoracic aorta. The procedure was performed with the patient in the right lateral decubitus position, and TEE was used to guide proper stent placement. General anesthesia provides greater patient comfort when adenosine is used to induce sinus arrest and temporary interruption of CO during thoracic aortic stent deployment. The stent - graft technique not only makes the task of the surgeon easier but eases the work of the anesthesiologists. It is important to note that considering the high risk patients we cannot lax th tight monitoring end technical equipment which encure the patient's safety and well being.

5.5 Endovascular technique for ruptured aortic aneurysm: RAAA

The decision of using endograft configuration in the RAAA depends of several factors. For the anesthesia the most important is the hypotension. We are in the position to use intra-aortic occlusion balloons in hemodinamically unstable patients, after the unsuccesfull volumen resuscitaion. It seems to be the hemodinamical instability is the most important factor of the survival in the patients with RAAA undergoing endovascular aortic aneurysm repair.

5.6 Hybrid solutions in aortic surgery

Hybrid solutions are called for vascular interventions, which are the traditional methods of open vascular surgery and insertion of the endograft are combined in order to reduce the risk of interference. The anesthesiologist must be always ready for a planned change in surgical technique, and the situation has changed to provide the surgeon and the patient to the optimal situation.

5.7 Peripheral vascular disease

1. Acute arterial obstruction: most commonly caused by thrombosis and embolisation.

The majority of patients are elderly people with chronic atrial fibrillation. Operation must be performed within 4 -6 hours after the acute ischemia, revascularization must be made as soon as possible. The longer the ischemic period, the less chance for limb survival. Preoperative lab test should routinely contain liver and kidney function and the creatine phosphokinase value (CK). Trends of CK level can indicate the length of ischemia. In case of significantly high level of CK, careful attention should be paid to the subsequent myoglobinuria and adequate fluid intake should be provided. Monitoring hourly diuresis is essential. Acid waste metabolites released from the ischemic, necrotic area impair the circulation, and upsets the acid-base and electrolyte metabolism of the body. Type of anesthesia is determined by the site of obstruction, which can range from narcosis to local anesthesia. If the patient is anticoagulated (e.g because of chronic atrial fibrillation), the regional technique cannot be performed. After the revascularization the impaired circulation is restored, which is followed by the release of large amount of acid waste metabolites from the necrotic areas which were accumulated during the ischemic period. Necroenzymes and myoglobin from the necrotized muscle are also released. These can results in further kidney failure and circulatory impairment. Thus, careful monitoring and lab control is necessary. In case of delayed revascularization, the so called revascularization syndrome develops, which can be life-threatening. Fast decision making becomes essential to determine whether to save the limb or the life. In case of revascularization syndrome despite the anatomically perfect revascularization, further increase of CK level, and rapid progression of kidney failure caused by the myoglobinuria are presented. Hypekalemia also develops. If CK level, during the monitorization reaches the 10.000 U/l , repeated surgical consultation should be organized to determine the further steps. Based on clinical experiences immediate amputation can save the patient's life in these cases. Hemodialysis becomes necessary if CK level exceeds the above mentioned value and if hourly diuresis decreases despite the forced diuretic therapy.

2. In case of chronic obstruction, the patient is referred to the operation after having performed an angiography, thus selecting the most appropriate anesthetic technique is easier. The principles are the same with the acute operation.

In case of peripheral vascular surgeries the anesthetic technique can be take into consideration. In patients with no anticoagulation, neuroaxial technique is widely used. Epidural cannulation at the level of L4 - L5 vertebrae provides appropriate anesthesia for peripheral vascular procedures and has great significance in postoperative analgesia.

Epidural anesthesia has several advantages in the preoperative period, as well, since it can use not only to alleviate the ischemic pain, but it can improve the impaired perfusion of the affected limb by its vasodilation causing effect. Intra-operative systemic heparinization does not increase the risk for epidural hematomas in case of preoperatively inserted epidural catheters. Nevertheless, particular care must be taken when administering unfractioned or low molecule weight heparins. According to the latest guidelines in case of LMWH therapy insertion and removal of the epidural catheter should be performed 12- 24 hours later after the last administration of heparin i.e. before the repeated dose. Significance of catheter removal should not be neglected, since in the formation of epidural hematoma, removal has the same role than the insertion. Intra-operatively 0.5 % bupivacain solution supplemented with opiates is administered, while postoperatively 0.125 % bupivacain can be used as continuous infusion or bolus doses.

Conditions of spinal anesthesia are similar to the epidural and this technique can also be effectively used in peripheral vascular procedures. Both neuroaxial techniques are particularly advantageous in patient with chronic bronchitis and impaired pulmonary function. As previously mentioned the majority of patient with generalized vascular disease smoke, thus these conditions are often presented in the preoperative examination.

Our patients are usually polyglobulic, has high blood viscosity and slow circulation, thus the risk for early graft occlusion is high. Monitored parameters at each anesthetic techniques are the same. These are the following: 5 leads ECG with ST segment analysis, pulse oximetry, hourly diuresis and in case of known renal dysfunction or oliguria central venous pressure.

5.8 Carotid artery revacularization

Indications for carotid artery operations:

Significant stenosis of the common and internal carotid artery and the carotid bifurcation, significant poststenotic flow reduction, in case of an ulcerated plaque which holds increased risk for embolisation, flow direction inversion, subclavian steal syndrome

Patients undergoing carotid artery surgery like other vascular surgical patients suffer from generalized vascular disease. The ACC/AHA 2007 guidelines consider carotid artery endarterctomy an intermediate risk procedure. Since the incidence of ischemic heart disease among these patients is 28 - 32 % the operative risk is also remarkably high. An international study (GALA -General Anesthesia contra Local Anesthesia) covering large patient population has been being performed to determine whether local or generalized anesthesia is preferable for patients requiring carotid endarterectomy. Careful preoperative examination and evaluation of the preoperative neurological status is important. Preexisting medication of the patient should not be changed, even the platelet aggregation inhibiting therapy should be maintained in the preoperative period. Establishing arterial line and registering blood pressure beat by beat is necessary for the monitoring of carotid operations. Pressure fluctuation should be treated by administering short-acting agents (ephedrine, phenilephrin or nitroprussid, urapidil). Increasing mean arterial pressure before carotid clamping is essential to ensure adequate blood flow in the opposite carotid and vertebral artery. Target pressure during operation should be 15 - 20 percent higher than the preoperative blood pressure.

Features of the cerebral circulation:

- Cerebral perfusion is determined by the mean arterial blood pressure
- The carotid stenosis is usually bilateral, only the extent of it may vary between the opposite sides
- 3.The blood distribution is unequal due to the stenosis
- The capacity of compensatory collateral circulation is difficult to estimate.
- The vascular response for alteration in perfusion is impaired due to the diseased vascular wall, which fact can further aggravates the inequality of circulation between areas with normal and abnormal blood supply.
- Intra-operative blood supply during carotid clamping cannot be estimated

Infiltration the carotid body with 1 % Lidocaine after the exposition can prevent blood pressure fluctuation caused by the mechanical manipulation (baroreflex response). Blood pressure elevation can increase the risk for myocardial ischemia.

Numerous studies have been carried out to determine the most suitable drug for induction and maintenance the anesthesia during intubation narcosis, however, after comparison the data, providing adequate perfusion pressure and oxygenation seems to be the most important factor.

Intraoperative monitoring:	Criteria for shunting:
Cooperation test	Uncertain responses, unconsciousness
Carotid stump pressure	< 50 mmHg
Stump pressure index (Carotid stump pressure x 100/mean arterial pressure)	< 33
Transcranial Doppler (TCD)	MCAV drop by 60 -70%
Cerebral perfusion (CBF) Xe133	< 18 ml/100 g/min
EEG	Reduction of the α, β activity by 50%, increased δ activity, asymmetry
Somatosensory Evoked Potential Conduction Time (SSEPS)	> 1 ms, reduction of amplitude by > 50%
Near-infrared spectroscopy	drop of cerebral saturation is more than 5%
Continuous Jugular Venous oxymetry	SJVO2 < 50%

The above scale describes the different options for intra-operative monitoring and criteria for shunting. Continuous jugular venous oxymetry and near-infrared spectroscopy in patient undergoing general anesthesia are the most commonly used techniques, but none of them are sensitive enough to determine cerebral hypoperfusion, thus combination of several techniques is necessary. Applying surgical criteria for shunting is widely accepted, but it is worth to mention that besides it can prevent the intra-operative hypoperfusion, shunting can cause complication, as well. During general anesthesia numerous drugs can be used for induction. Formerly the barbiturates were administered preferably because of its oxygen demand decreasing effect, but either propofol or ethomidat can be used effectively. During induction care must be taken of maintaining the hemodynamic stability of the patient. For maintaining the anesthesia oxigen 50% and isoflurane or sevoflurane with low MAC value is recommended. (ischemic EEG abnormalities were registered during administration of enflurane). During ventilation particular attention must be paid to the PaCO2 value, since the cerebral CO2 reactivity is an important part of the cerebral autoregulation. This is because hypocapnia can decrease, whilst cerebral vasodilatation caused by hypercapnia can increase the cerebral perfusion. In case of patients with preexisting significant cerebral stenosis hypercapnia can further diminish the perfusion in the already hypoperfused area because of steal phenomenon. Thus maintaining normocapnia or minimal hypocapnia is recommended during carotid operations.

The best monitorization can be achieved in case of awake patient and administration of locoregional anesthesia. In these patients preoperative evaluation should include the determination of the dominant brain hemisphere, which is usually corresponds with the patient's handedness. It can be different among elder people, since formerly left-handedness was inacceptable. Determination of the dominant hemisphere is important because of the localization of the speech center. During locoregional technique C2 - C4 spinal roots are deeply whilst the dermatomes are superficially anesthetized by infiltrating them with 7.5 % naropin or 0,5 % bupivacain solution.

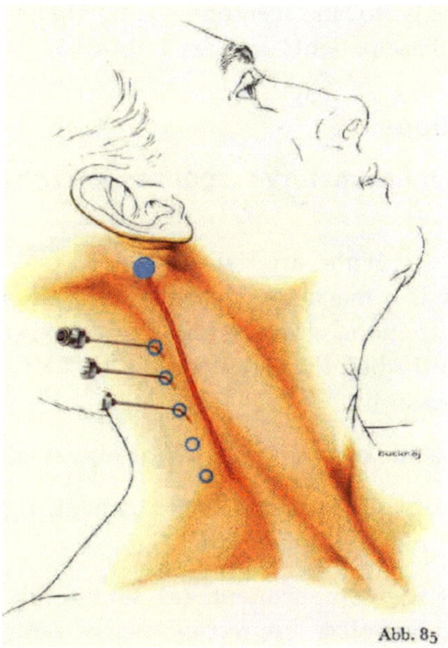

Fig. 1. Infiltration sites of cervical roots

During locoregional anesthesia blood pressure fluctuation is less remarkable. After carotid clamping continuous talking with the patient for 3 minutes should be performed during which the patient should continuously move his/her extremities. If no abnormalities of the sensory or motor function are registered the essential part of the operation can be commenced. If the patient's level of consciousness begins to decrease, aphasia or disability of limb movement develops immediate shunting becomes necessary.

What are the advantages of local anesthesia?

Cerebral ischemia can be early recognized.With the use of intra-operative shunt: patients' consciousness gives a chance for continuous neurological monitoring.Shunting is used only if needed. Blood pressure drops that are dangerous for cerebral and coronary perfusion are less likely to develop than in case of narcosis due to the maintained regulation. Consciousness facilitates the post-operative observation.

What are the disadvantages of local anesthesia?

Hoarseness, difficulty swallowing, numbness of the hand at the opposite side, movement difficulties, dysarthria, confusion, loss of consciousness (if the local anesthetic diffuses or directly gets into the epidural space).Preparation must be made to handle the complications. Local availabilities must be taken into consideration.

5.9 Carotid artery stenting techique

Requires minimal moderate sedation and standard monitoring technique. In both tecnique we have to listen to the postoperative stroke, it mostly embolic origin. The increase sensitivity of the baroreceptors after the plaque removal can cause bradycardia and hypotension. At the other hand hypertension can lead to hyperperfusion - hyperperfusion syndrome -which may leads to intracerebral hemorrhage. So the neurological and haemodinamical controll of these patients are very important.

6. Postoperative evaluations

6.1 Reperfusion injury and inflammatory responses following acute revascularization surgery

After revascularization of an acute arterial occlusion the development of a serious ischaemic-reperfusion injury is a menacing challenge and a hard task in vascular surgery. The clinical phenomenon with increase in the lower limb compartment pressure leading to circulatory deterioration and therefore inadequate tissular oxygenation is known as compartment syndrome of lower limb

The most frequent causes of acute compartment syndrome would be classified as:

1.1. Decrease in the volumetric size of the compartment: tight bandages or casts, tight closure of the fascia, burn or frostbite injuries.

1.2. Increase in the size of the compartment: (a) as a result of edema: arterial injuries, arterial thrombosis and embolization, reconstructive vascular operations, replantation (revascularization), long tourniquet time, arterial spasm, angiography, ergotamin intoxication, prolonged immobilization with limb compression, narcotic influence, high strain, venous insufficiency, snake bite; (b) as a result of a hemorrhage. According to the progression, compartment syndrome can also be classified in the following manner:

- First degree: pain, swelling, paresthesia.
- Second degree: neurological changes, absence of pulse and early focal necrosis in muscles..
- Third degree: complete muscular and dermal necrosis.

To set the diagnosis of classic compartment syndrome, the observation of the following six signs and symptoms are of great importance.

- Disproportional higher pain compared to clinical findings.
- Pain in the affected compartment with passive movement of the limb.
- Paralysis or paresis of the muscles of the concerned compartment.
- Hypaesthesia or paresthesia in the affected compartment.
- Induration and inflammation in the affected compartment.
- Absence or diminished distal pulse.

To prevent neuromuscular ischemia and necrosis, fasciotomy must be performed, in order to decompress the rigid osteofascial compartments of the lower limb, thus, to relieve the muscles and neurovascular bundles. Revascularization syndrome is undoubtedly one of the most common causes of compartment syndrome requiring urgent fasciotomy.

6.2 Pathomechanism of compartment syndrome

Interruption of circulation in muscle tissue results in a series of biochemical changes, starting with cellular dysfunction, followed by cellular and tissular edema, leading to reversible and then irreversible impairment of the cells. Ischemic injury to tissue leads to decreased energy supply needed for membrane function and electrolyte homeostasis, leading to enzyme system impairment and finally irreversible changes at the cellular level. Therefore, the fine balance between homeostasis and microcirculation becomes upset. Anaerobic metabolism then starts in muscle tissue due to ischemia resulting in accumulation of acidic metabolites including lactic acid. Due to the impairment of membrane functions, among the others, Na^+-K^+ pump dysfunction is the most important as it causes intracellular uptake of Na^+ and water and release of K^+. Intracellular Na^+ and water will generate swelling and edema and, therefore, the compartment pressure increases (above 40 mmHg). This leads to secondary arterial compression, thus, despite established patency, the oxygen transport remains disturbed. Many authors reported on necessity of amputation after successful embolectomy because of serious, generalized life-threatening symptoms]. In a revascularized limb reactive hyperaemia is one of the first signs, which occurs due to dilation of capillaries and arteriovenous shunts. Capillary dilation along with products of anaerobic metabolism causes increase in the permeability of capillaries and worsening edema, leading to a secondary hypovolaemia.

Apart from the vascular lesion, impairment of circulation is on of the most important factors by which a series of hemodynamic disorders can be started, leading to capillary nutritional impairment and muscular edema. Muscle fiber swelling and edema causes elevation of compartment pressure. Then retention of intracellular fluid and microbleedings will develop, leading to further impairment in circulation as the process rapidly advances. At this level fasciotomy must be performed immediately to prevent serious myopathy and muscle necrosis. Arterial or venous occlusion alone, cannot explain the pathogenic background of compartment syndrome, since this complex of signs of vascular occlusion may develop even in the absence of vascular injury. Phenomenos as "chronic exertional compartment syndrome" or "overuse syndrome" are pieces of evidence proving that many other mechanisms are also involved in the development of compartment syndrome. Irrespective of origin of injury and ischemia, the end point of this process is swelling of muscle bundles in the compartment space and elevation of intracompartmental pressure (ICP). If intracompartmental pressure exceeds the critical level of 35-40 mmHg, the nutritional function of capillaries would cease and perfusion of muscles fail. If this process is not interrupted by performing fasciotomy, ischemic changes will ultimately develop resulting in irreversible injuries.

6.3 The role of oxidative stress in the pathogenesis of compartment syndrome

At the beginning of compartment syndrome, ischemic-reperfusion signs are present only at the cellular level. The reasons behind elevation of capillary permeability are not well known yet, though many biochemical changes observed may give partial explanation. During ischemia–reperfusion, well-known reactive oxygen-derived intermediators are formed. Toxic action of free radicals would affect intracellular matrix and cell membranes. Due to the above mentioned mechanism, antioxidant enzymes and different types of scavengers like allopurinol, mannitol, catalase, dimetylsulfoxide and superoxide dismutase (SOD), which block cytotoxic free radicals procreation, may also play an important role in stopping compartment syndrome evolution.

By monitoring ischemia–reperfusion, Lee et al. have presented further proves about the role of free radicals. During ischemia, the calcium transport in the sarcoplasma reticulum of skeletal muscles is significantly depressed. Lee has monitored physiologic alterations during and after ischemia by strangulation of back limbs in rat models. These observations have shown that in the group of rats treated previously by superoxide dismutase and catalase, calcium uptake in the sarcoplasma network is appreciably higher comparing to the non-treated group, though, treatment by antioxidant enzymes does not elevate the calcium uptake level to non-ischemic range. This might lead to conclusion that, possibly other mechanisms are also involved in development of compartment syndrome.

6.4 Main points

Indications for surgery for compartment syndrome, used to happen decisively on the basis of clinical findings, which was mostly subjective, and therefore leads to delayed surgical intervention in many cases. By monitoring of elevated compartment pressure, microcirculation impairment and tissular oxygen saturation (StO2), we tried to observe the progression of compartment syndrome. We also tried to choose a fast, practical and reliable method that can also be performed at bed-side, providing us with objective data supporting the foregoing subjective indication of fasciotomy. Using a non-invasive oxygen saturation detector and by minimally invasive measurement of compartment pressure, the stage of the disease progression and its reversibility can be assessed objectively. Using literature references, we measured intracompartmental pressure (ICP) and tissular oxygen saturation (StO2) to evaluate the circulation of the extremity. We applied these two methods abreast, in patients suffering from clinically proved compartment syndrome, thus, our data might help in diagnosing of compartment syndrome due to reperfusion injury and deciding whether the patient should undergo conservative versus surgical treatment.

6.5 Determination of tissue oxygen saturation

For determination of tissular oxygen saturation, we used InSpectra Tissue Spectrometer (Model 325; Hutchinson Technology Inc., Arnhem, The Netherlands). InSpectra tissue spectrometer can detect light absorption characteristic of hemoglobin in a near-infrared range (near-infrared spectroscopy-NIRS; wavelength: 680–800 nm). Deflected light from tissues and its absorption by sensor device decisively indicates the level of oxyhemoglobin and deoxyhemoglobin concentration. We placed the detector part on gastrecnemius muscle, and after calibration a continuous monitoring of saturation values could be obtained. NIRS is a non-invasive method for monitoring tissular perfusion. Former studies also intended to apply tissular oxygen monitoring methods like as Doppler, thermometry and application of optochemical oxygen sensors. The detector part is able to emit near-infrared light, and absorb deflected rays from different layers of tissues. Tissular Hgb–oxygen saturation would appear in 4 dissimilar wavelengths. Near-infrared light can easily penetrate skin, muscles and even bones, thus it would be absorbed in distinct ways in layers containing different concentration of blood and Hgb. The near-infrared emitter and the deflected light absorber optical cable are placed 25 mm away from each other. Depth of measurement can be set on 12, 15, 20, 25 and 35 mm. These will be the depths of the tissue where we received our data from. (Emitted light, minus absorbed light is equal to reflected light.) During measurement by NIRS we could register arterioles, capillaries, veins and tissular bed Hgbconcentrations of different depth. This is the main difference between NIRS and pulsoxymeter, which can only detect Hgb-concentration of pulsating layer. This technique is appropriate for single or continuous non-invasive monitoring of tissular perfusion]. It is therefore very convenient to detect perfusion alterations occuring in the area under detector, and practically can be used to diagnose peripheral obliterative atherosclerosis (measurement of perfusion changes under strain), operative perfusion and reperfusion perception. And finally, it can be used as a reliable tool in making correct diagnosis and treatment.

6.6 Results

The cut-off ICP pressure was 40 mmHg above which fasciotomy was considered to be an absolute indication- we assumed normal oxygen saturation level to be 87%.(Arató et al) Undoubtedly, clinical diagnosis and surgical treatment of compartment syndrome in a timely manner requires a great attention and co-evaluation of many parameters. Complications are usually due to a delayed or inadequate fasciotomy ("too little and too late" phenomenon). Measurements performed in limited numbers are not suitable for statistical analysis. According to literature data and our experiments, measurement of limb saturation significantly correlates with compartment pressure alterations.

We emphasize that only a parallel observation of the patient's clinical status, laboratory data, ICP and limb StO2 may lead to correct and reliable diagnosis resulting in determining the optimal time of fasciotomy and proper evaluating of efficiency of surgery. We believe that measurements of compartment pressure and tissular oxygen saturation both can be helpful in making accurate diagnosis, indication of fasciotomy and also during postoperative follow-up. A novel method of our team that we used objective parameters as basis of a new interventional indication strategy in making decision for fasciotomy along with empirical treatment guidelines applied generally in clinical practice (evidence-based medicine). We were the first to study lower limb compartment syndrome by parallel monitoring of non-invasive tissular oxygen saturation and by minimal invasive measurement of compartment pressure. The pressure and oxygen saturation cut-off values defined by our team can be beneficial in making decision regarding operative versus conservative treatment.

The long time monitoring of the oxidative and inflammatory changes in reperfusion helps to understand the pathology and to develop a more effective therapy. During exclusion of blood from the circulation ischemia and acidosis appear in the surrounding tissues of the occluded vessels, which try to adapt to the absence of oxygen by switching their metabolism from aerobic to anaerobic, but finally these strategy will lead to tissue damage and loss. In the chronic or acute occlusive diseases the tissue injuries depend on the duration of hypoxia, the mass of tissues involved and the blood pressure of the patients. Reconstruction of the occluded vessels is not without risk, because it can cause volume, pressure and metabolic load, with further tissue damage resulting in the so-called reperfusion injury. Peripheral arterial diseases are a seriously under-diagnosed disorder affecting up to 20 % of the adult population worldwide. Atherosclerotic involvements frequently are in the background, thrombosis or embolization can occur within the narrowed or calcified vessels, or within the aneurismal sites, resulting in serious tissue ischemia. It is very difficult to monitor the cellular processes, which influence the outcome of the surgical manoeuvres or serve as a marker of the following events. A huge amount of data emerged for the characterization of ischemia reperfusion injury, but function of thrombocytes has been hardly investigated by Kürthy M et al. In their study showed that the duration of hypoxia basically influenced the degree of reperfusion injury in revascularization surgery, resulting in a different outcome in ADP and collagen induced platelet aggregation in whole blood even one week after surgery. Platelet aggregation highly and significantly elevated , in spite of the intensive antiplatelet and antiaggregation therapy. Sinay et al. measured in an in vivo animal model the serum total peroxide concentration during infrarenal aortic cross clamping ischaemia and reperfusion. Reperfusion injury is an integrated response to the restoration of blood flow after ischaemia, and is initiated at the very early moments of reperfusion, lasting potentially for days. The extent of the oxidative stress and the consecutive generalized inflammatory response depends on the ischaemic-time, the ischaemic tissue volume, and the general state of the endothelium-leukocyte-tissue functional complex (diabetes, chronic ischaemia, drugs).

The pathogenesis of reperfusion injury is a complex process involving numerous mechanisms exerted in the intracellular and extracellular environments. Hypoxia leads to intracellular ATP depletion with a consecutive hypoxanthine elevation.(Jancsó et al) In the early seconds of reperfusion, when the molecular oxygen appears in the cell, the - xanthine oxidase catalised -hypoxanthine-xanthine conversion will produce a mass of superoxide radicals. Superoxide radical and the other reactive oxygen intermediates will damage the membrane-lipids (through lipidperoxidation), the proteins (causing enzyme defects and ion channel injury) and the DNA. These are the main pathways of the cellular oxidant injury. The endogenous antioxidant system defends against these radical injuries Reactive oxygen species (ROS) will also induce local and systematic inflammatory responses through the inducing of cytokine expression and leukocyte activation. Inflammatory process leads to increased microvascular permeability, interstitial edema, and capillary perfusion depletion. The oxidative and inflammatory pathways will lead to a complex reperfusion injury (Fig.2).

While these pathways are well known in vascular surgery, there is no real effective tool in the hand of the surgeons to treat or to prevent them. As we know how to limit ischemic damage (mostly by reducing the ischemia time via an early reperfusion, and improving O2 demand/supply balance), postconditioning might be the way to prevent or reduce reperfusion damage. Postconditioning has the advantage of being a way to influence and modify ischaemia-reperfusion injury after it has occurred. This may open a therapeutic alternative in situations of unexpected and uncontrolled ischaemic injury, for instance in the situation where complications occur during surgery, making a simple procedure into a complicated one, and making aortic cross-clamping longer than anticipated.

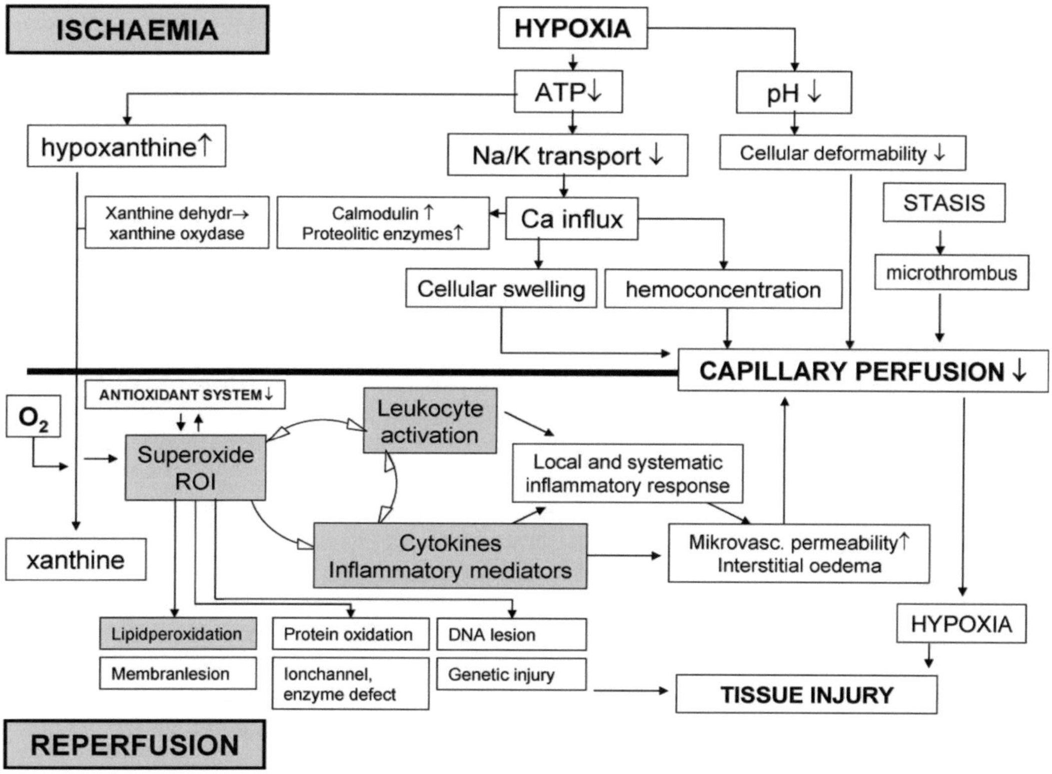

Fig. 2. Simplified presentation of the mechanism of ischaemic-reperfusion injury. Emphasizing, that the engine of reperfusion injury is the ROI-cytokine-leukocyte positive feedback circle (ROI: reactive oxygen intermediers; ATP: adenosine triphosphate; DNA: deoxyribonucleic acid).

7. Summary

In the postoperative period the most important factor is the stress response. This includes preventing the triggers for myocardial ischaemia . These triggers are the pain, the anemia, haemodynamic instability , hypothermia and the oxigen demand. The important task of the anesthesiologist to optimization of cardiac risk , implications of anesthetic technique, diagnosis and prevent the myocardial ischaemia . It is a great challange to keep balance on a relative elderly patients with high incidence of coexisting disease. Our job is ti do everything for vascular surgery patients to reduce the morbidity and better ocerall outcome.

8. References

Arató E, Jancsó G, Sinay L et al: Reperfusion injury and inflammatory responses following acute lower limb revascularization surgery Clin Hemorheology and Microcirculation 39 (2008) 79–85 79

Drake AR, Arko FR, Filis KA et al: Intrasac flow velocities predict sealing of type II endoleaks after endovascular abdominal aortic aneurysm repair. J Vasc Surg. 2003 Jan;37(1):8-15

Eagle K, Coley CM,Newell JB, et al: Combining clinical and thallium data optimizes preoperative assessment of cardiac risk before major vascular surgery . Ann Intern Med 110:859-866,1989

Fleisher LA, Beckmann JA, Brown KA at al. : ACC/AHA 2007 guidelines on perioperative cardiovascular evaluation and care for noncardiac surgery: a report of the American Heart Associaton Task Force onPractice Guidelines (Writing Comittee to revise the 2002 Guidelines on Perioperative Cardiovascular Evaluation for Noncardiac Surgery) J Am Coll Card 2007.50. 159-241

Fleischmann KE, Beck,am JA, Buller CE et al: 2009 ACCF/AHA Focused Update on Perioperative Beta Blockade .American College of Cardiology Foundation, America Heart Association Task Force on Practice Guidelines, American Society of Echocardiography, American Society of Nuclear Cardiology, Heart Rhytm Society, Society of cardiovascualar Anethesiologists, Society for Cardiovascular Angiography and Interventions, Society for Vascular Surgery J.Am Coll Cardiol 2009, 07.004

GALA Trial Collaborative Group General anaesthesia versus local anaesthesia for carotid surgery (GALA): a multicentre, randomised controlled trial. Lancet. 2008 Dec 20;372(9656):2132-42. Epub 2008 Nov 27

Goldman L, Caldera DL, Nussbaum SR, et al.: Multifactorial index of cardiac risk in noncardiac surgical procedures N.Engl.J Med 297:845-850,1977

Jancsó G , Cserepes B, Gasz B et al: Expression and protective role of heme oxygenase-1 in delayed myocardial preconditioning Ann N Y 2007 Jan, 1095:251-61

Kumar N, Cowlishaw P , Telford R: Anesthesia for Abdominal Aortic Surgery www.frca.co.uk

Kürthy M, Arato E, Jancso G et al.: Duration of hypoxia influences platelet function due to free radical production in revascularization surgery of lower limb Perfusion 2007, 20:187-199

Lee TH, Marcantonio ER, Mangione CM, et al: Derivation and prospective validation of a simple index for prediction of cardiac risk of major non-cardiac surgery .Circulation 100:1043-1049, 1999.

Manago DT: Perioperative cardiac morbidity. Anesthesiology 72:153-184,1990

Poldermans D, Boersma E, Bax JJ, et al: Bisoprolol reduced cardiac death and myocardial infarction in high risk patients as long as two years after succesful major vascualr surgery. Eur. Heart J 22: 1353-1358, 2001.

Sinay L, Kürthy M,. Horváth Sz, et al: Ischaemic postconditioning reduces peroxide formation, cytokine expression and leukocyte activation in reperfusion injury after abdominal aortic surgery in rat model Clinical Hemorheology and Microcirculation 40 (2008) 133–142 133

Walsh SR: Eur Anaesthetic specialisation leads to improved early- and medium-term survival following major vascular surgery. Eur J Vasc Endovasc Surg. 2010 Jun;39(6):719-25. Epub 2010 Mar 11.

White CJ, Gray WA: Endovascular therapies for peripherial arterial disese: An evidence-based review.Circulation 2007, 116:2203

10

Intraoperative Anesthetic Management for Vascular and Endovascular Abdominal Aortic Surgery

Maria J. Estruch-Perez, Josep Balaguer-Domenech, Angel Plaza-Martinez and Cristina Solaz-Roldan
Dr. Peset University Hospital, Valencia, Spain

1. Introduction

Management of patients undergoing vascular surgery concerns elderly patient, high incidence of coexisting disease as coronary artery disease, hypertension, and diabetes mellitus, acute changes in arterial pressure or metabolic stress associated with arterial ischemia or arterial cross-clamping. As a result, the ischemic insults to vital organs (heart, kidneys, and spinal cord) cause more frequent perioperative morbidity and mortality than other surgical procedures. Cardiovascular instability is more common and marked in patients with cardiovascular disease or those receiving vasoactive medications and undergoing cardiovascular surgical procedures.

The care must focus on preservation of vital organ, specially on the heart, which is the most important cause of morbidity after vascular surgery.

Major vascular surgery is particularly challenging to the anaesthesiologist because these are high-risk operations in a patient population with a high prevalence of either overt or occult coronary artery disease, which is the leading cause of perioperative and long-term mortality after vascular surgery. The last decade the multidisciplinary field of endovascular surgery has provided less invasive approaches or alternatives to conventional vascular reconstruction. These less invasive procedures, initially offered to patients traditionally considered unfit for open surgery, are being widely applied to the larger cohort of patients undergoing vascular surgery.

2. Preoperative improvement

Perioperative risk is multifactorial and depends on the interaction of anaesthesia, surgery and patient-specific factors. The fundamental purposes of preoperative evaluation are firstly, the identification of those patients for whom the perioperative period may constitute an increased risk of morbidity and mortality, aside from the risks associated with the underlying disease through the medical history information and, secondly, to design perioperative strategies for optimizing the patient's condition in case of presence of risk factors and reducing additional perioperative risks. Age per se, however, seems to be responsible for only a small increase in the risk of complications; greater risks are associated with urgency and significant cardiac, pulmonary, and renal disease.

An interesting question of who should - at a certain point in the pre-operative trajectory - in close cooperation with the patient - decide whether or not the surgical intervention should be performed. The decision is not only a surgical one and should be based on knowledge of risk but also on the close knowledge of the individual patient, the planned procedure and also of alternative procedures. The increasing burden that expensive technical investigations put on social health care systems will oblige us to consider this aspect of the preoperative management of the patients in the near future.

Cardiac complications are a major cause of perioperative morbidity and mortality. Perioperative cardiac complications can occur in patients with documented or asymptomatic ischaemic heart disease, ventricular dysfunction and valvular heart disease. It has been estimated that in non-cardiac surgery major perioperative cardiac events may occur in up to 4% of cardiac patients, and 1.4% of an unselected patient population. In particular, vascular surgery patients are at increased risk with reported mortality rates of 1.5-2% for endovascular and 3-4% for open procedures. Mortality is mainly caused by perioperative myocardial infarction (accounting for 10-40% of postoperative deaths), in addition non-fatal perioperative myocardial infarction is associated with an increased risk of late mortality. Because of the systemic nature of atherosclerotic disease, vascular patients frequently have arterial disease affecting multiple vascular territories. It is not clear whether any specific category of vascular disease is associated with a greater likelihood of coexisting CAD. Perioperative cardiac complications are either caused by myocardial ischemia resulting from an increase in myocardial oxygen demand (tachycardia, hypertension, pain) or decreased supply (hypotension, vasospasm, tachycardia, hypoxia, anaemia) or, by acute coronary plaque rupture caused by factors that increase intra-coronary wall stress and the presence of a hypercoagulable state, leukocyte activation, and activation of the inflammatory response may contribute.

In 2009, the European Society of Cardiology published guidelines for pre-operative cardiac risk assessment and perioperative cardiac management in non-cardiac surgery, which were endorsed by the European Society of Anaesthesiology (www.escardio.org/guidelines). It shows the present evidence (and lack of evidence) in this field that is so important for the specialty. The European guidelines should not overrule the national ones but should be seen as a help to create harmonization of practice. Not all of these can be covered by recommendations. In addition, evidence on many issues is scarce and of low quality. Therefore, where possible, recommendations will be provided based on the best available evidence and when this is not possible, the recent available evidence will be summarized.

As surgical techniques become increasingly complex, the physical fitness required of the patients as well as the surgical impact on perioperative risk increases. Depending on duration of procedure, estimated blood-loss, estimated fluid shifts and anatomical region, the risk of surgery may vary tremendously. Surgical risk for cardiac events has been described by a 3 part classification that distinguishes between low, intermediate and high risk procedures according to the AHA/ACC-guideline and the guideline of the European Society of Cardiology (ESC). Therefore, in order to stratify overall perioperative risk, it is essential to consider the nature and duration of a surgical procedure. The cardiac risk can also influence the type of operation and guide the choice to less invasive interventions, such as peripheral arterial angioplasty instead of infra-inguinal bypass, or extraanatomic reconstruction instead of an aortic procedure, even when these may yield less favourable results in the long term.

A key component in the preoperative assessment is the evaluation of the presence of active or unstable cardiac conditions (table 1), the surgical risk factors (table 2), the functional capacity of the patient (< or > 4 METs), and the presence of cardiac risk factors (table 3). Decision for further testing and possible treatment should be performed in close cooperation with the cardiologist.

2.1 ESC Guidelines

The ESC guidelines propose a step-wise approach for perioperative cardiac assessment and management of cardiac patients scheduled for non-cardiac surgery.

1. The first step determines the urgency of the operation. The necessity for immediate surgery is such that no time is left for further cardiac assessment and/or treatment. Adequate measures for perioperative surveillance and treatment should be taken. Further risk stratification and risk factor management will be planned during the postoperative period.
2. The second step if there is no need for emergency surgery is to screen the patients for the presence of active cardiac conditions (Table 1). If one of these conditions is present, they should be evaluated and treated. For all these conditions, the potential benefits of delaying surgery to optimize the effects of treatment must be weighed against the risk of delaying the surgical procedure. With respect to a previous recent myocardial infarction, it is recommended to wait 4-6 weeks before performing elective surgery, even if there are no adequate clinical trials on the subject.
3. The third step if no active cardiac conditions are present is to assess the risk of surgery (Table 2). Many surgical procedures are associated with a low risk of perioperative complications even in high-risk patients. In such cases it is recommended to proceed with planned surgery.
4. The fourth step in the case of intermediate or high risk surgery evaluates whether the patient can sustain a functional capacity equal or greater than 4 metabolic equivalents (METs) without symptoms. If so, the recommendation is to proceed with surgery. In patients with coronary artery disease or risk factors, statin therapy and a titrated low-dose beta-blocker regimen can be initiated prior to surgery.
5. The fifth step in patients with a poor functional capacity or it is unknown consider the risk of the surgical procedure. When patients are scheduled for intermediate risk surgery statin therapy and a titrated low-dose beta-blocker regimen appears appropriate prior to surgery. In patients with systolic left ventricular (LV) dysfunction (ejection fraction <40%) ACE-inhibitors are recommended prior to surgery.
6. The sixth step in patients undergoing high risk surgery clinical risk factors (Table 3) are noted. In patients with up to two clinical risk factors, statin therapy and a titrated low-dose b-blocker regimen are recommended prior to surgery. In patients with systolic LV dysfunction ACE inhibitors (or ARBs in patients intolerant of ACE inhibitors) are recommended before surgery.
7. The step seventh consider non-invasive testing in patients with ≥ 3 clinical risk factors (Table 3). Patients without stress-induced ischemia, or mild to moderate ischemia suggestive of one- or two-vessel disease, can proceed with the planned surgical procedure.

It is recommended that statin therapy and a titrated low dose b-blocker regimen be initiated. In patients with extensive stress-induced ischemia, as assessed by non-invasive testing, an individualized perioperative management is recommended considering the potential benefit of the proposed surgical procedure compared with the predicted adverse outcome, and the effect of medical therapy and/or coronary revascularization not only for immediate postoperative outcome, but also for long-term follow-up. In patients referred for percutaneous coronary artery intervention, the initiation and duration of antiplatelet therapy will interfere with the planned surgical procedure.

In patients referred for angioplasty, non-cardiac surgery can be performed within 2 weeks after intervention with continuation of aspirin treatment.

In patients with bare metal stent placement, non-cardiac surgery can be performed after 6 weeks to 3 months following intervention. Dual antiplatelet therapy should be continued for at least 6 weeks, preferably for up to 3 months. After this period, at least aspirin therapy should be continued.

In patients with recent Drug-eluting stent placement, non-cardiac surgery can be performed after 12 months following intervention, before which time dual antiplatelet therapy is recommended. After this period, at least aspirin therapy should be continued.

If applicable, discuss the continuation of chronic aspirin therapy. Discontinuation of aspirin therapy should be considered only in those patients in which haemostasis is difficult to control during surgery (intracranial neurosurgery, medular surgery, posterior chamber of the eye) that not concerns vascular surgery.

2.2 Recommendations

1. If active cardiac disease is suspected in a patient scheduled, the patient should be referred to a cardiologist for assessment and possible treatment (grade of recommendation: **D**).
2. In patients currently under b-blocking or statin therapy:
   a. should not be stopped preoperatively (grade of recommendation: **A**);
   b. is recommended to high risk patients;
   c. low and intermediate risk patients should not routinely be subjected to beta-blockade.

   An important point is that especially when heart failure has not been excluded, the beta-blockade should be started slowly titrating the dose, which implies that the treatment should ideally be started between 30 days and at least 1 week before surgery. Therefore these should be interpreted within the constraints of logistics and infrastructure that allow to see the patient sufficiently long in advance preoperatively.

   In general terms, patients should be maintained on their usual cardiovascular medications throughout the perioperative period. Antiplatelet therapy requires special consideration and must be individualized to each patient.

3. Guidelines on perioperative cardiovascular evaluation and care suggest that coronary intervention is rarely necessary to simply lower the risk of surgery unless such intervention is indicated irrespective of the preoperative context. Current evidence does not support the role of prophylactic coronary revascularization as a means to reduce perioperative or long-term morbidity after major vascular surgery.

   Caregivers will increasingly be reminded that additional testing of the patient is only relevant if they may lead to substantial alterations of perioperative management.

4. Non-invasive testing can also be considered prior to any surgical procedure for patient counselling, or change of perioperative management in relation to type of surgery and anaesthesia technique.

1. Unstable coronary syndromes 1.1 unstable or severe angina 1.2 recent myocardial infarction (within 30 days)
2. Decompensated heart failure
3. Significant arrhythmias 3.1 high-grade atrioventricular block 3.2 symptomatic ventricular arrhythmias 3.3 supraventricular arrhythmias with uncontrolled ventricular rate (> 100 bpm at rest) 3.4 symptomatic bradycardia 3.5 newly diagnosed ventricular tachycardia
4. Severe valvular disease 4.1 severe aortic stenosis (mean pressure gradient > 40 mm Hg, area < 1 cm2 or symptomatic) 4.2 symptomatic mitral stenosis

Table 1. Active cardiac conditions that necessitate further evaluation and treatment before non-cardiac surgery

A. High risk (cardiac risk > 5%) A.1 Aortic surgery A.2 Major vascular surgery A.3 Peripheral vascular surgery
B. Intermediate risk (cardiac risk 1 – 5%) B.1 Abdominal B.2 Carotid B.3 Peripheral arterial angioplasty B.4 Endovascular aneurysm repair B.5 Head and neck surgery B.6 Major neurologic/orthopedic B.7 Pulmonary B.8 Major urologic
C. Low risk (cardiac risk < 1%) C.1 Breast C.2 Dental C.3 Endocrine C.4 Eye C.5 Gynecology C.6 Reconstructive C.7 Minor orthopedic C.8 Minor urologic

Table 2. The risk of cardiac death and non-fatal myocardial infarction for non-cardiac operations.

1. History of ischemic myocardial disease or angina pectoris
2. Current stable or history of heart failure
3. History of cerebrovascular disease / transient ischemic attack
4. Diabetes requiring insulin therapy
5. Renal failure (serum creatinine > 2 mg / dL or a creatinine clearance <60 ml/min)

Table 3. Clinical risk factors

3. Intraoperative management of Abdominal Aortic Aneurysm

An important part of perioperative patient care resides in the possible impact of intra-operative patient care on the outcome. However, strong evidence remains to be gathered of the influence of intra-operative anaesthetic management on short and long-term postoperative outcome. For instance, while epidural analgesia is generally considered a valuable tool in the perioperative pain treatment it remains to be proven that the treatment positively affects perioperative morbidity and mortality. But, the increasing preoperative use of antiplatelet and anti-coagulant drugs will interfere with the possibilities to freely apply neuro-axial techniques. It is mandatory to realize that the choice of anaesthetic techniques will influence the potential for starting and / or continuing anti-coagulant therapy. Thus, the anaesthesiologist is required to consider his/her work in the context of the total perioperative course. Further, the important question of fluid management has not resulted in specific recommendations due to the combination of conflicting and lacking evidence.

The importance (lack of) of perioperative respiratory interventions is not evident. Several studies have shown that postoperative pulmonary complications are associated with worse outcome. However, there has been conflicting evidence to which degree preventive measures have been effective, a fact which is mirrored in the Guidelines. There are studies reporting effectiveness of early application of non invasive continuous positive airway pressure in presence of acute lung injury.

Infrarenal abdominal aortic aneurysms (AAAs) are more common (70%). The abdominal aorta is aneurismal when its diameter is greater than 3.0 cm. The disorder is more common in men than in women. Sakalihasan reports that the prevalence of AAAs is rising and is between 1.3% and 8.9% in men and between 1.0% and 2.2% in women over the age of 65.

Sakalihasan et alt. also refer that most deaths due to ruptured AAAs are potentially preventable since elective repair can be performed with an perioperative mortality rates in the 2% to 4% range even in contemporary experience due to cardiac complications. Population-based series employing state wide or national databases indicate higher mortality, in the 4% to 8% range. By contrast, with the progress in elective repair mortality, no improvement in operative mortality of ruptured aneurysms has been reported during the past decades remaining as high as 30–70%. Mortality depends on the haemodynamic status of the patient at the time of surgery. Overall mortality from ruptured abdominal aortic aneurysms is about 80% associated to hypovolemic shock with an operative survival of 50%. Mortalities occurring at the scene of rupture, during transfer, shortly after admission to the emergency department, and during surgery are combined, then only 18% of patients with ruptured aortic aneurysms survive.

Most patients with AAAs are asymptomatic and are discovered incidentally when other examinations are performed. Patients presenting with back, abdominal or groin pain in the presence of a pulsatile mass require urgent evaluation to exclude a rupture or dissection. The main risk factors for developing AAAs are advancing age, family history, smoking and hypertension.

3.1 Surgical indication

Current guidelines of American Association for Vascular Surgery for the treatment of abdominal aortic aneurysms are to offer operative intervention when the aneurysm exceeds 5.5 cm. The risk for rupture of a 5.5-cm aneurysm (per year) is equal to or greater than the risk for perioperative mortality. The risk of rupture of a 6 cm or greater exceeds 20%. The bigger the aneurysm is, the more tendency to the rupture is.

The incidence of rupture in small aneurysms less than 5 cm is 2%. There is no survival benefit from early surgical intervention. Patients with small aneurysms should undergo regular ultrasound scanning to monitor the aneurysm size.

Open repair remains the gold standard treatment. Endovascular aneurysm repair (EVAR) is emerging as a minimally invasive treatment for some AAAs that are anatomically suitable.

3.2 Preoperative evaluation

We must search risk factors and co-morbidities. Patients presenting for abdominal vascular surgery have a high incidence of co-morbidities:

- Coronary artery disease often with impaired ventricular function is observed in the 80% of patients scheduled for vascular surgery
- Cerebrovascular disease
- Hypertension
- Pulmonary disease (often related to smoking)
- Renal impairment
- Diabetes mellitus
- Obesity
- Dislipemy

Careful preoperative assessment is required by the surgeon and anaesthetist to identify high risk patients and to optimise medical management according the guideline in previous section:

- Lifestyle advice should be given.
- Cessation of smoking and structured exercise programmes may improve cardio-respiratory fitness.
- Patients should receive antiplatelet medication to protect against thromboembolic complications.
- Statins should be prescribed due to plaque stabilisation.

Patients with inducible ischemia on pharmacological stress testing have improved outcomes if prescribed b blockers. The success of modern medical treatments in coronary artery disease offers benefits over coronary revascularisation prior to non cardiac surgery. Preoperative coronary artery bypass surgery should only be performed if indicated on prognostic grounds (severe left main stem disease or severe triple vessel disease with impaired left ventricular function). This should be performed 1-2 months prior to surgery.

- Patients should receive all their regular medication on the day of surgery.
- Correct premedication to decrease anxiety
- Antibiotic prophylaxis
- Intestinal cleanse to ensure vascular prosthesis viability.

3.3 Anaesthetic management of open surgery repair (OSR)

3.3.1 Aims

Haemodynamic stability, according to the patient with CAD preventing tachyarritmies, high and low blood pressure, sympathetic stimulation, myocardial depression or coronary steal.

Normothermia. Perioperative hypothermia is associated with myocardial ischemia and dysrhythmias. It contributes to a coagulopathy and increases wound infections. Shivering can increase oxygen consumption up to six fold placing excessive demands on the cardiovascular system. Forced air warming devices, fluid warmers and increasing ambient theatre temperatures are used to minimise heat loss. The legs should not be actively warmed during cross clamping.

Pain free patient on completion of surgery.

Balanced general anaesthetic technique is usually used (high dose opioid, oxygen, air, low dose volatile agent) with a thoracic-lumbar epidural oriented to haemodinamic management with deep neuromuscular relaxing. Epidurals ameliorate the stress response to surgery, reducing cardiovascular demands and provide high quality postoperative analgesia, facilitating early extubation and reducing the incidence of pulmonary complications. But, there is no evidence that epidurals reduce mortality. It is safe to insert epidurals on patients taking aspirin and less clear with clopidogrel. Patients should be monitored closely for the symptoms and signs of spinal haematoma (back pain, bladder dysfunction, leg weakness)

3.3.2 Monitoring

Regular observations of the patients and the information provided by monitoring devices must be undertaken and documented. Electronic record keeping is recommended. Monitoring itself cannot prevent adverse reactions during anaesthesia, but basic monitoring reduces the risk of incidents by providing an early warning if the patient's condition worsens. However, human error is inevitable and a number of studies of critical incidents and mortality associated with anaesthesia have shown that adverse events are often attributable to this type of error.

Basic physiologic monitoring in anaesthesia includes continuous display of the electrocardiogram (ECG), intermittent non-invasive measurement of blood pressure (NIBP), pulse oximetry and capnography. Sensitivity increases when a five-lead ECG is used and leads II and V5 are continuously monitored and routine use of a five-lead ECG is strongly recommended in patients with known or suspected coronary artery disease. In patients with one or more cardiac risk factors a pre-operative baseline ECG is recommended to monitor changes during the perioperative period.

Monitoring of anaesthetic equipment comprises the use of an oxygen analyser, capnography, and a disconnection alarm. The use of a vapour analyser is essential if a volatile anaesthetic agent is used.

Then, basic physiologic monitoring with a 5 lead ECG will aid detection of ST segment changes.

In addition to standard monitoring, direct measurement of arterial and central venous pressure, temperature and urine output is mandatory.

Cardiac output during AAA surgery with pulmonary artery flotation catheters, transoesophageal echocardiography (TOE), oesophageal doppler monitoring or pulse contour analysis cardiac output monitoring (LiDCO™ and PiCCO ™) can be considered.

3.3.3 Heparinisation

A dose of 100units/kg of heparine prior to crossclamping has reduced thrombotic and embolic events in the prothesis. Heparin needs to be available five minutes before aortic crossclamping. We must check ACT (activated clotting time) baseline, 3 minutes after heparin given and every 30 minutes thereafter while cross-clamped. Additional heparin may be required in the presence of prolonged clamp times. Heparin can be reversed by protamine if bleeding. Protamine should be used with caution as it may lead to myocardial depression, anaphylaxis and pulmonary hypertension.

3.3.4 Fluid replacement - haemorrhage and blood product management

We have fluid negative balance due to, intestinal cleanse, fasting, osmotic diuresis by previous contrast, intestinal oedema and big lost due to evaporation. We must manage this balance according to aortic crossclamping and diuresis (1,25ml/kg/h).

Blood loss during AAA surgery is highly variable from 500ml to various litters. It is greater in suprarenal aneurysms. Significant bleeding can occur when opening the native aorta due to backbleeding from the lumbar arteries. Blood loss can also result from malpositioned clamps, from leaking anastomosis, excessive heparine or coagulopathy. Homologous blood transfusion can be minimised by intraoperative cell salvage (ICS). Since vascular patients have a high incidence of coronary disease the haematocrit should be kept greater than 27% (Hb > 9g/dl).

Massive haemorrhage more than 2000ml results in a dilutional coagulopathy requiring fresh frozen plasma, cryoprecipitate and platelet transfusions and calcium. Appropriate administration of clotting factors is best guided by near patient testing using a thromboelastograph if possible. Laboratory based coagulation tests which often lag behind the clinical picture. Appropriate goals are an International Normalised Ratio (INR) of less than 1.5, a platelet count of greater than $50 \times 10^9/l$ and fibrinogen levels greater that 1g/dl.

3.3.5 Crossclamping

Aortic cross clamping is necessary in open AAA surgery. The increased vascular resistance results in arterial hypertension. Higher the crossclamping is, higher haemodinamic repercussion and higher hypoperfussion on vital organs. Blood pressure typically rises by 7-10%and until 50% if supraceliac aortic crosscalmping. Blood pressure decreases under the crossclamping about 80%. Aortic crossclamping also increase intracranial pressure.

A diseased coronary system may be unable to respond to increases in cardiac workload resulting in cardiac failure. This may be exacerbated by over fluid administration prior to cross-clamping. Studies show reductions of cardiac output of between 9-33% after infra-renal cross clamping.

We must minimize these haemodinamics effects with: 1.Vasodilators (e.g. urapidil, glyceryl trinitrate, sodium nitroprusside) that may exacerbate organ ischaemia by reducing perfusion pressure in the collateral circulation. 2. Deeper anaesthesia. 3. Small hypovolemia. Aortic crossclamping has compensatory changes as liberation of vasoactive substances due to intestinal ischemia, prostaglandins liberation due to aortic dilatation, hormonal liberation due to ventricular dilatation and vasoactive intestinal peptides and prostaglandins released by the mesenteric traction and evisceration.

Patients with severe aorto-occlusive disease often have a well developed collateral circulation and show minimal response to cross clamping.

3.3.6 Unclamping

Unclamping may result in a dramatic reduction in blood pressure. The causes for this are: a decrease in systemic resistance due to the removal of the cross clamp and the release of vasoactive cytokines and metabolites from ischaemic tissues; central hypovolemia due to sequestration of blood in the reperfused organs and the release of myocardial depressant factors.

The severity of hypotension is proportional to cross clamp time. It also depends on the level of clamp. We must prepare the patient: optimizing and ensuring adequate fluid resuscitation (fluids and blood); with a gradual release of the cross clamp; vasopressors may with the potential disadvantage of preferential vasoconstriction of the vasculature above the clamp; increasing $F_i O_2$; with lighter anaesthesia; reducing metabolic acidosis with HCO_3^- or $CaCl_2$. Reclamping may be required in resistant hypotension.

We must hyperventilate the patients due to metabolic acidosis and also because there are an increase of CO_2. During clamp the arterial CO_2 decreases secondary to deep anaesthesia, no venous return from the inferior part of the body and hypothermia.

3.3.7 Regional circulation

3.3.7.1 Renal system

The incidence of renal failure after AAA surgery is from 0.2% to 5.4% for infrarrenal crossclamping (up to 40% renal blood flow decrease) and 13% for suprarenal crossclamping (80% renal blood flow decrease). The level of aortic crossclamping is the more important risk factor. Other renal risk factors are: Pre existing renal disease; Prolonged clamp time;

Hypotension; Massive haemorrhage; Severity of renal artheriosclerosis; The type of Aortic reconstruction; Increasing age; Contrast nephropathy or Drugs (NSAID's ACEI, aminoglycosides)

Loop diuretics (e.g. furosemide), dopamine, mannitol, fenoldapam and N-acetylcysteine are proposed renal protective agents. There is no Level 1 evidence to support their use. The mainstay of renal preservation is by adequate fluid resuscitation, to diminish clam time, and, the avoidance of nephrotoxins (NSAID's, ACEI, aminoglycosides). Intraoperative diuresis can led fluid therapy but is a bad predictor of the renal perfusion and the postoperative renal function.

3.3.7.2 Digestive system

Bowel complications as intestinal ischemia increase the postoperative mortality in 25%. In the majority of surgeries the inferior mesenteric artery is removed causing ischemic colitis of descendent colon and sigma that can reache 6% if there are not collateral flow. The diagnosis is late due to a high incidence of paralytic ileus. The infrarenal clamp also decreases mesenteric flow due to a regulatory vasoconstriction.

Predisposing factors are: previous medical condition; renal insufficiency; high degree of artheriosclerosis, the level of clamp; time of clamp; hypoblood pressure.

During the clamp ischemia disturbs intestinal permeability and favours bacterial translocation.

3.3.7.3 Nervous system and medullary ischemia

The patient has increased risk of neurological complication if the aorta is clamped above the Major Anterior Segmental Medullary Artery (Artery of Adamkiewicz) which has variable origin: T5-8 15%, T9-12 60%, L1-2 25%.

Anterior spinal syndrome caused by anterior motoneurons ischemia consists of loss of motor (different degree of paraplegia) and pinprick sensation but preservation of vibration and proprioception. In men is frequent unnoticed erectile dysfunction

We can improve ischaemia with a small time of clam; fast surgery; increasing blood perfusion pressure; decreasing CSF; decreasing medullar metabolism by barbiturics or hypothermia.

3.3.8 Postoperative care

Patients require close monitoring after abdominal vascular surgery. Traditionally this has been provided in an Intensive Care Unit. However, careful patient selection coupled with improvements in anaesthetic and surgical techniques allow early extubation and transfer to a High Dependency Units (HDU). Early enteral nutrition is encouraged to maintain gut mucosal integrity and reduce bacterial translocation. Nasogastric tubes are not routinely required. Tight glycaemic control, temperature and analgesia are important. Appropriate antacid and thromboembolic prophylaxis must be prescribed.

3.4 Emergency AAA surgery

Ruptured AAA classically presents with back or abdominal pain, shock and an expanding pulsatile abdominal mass. If the patient is stable the diagnosis can be confirmed by CT scanning. Shocked patients require immediate transfer to the operating theatre and laparotomy. Surgery may be futile in patients with severe pre-existing co-morbidity.

Emergent EVAR should be considered for treatment of a ruptured AAA, if anatomically feasible. Endovascular aneurysm repair (EVAR) is increasing in popularity as it avoids the need for a laparotomy in a group of patients who usually have significant co-morbidity. At present, there are no large, multi-centre, prospective, randomized data assessing the efficacy of EVAR in the treatment of ruptured AAA but many small series have demonstrated a trend towards decreased mortality compared with open repair.

3.4.1 Anaesthetic management

Insertion of two wide bore cannulas. Rapid fluid infusor. Cell salvage blood equipment. Aggressive preoperative fluid resuscitation is contraindicated as it will only serve to increase bleeding and dilute clotting factors.

- Baseline bloods (blood count, electrolytes, coagulation screen).
- Insertion of urinary catheter.
- Forced air warming device.
- Drugs and Fluids: 6 - 10 units of cross matched blood, FFP and platelets; Routine anaesthetic drugs, crystalloids and colloids; Inotropes and vasopressors.

The patient is draped and skin prepared prior to a rapid sequence induction. Loss of abdominal tone combined with the negative inotropic and vasodilatory effects of the anaesthetic agents may result in severe hypotension post induction. Skin incision is made as soon as the airway is secure. Aortic cross clamping is a life saving manoeuvre. For EVAR: Do not induce anaesthesia until aorta is occluded by the balloon, if possible.

After the aorta is cross clamped aggressive fluid resuscitation can be instituted with blood and colloid solutions. A dilutional coagulopathy should be anticipated and FFP and platelets ordered.

Heparinization is not required.

Once haemodynamic stability is obtained arterial and central venous catheters can be inserted, a nasogastric tube passed, and temperature monitoring commenced.

3.4.2 Postoperative care

All patients should be transferred to ICU postoperatively where supportive care includes optimization and maintenance of circulating volume. Re-warming will continue until normal body temperature is achieved and respiratory support is usually required for up to at least 24 h and frequently several days. Renal function, coagulation, haemoglobin, and acid-base balance are monitored closely. There is a high incidence of myocardial ischemia and renal failure. Renal replacement therapy is required in a significant proportion of patients and those with a coagulopathy may require continuing blood product transfusion. Other important issues include an anticipated prolonged ileus and analgesia. Prolonged stays are common due to multi-organ failure.

Patients are particularly prone to developing intra-abdominal hypertension (intra-abdominal pressure> 12 mmHg) and abdominal compartment syndrome (ACS, defined as

IAP > 20 mmHg). Factors which contribute to the development of ACS include anaemia, prolonged hypotension, cardiopulmonary resuscitation, hypothermia, severe acidosis (base deficit > 14 mEq) and aggressive fluid resuscitation (>4 l/h). The International Conference of Experts on Intra-abdominal Hypertension and Abdominal Compartment Syndrome recommends that decompression should be considered at the time of laparotomy in patients who demonstrate multiple risk factors for IAH/ACS (grade 1C) as patients with ruptured abdominal aneurysm. These patients may benefit from laparastoma or mesh closure of the abdominal wall with delayed secondary surgical closure after 2–3 days. No prospective randomized studies are available to validate the concept of the open abdomen protocol. However, retrospective data in the form of case and cohort studies do exist as Rasmussen et al. report. Performing a mesh closure initially in these patients reduces the incidence of multiorgan failure when compared with patients who require a second operation for ACS in the postoperative period. Monitoring of IAP should be considered in all patients and consideration given to parenteral nutrition if ileus is prolonged.

Predictors of survival to discharge include patient age, total blood loss and postoperative hypotension.

3.5 Endovascular aortic aneurysm repair (EVAR)

EVAR was developed as a less invasive alternative to open repair. Modular bifurcated stent grafts are placed via open femoral arteriotomy. This is a combined surgical and radiological procedure which may be performed in theatre or the angiography suite.

Physiological disturbances are reduced as there is no requirement for laparotomy or crossclamping of the aorta. The last guideline for the care of patients with abdominal aortic aneurysm of The Society for Vascular Surgery points the EVAR technique, as a minimally invasive technology that would be associated with lower inhospital and 30-day mortality rates as compared to OSR. Specifically, in-hospital mortality rates were 1.7% - 1.2% for EVAR and 6% - 4.6% for OSR. Procedural blood loss is less for EVAR (414 mL) when compared to OSR (1,329mL), with reductions in ICU (0.7 vs 1.6 d) and hospital (4.2 days vs 9.9 days) stays.

The society of Vascular Surgery also refers that major medical complications are lower after EVAR than OSR. A meta-analysis of observational studies conducted prior to 2002 demonstrated an incidence of systemic complications of 9% after EVAR, as compared with 22% after OSR, largely attributable to fewer cardiac and pulmonary events. It has been observed a lower incidence of cardiac complications in a statewide review of patients treated by EVAR in 2002 (3.3% vs 7.8%). In addition, the latter study noted a reduction in the incidence of pneumonia (9.3% vs 17.4%), acute renal failure (5.5% vs 10.9%), and need for dialysis (0.4% vs 0.5%) among those treated by EVAR.

3.5.1 Indications

A number of reports have documented that EVAR can be performed with low rates of perioperative mortality and morbidity in patients at high risk for open surgery repair (OSR). Additional research is needed to define objective criteria that identify patients who are unfit for OSR and whose anticipated life expectancy limits benefit from EVAR. At present EVAR should be reserved for fit elderly patients (age > 80) and those patients in whom previous abdominal surgery may make open access to the abdominal aorta difficult. The inclusion criteria also depends on the anatomy of the aneurism.

3.5.2 Anaesthetic management of EVAR

EVAR can be safely performed under general, epidural, or local anaesthesia. Lesser degrees of anaesthesia may be of benefit. Mortality differences have not been observed. Local anaesthesia was associated with shorter operative times, reduced ICU admission, shorter hospital stay, and fewer systemic complications. However, the anaesthetist should consider: the problems of anaesthesia in the angiography suite; the requirement for short periods of apnoea; prolonged bilateral femoral occlusion resulting in ischemic pain; the risk (1%) of conversion to an open procedure and the average surgical time of 3 hours with the necessity of an immobile patient.

3.5.3 Monitoring

Basic physiologic monitoring with a 5 lead ECG will aid to detect ST segment changes. In addition to standard monitoring, direct measurement of arterial, temperature and urinary catheterisation is required as the high contrast load may result in nephropathy.

Large bore venous access is necessary as rupture of the aorta or of an iliac artery are reported complications.

3.5.4 Heparinisation

Anticoagulation is recommended. Heparin can be reversed by protamine if bleeding. Protamine should be used with caution as it may lead to myocardial depression, anaphylaxis and pulmonary hypertension.

3.5.5 Fluid replacement - haemorrhage

We must consider fasting and osmotic diuresis by contrast specially in the postoperative cares that can led to a prerenal failure.

Blood loss during is less for EVAR (414 mL) when compared to OSR (1,329mL). We must be aware to the unnoticed blood lost under the drapes and sometime they are important.

Massive haemorrhage can arrive after a vascular rupture.

3.5.6 Radio-contrast injection

Radio-contrast injection can cause allergic reactions in patients with history of asthma, atopy, allergy or previous exposition to up than 20gr of contrast. We can do prophylaxis with dexchlorpheniramine, ranitidine and prednisone.

Contrast is nephrotoxic and can cause acute tubular necrosis. We must prevent it with adequate hydration and n-acetylcysteine 600mg 12h before and the day of surgery.

Radio-contrast can induce osmotic diuresis and polyuria with secondary hypovolemia.

3.5.7 Critical moments during surgery

During surgery we must pay attention to some events: Skin incision, prothesis introduction, device implantation where migration must be prevented by severe bradichardia and hypotension and ballon insuflation to fix the device that results similar to crossclamping but much shorter in time.

3.5.8 Complications

Endoleak, or persistent blood flow in the aneurysm sac outside of the endograft, is the most frequent complication after EVAR and has been reported in nearly one in four patients at some time during followup. It is one of the most common abnormalities identified on late imaging and used to justify lifelong followup of these patients. Type I endoleak occurs in the absence or loss of complete sealing at the proximal (Type IA) or distal (Type IB) end of the stent graft. Type I endoleak is associated with significant pressure elevation in the sac and has been linked to a continued risk of rupture. It should be made to resolve Type I endoleaks noted at the time of EVAR before the patient leaves the intervention suite. On occasion, small persistent Type I endoleaks may be observed and if endovascular intervention has been unsuccessful, the only alternative is surgical conversion. Type II endoleaks are the most common form of endoleak and arise from retrograde filling of the sac by lumbar branches or the inferior mesenteric artery. For those detected at the time of EVAR, further treatment is not indicated, since spontaneous resolution is possible. Type III endoleaks arise from poorly seated modular connections or from disconnection and separation of components. All Type III endoleaks should be treated, typically with limb components, as they represent a lack of exclusion of the aneurysm with repressurization of the aneurysm sac. Type IV endoleaks represents self-limiting blood seepage through the graft material due to porosity and treatment is not required. Typically, this form of endoleak is only noted at the time of repair on post-implantation intra-operative angiography. An endoleak noted on follow-up imaging should not be considered a Type IV endoleak.

Vascular rupture

Technical difficulties for putting the endoguide with the endograf to the right position through the aorta artery.

Device migration

Contrast-induced nephropathy occurs infrequently after EVAR.

The incidence of local vascular or device related complications, as well as the 30-day re-intervention rate is greater after EVAR than OSR. Similar findings have been reported in several observational studies with local or vascular complications occurring in 9% to 16% of patients after EVAR. In the EVAR-1 and EVAR-2 trials, reintervention within 30 days of EVAR occurred in 9.8% and 18% of patients, respectively. Groin and wound complications are the most frequent event. Stents, endografts, or surgical repair may be required if severe vascular access injuries occur.

Distal embolization is now rare with lower profile introducer systems. Limb occlusion occurs more frequently in patients with aortoiliac occlusive disease, a small (<14 mm) distal aorta and tortuous vessels and when unsupported endografts are used.

Post-implantation syndrome, characterized by fever, malaise, back or abdominal pain after EVAR, may last up to 10 days, but appears to be a relatively rare phenomenon. It has been attributed to the release of cytokines after aneurysm sac thrombosis.

3.5.9 Postoperative care

Patients can be transferred to the ward after a brief period of observation in a HDU. Hospital stay is reduced to 24-48h. The Pain is minimum and patient can food almost immediately. We must watch the diuresis and the blood lost. There is a 65% absolute reduction in early (30 day) mortality compared to open repair. This early survival advantage must be balanced against the risk of endograft related complications, in particular endoleak which necessitates annual CT surveillance.

In summary, the recognized benefits of EVAR, including reduced morbidity, ICU and hospital length of stay, as well as observed lower perioperative mortality rates, especially among elderly patients, has led to widespread adoption of this technology. Nonetheless, it is recommended that elective EVAR is best performed at centers that have a documented in-hospital mortality of less than 3% and a primary conversion rate to OSR of less than 2% for elective repair.

Further research is needed to improve EVAR devices and related techniques to reduce complications and long-term follow-up; to identify whether EVAR outcomes vary with respect to endograft type or aneurysm features; and to define the relationship of hospital and physician volume to outcomes after EVAR.

4. References

Anton Leonard, Jonathan Thompson. 2008. Anaesthesia for ruptured abdominal aortic aneurysm. *Continuing Education in Anaesthesia, Critical Care & Pain*, 8,1:11-15.

Brewster DC, Cronenwett JL, Hallett Jr JW, et al. 2003. Guidelines for the treatment of abdominal aortic aneurysms. Report of a subcommittee of the Joint Council of the American Association for Vascular Surgery and Society for Vascular Surgery. *J Vasc Surg*, 37:1106-1117.

Edward J. Norris. 2007. Anesthesia for Vascular Surgery, In: *Miller´s Anesthesia,* Ronald D. Miller,2051-2126, Natasha Andjelkovic, ISBN 978-0-443-06959-8, New York.

Elliot L. Chaikof, David C. Brewster, Ronald L. Dalman, Michel S. Makaroun, Karl A. Illig, Gregorio A. Sicard, Carlos H. Timaran, Gilbert R. Upchurch Jr, Frank J. Veith. 2009. The care of patients with an abdominal aortic aneurysm: The Society for Vascular Surgery practice guidelines. *Journal of Vascular Surgery,* 50, 8S:2S-49S.

Munter Sellevold OF, de Hert S, Pelosi P. 2010.A major step forward: Guidelines for the management of cardiac patients for non-cardiac surgery - the art of anaesthesia. *European Journal of Anaesthesiology*, 27:89-91.

Poldermans D, Bax JJ, Boersma E, et al. 2009. Guidelines for pre-operative cardiac risk assessment and perioperative cardiac management in non-cardiac surgery: The Task Force for Preoperative Cardiac Risk Assessment and Perioperative Cardiac Management in Non-cardiac Surgery of the European Society of Cardiology (ESC) and endorsed by the European Society of Anaesthesiology (ESA). *European Journal of Anaesthesiology,* 27:92-137.

Rasmussen TE, Hallett JW, Jr, Noel AA et al. 2002. Early abdominal closure with mesh reduces multiple organ failure after ruptured abdominal aneurysm repair: guidelines from a 10-year case-control study. *J Vasc Surg,* 35: 246–53

Sakalihasan N, Limet R, Defawe O D. 2005. Abdominal aortic aneurysm. *Lancet*, 365:1577–89.

11

Parametric Stochastic Modelling of Uncertainties in the Mechanical Study of the Abdominal Aneurysm Aorta

Anissa Eddhahak[1], Faîza Mohand Kaci[2] and Mustapha Zidi[2]
[1]*Ecole Spéciale des Travaux Publics, du Bâtiment et de l'Industrie (ESTP), Institut de recherche en constructibilité (IRC),*
[2]*CNRS EAC 4396, Université Paris-Est Créteil Val de Marne, Faculté de médecine, Centre de Recherches Chirurgicales, France*

1. Introduction

1.1 Abdominal Aortic Aneurysm (AAA)

Human body is subjected to many cardiovascular diseases (CVDs) claiming 17.1 million lives a year. Abdominal aortic aneurysms (AAAs), for instance, are the 3th leading cardiovascular cause of death (Sakalihasan et al., 2005; Allaire et al., 2009). The AAA represents a widening of the abdominal aorta generally caused by the hardening of the arteries known as the atherosclerosis. The accumulation of the plaques on the arterial wall leads to its weakness. The blood flow pressure can therefore cause the expansion of the weak arterial part leading thereby to abdominal aneurysm rupture. The AAA can affect either men and women, however statistics have shown that male are five times more likely than female to get AAA. Apart from atherosclerosis, there are many factors which may contribute to the AAA development such as smoking, high blood pressure (hypertension), diabetes, aging, etc.

1.2 Actual pathology solutions

The surgical treatment has been developed in order to avoid aneurysm rupture. Until now, the management of AAAs is instrumental, with intervention decided once the risk of aortic rupture exceeds the risk of elective repair. Traditionally, there are currently two modes of repair available for AAAs, open aneurysm repair, and endovascular stent grafting repair. The first repair consists of opening the abdomen in order to remove the aneurismal aorta part and replace it by a synthetic Dacron tube sewn in place. The second method is less invasive than the open surgey and consists on guiding a graft (stent) within the blood vessel by a catheter just above the damaged aorta section and fastening it to the vessel wall. This technique aims to strengthen the aorta wall and therefore to prevent aneurysm bursting.

It must be noted that the surgical treatment of AAAs carries a high mortality rate of 6 to 14% (Teufelsbauer et al., 2002). No proved cellular or gene therapy exists to inhibit growth or promote healing human AAA. For this reason, fundamental studies were developed *in-vivo* in animal models to recapitulate features of human aneurysms in the hope of finding treatments which could stop AAA expansion (Dobrin et al., 1984) or promote repair. Thus, different experimental approaches have been used like elastase perfusion (Anidjar et al., 1990) or xenograft implantation (Allaire et al., 1994). Elastase perfusion targetting elastin provides vessels which have some characteristics similar to those observed in human AAAs and has been used to study *in-vitro* the "pressure - diameter" response in canine carotids and human iliacs (Dobrin et al., 1984). O'Connell et al. (2003) employed a rat elastase AAA model to investigate the correlation between arterial mechanical properties and tissue microstructure of AAA. Nevertheless, the clinical relevance of the elastase model is not sufficient since it doesn't create the thrombus as observed in the human AAA.

1.3 AAA Cell therapy (endovascular gene) and biomechanical approach

Apart from surgey and endoprothesis treatments, clinical solutions based on cell therapy have been developed. These approaches are based on the finding that AAAs develop because of extracellular matrix destruction and wall atrophy. The xenograft model, for example, consists in decellularizing an abdominal aorta of a particular animal species (i.e. guinea pig), and to graft it orthotopically into a different species (i.e. rat). This process was used by Allaire et al. (2004) in order to evaluate the impact of the injection of smooth muscle cells into formed AAAs and to determine the proportions of elastin, collagen, and nuclear density in the three layers of the graft wall by morphometric methods after diameter stabilization. The authors investigated the efficiency of endovascular smooth muscle cell seeding in promoting endovascular healing and stability in already-developed AAA by matrix metalloprotease-driven injury. In the same experimental model Dai et al. (2005) have developed an endovascular gene therapy approach and showed that a time-limited expression of TGF-ß1 is sufficient for diameter stabilization.

So far no mechanical approach has been developed to evaluate the impact of gene therapy on AAA stabilization. In fact, one of the challenges is to investigate this experimental approach to estimate the variation of stress distributions in the AAA during its expansion and stabilization.

Thus, much attention has been focused over the years on the biomechanics of aneurysms especially to wall stress assessment and constitutive models (Raghavan et al., 1996; Li and Kleinstreuer, 2005; Di Martino et al., 2006; Watton and Hill, 2009). Accordingly, numerous analytical and numerical models have been developed for this objective (Humphrey, 2002; Vorp, 2007) but none in endovascular biotherapies of expanding AAAs using the Xenograft model.

2. Xenograft model

In order to validate concepts of an endovascular gene therapy developed in surgical research laboratory (Allaire et al., 2004; Dai et al., 2005; Allaire et al., 2009), the experimental xenograft model of AAA was used. First, the abdominal aorta of male guinea pigs was removed and decellularized with a detergent, 0.1% sodium dodecyl sulfate (SDS). Then, the aorta was grafted orthotopically into male Lewis rats (200g). Two weeks after xenotransplantation, the aneurysm was formed. The rats were reoperated in order to exclude the xenograft from the blood flow by clamps. An aortectomy performed in the healthy aorta so that a PE10 catheter was introduced into the lumen of AAA. A suspension of viruses representing the gene of interest, TGF-ß1 (Ad-sTGF-ß1), or a control gene, *Escherichia coli* ß-galactosidase (Ad-LacZ) was injected. Finally, the aortotomy was sutured and the blood flow reestablished (Figure 1). Both length and diameter of AAA were measured using an operative microscope under beating heart, before artery treatment or harvest. The measured length corresponded to the distance between the two suture lines of the xenograft. The diameter indicated the maximum dilatation level. Note that no tortuosity of the AAA was observed during measurement.

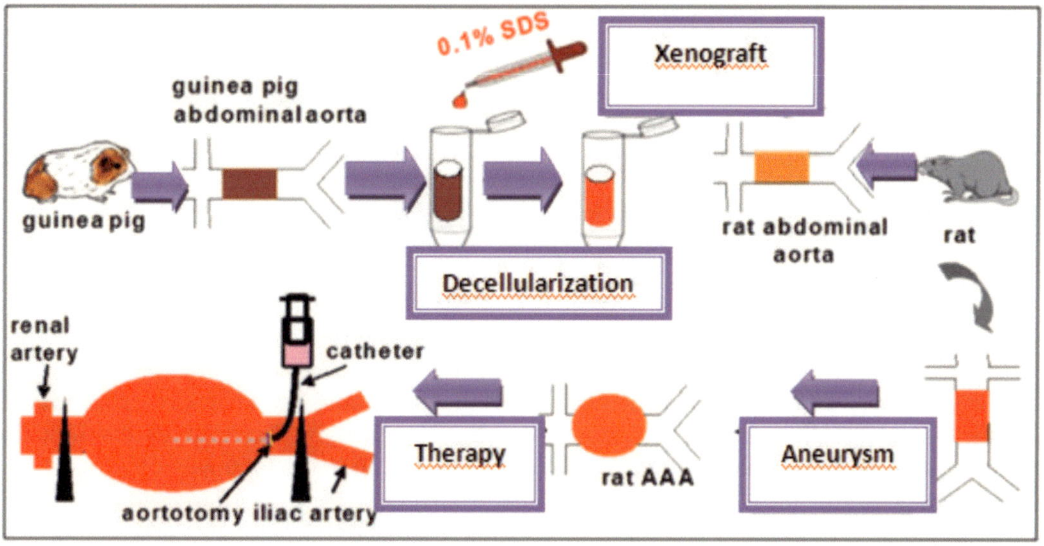

Fig. 1. Different stages of a Xenograft process

In order to study the mechanical behaviour of AAAs in rats during their expansion, , we have used here a membrane model (Humphrey, 2002) based on our experience in gene therapy as well as the xenograft model. Accordingly, it was assumed that the shape of aneurysms is a "parabolic-exponential" function (Elger et al., 1996; Rodriguez et al., 2008, Mohand-Kaci et al., 2011) depending on diameter and length measurements so that the mechanical problem can be solved analytically. Then, in order to investigate the influence of parametric random uncertainty on the growth of AAAs, experimental measurements performed in laboratory were used. A stochastic approach (Jaynes, 1957; Eddhahak et al., 2009) using the principle of maximum entropy is described here to investigate the effect of experimental uncertainties on the evaluation of aorta wall stresses.

3. Mechanical model

Note that the shape of AAAs represents a critical factor influencing the stress distributions in the aorta wall and the aorta rupture mechanism. It was revealed by imaging techniques (Sacks et al., 1999; Lu et al., 2007) that aneurysm can occur in a large variety of complex shapes and sizes. Nevertheless, for simplification reasons, we considered in the present study that the AAA of rats can be described by an axisymmetric "perfect" membrane (Figure 2). Thus, the AAA is defined with a « parabolic-exponential » shape (Elger et al., 1996; Rodriguez et al., 2008) with the parameters R_0, R_a and L_a which denote respectively the initial radius of the abdominal aorta, the radius and the length of the AAA measured during its expansion.

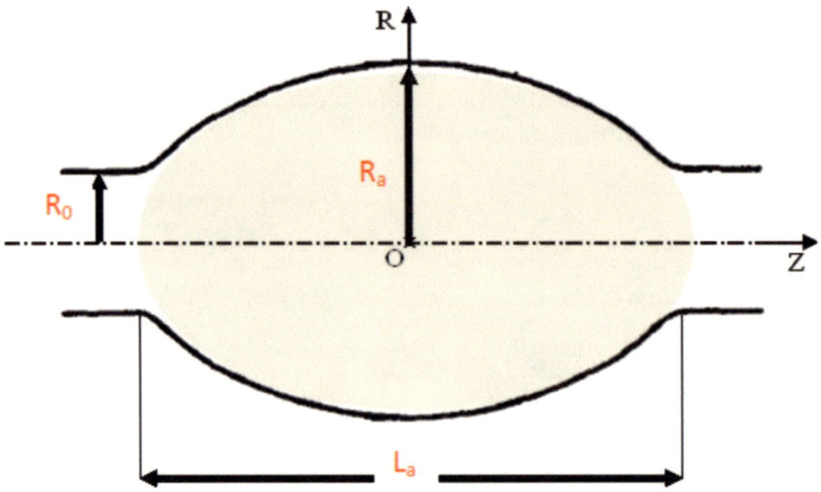

Fig. 2. AAA simplified shape

In the following, given the experimental uncertainties of aorta geometric variables, both radius R_a and length L_a of the aneurysm will be modelled respectively by the random variables $\mathbf{R_a}$ and $\mathbf{L_a}$ (in bold letters). Accordingly, the considered shape was defined by the following function

$$\mathbf{R}(Z) = R_0 + [(\mathbf{R_a} - R_0) - \boldsymbol{\alpha}_3 \frac{Z^2}{R_0}].\exp(-\boldsymbol{\alpha}_1 \left|\frac{Z}{R_0}\right|^{\boldsymbol{\alpha}_2}) \tag{1}$$

where p_1 is a constant whereas α_2 and α_3 are random functions since they depends on random variables. They are linked to $\mathbf{R_a}$ and $\mathbf{L_a}$ by

$$\boldsymbol{\alpha}_2 = \frac{4.605}{(0.5 \times \mathbf{L_a} / \mathbf{R_a})^{\alpha_1}}, \quad \boldsymbol{\alpha}_3 = \frac{R_0(\mathbf{R_a} - R_0)}{(0.5 \times \mathbf{L_a})^2} \tag{2}$$

Moreover, a mechanical study of AAAs has been suggested based on data derived from the xenograft rat protocol. For that, we considered the static membrane theory (Humphrey, 2002) which is independent of the AAA wall material properties. By assuming that the AAA is in equilibrium under a uniform intraluminal pressure, one can write the equilibrium equations for the membrane as

$$\begin{cases} \dfrac{d}{d\mathbf{R}}(\mathbf{R}\boldsymbol{\sigma}_1) = \boldsymbol{\sigma}_2 \\ \mathbf{K}_1\boldsymbol{\sigma}_1 + \mathbf{K}_2\boldsymbol{\sigma}_2 = 1 \end{cases}, \tag{3}$$

where $\boldsymbol{\sigma}_1$ and $\boldsymbol{\sigma}_2$ represent respectively the longitudinal and circumferential stresses. These stresses, normalized by the pressure, are given by

$$\boldsymbol{\sigma}_1(Z) = \frac{1}{2.\mathbf{K}_2} \qquad \boldsymbol{\sigma}_2 = (1 - \frac{\mathbf{K}_1}{2.\mathbf{K}_2}) \tag{4}$$

$\mathbf{K}_1$ and $\mathbf{K}_2$ represent the local curvatures functions obtained from Eq. (1) and expressed as

$$\mathbf{K}_1 = \frac{-d^2\mathbf{R}/dZ^2}{[1+(d\mathbf{R}/dZ)^2]^{\frac{3}{2}}}, \; \mathbf{K}_2 = \frac{1}{\mathbf{R}.[1+(d\mathbf{R}/dZ)^2]^{\frac{1}{2}}}. \tag{5}$$

In order to investigate the wall stresses variations, Von-Mises characteristic equivalent stress was also computed

$$\boldsymbol{\sigma}_{vm} = \sqrt{\boldsymbol{\sigma}_1^2 + \boldsymbol{\sigma}_2^2 - \boldsymbol{\sigma}_1\boldsymbol{\sigma}_2}. \tag{6}$$

Note that the normalized stresses given by Eq. (4) and Eq. (6) depend on geometric random variables characterizing the expansion of AAAs.

In Table 1, we present the measurements corresponding to 4 control and treated groups of rats sacrified at 3 or 28 days. All data are expressed as the average ± the standard error/deviation (SE). Statistical analysis was carried out by one-way ANOVA followed by the Mann Whithney U test. The information $p < 0.05$ was considered statistically significant. In addition, it must be also highlighted that the intraluminal pressure was taken constant and equal to the mean value during a cardiac cycle in AAA of rats. The days D0 and D14 correspond respectively to the Xenograft implantation and the endovascular gene therapy in the artificially formed AAAs.

	Radius (mm)		Length (mm)	
3 days after treatment	Control (n=4)	Treated (n=6)	Control (n=4)	Treated (n=6)
D0	0,75 ± 0,02	0,78 ± 0,02	10,33 ± 0,45	11,38 ± 0,39
D14	1,16 ± 0,12	1,22 ± 0,07	11,88 ± 0,75	13,67 ± 0,40
D14+3	1,18 ± 0,11	1,22 ± 0,07	11,95 ± 0,79	13,83 ± 0,33
Relative variation* (%)	1,32 ± 1,32	0,00 ± 0,00	0,85 ± 4,43	1,31 ± 0,83
p	0,24		0,90	
28 days after treatment	Control (n=5)	Treated (n=5)	Control (n=5)	Treated (n=5)
D0	0,77 ± 0,03	0,76 ± 0,02	11,36 ± 0,42	10,84 ± 0,26
D14	1,15 ± 0,05	1,56 ± 0,16	14,44 ± 0,76	15,70 ± 1,74
D14+28	1,82 ± 0,11	1,71 ± 0,24	16,50 ± 1,48	16,30 ± 1,58
Relative variation* (%)	59, 13 ± 11,24	8, 69 ± 6,80	13,62 ± 4,99	4,50 ± 2,98
p	0,02**		0,17	

*: Between D14 and after treatment
p : Mann Whitney U test for % of variation
**: p< 0,05

Table 1. Experimental measurements of aorta radius and length

The plots of figure 3 depict the longitudinal and circumferential membrane stresses σ_1 and σ_2 computed with respect to the mean (or deterministic) model. The stresses are corresponding to the observation days D0=14days, D3=D0+3days and D28=D0+28days. The notation "Dx Ly" in the graph denotes the measurement recorded at the day x and corresponding to the rats group y. The comparison with the initial AAA at D0 reveals that the membrane aortic stresses change very slightly after 3 days in both control and treated cases. On the contrary, a significant increase is noticed at D28. Furthermore, as consequence of a stress gradient due to the axial lesion one can also remark that the stress pick appears always at the maximum radius of the AAA and the medium axial position (Z = 0).

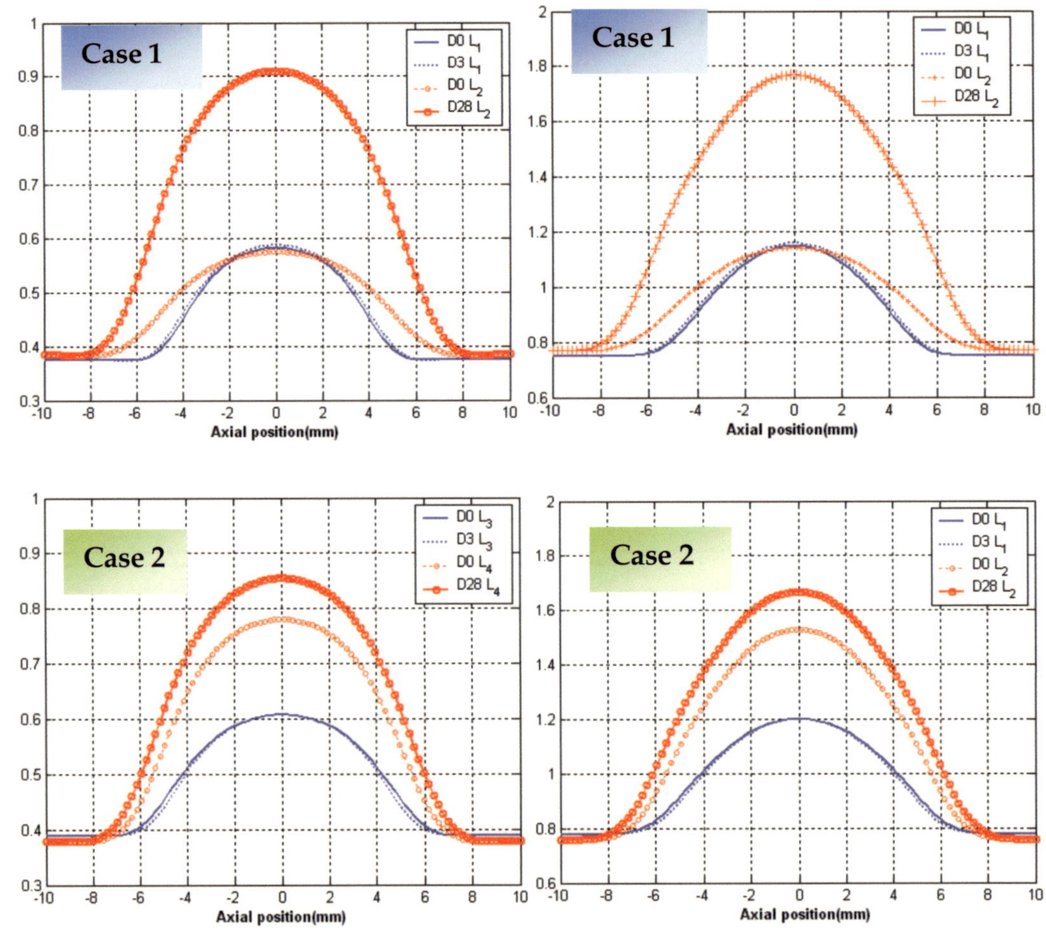

Fig. 3. Variation of normalized aortic stresses versus axial position (Right: σ_2, Left: σ_1).

Indeed, the expansion of AAA influences the magnitude of the peak stress in the aorta wall. The stress amplification is then evaluated to 58% and 55 % for respectively σ_1 and σ_2 as shown in the upper curves. In addition, one can note that the difference between the upper row curves corresponding to the control case (case 1) is more important that the one of the second row corresponding to the gene therapy case (case 2) notably at the axial position Z = 0. This first biological finding highlights the advantageous of the suggested gene therapy treatment which decreases the wall mechanical stresses in AAAs and improves therefore their mechanical behaviors. In Figure 4, we emphasize on this last finding by comparing the differences of membrane stresses in both treated and control cases.

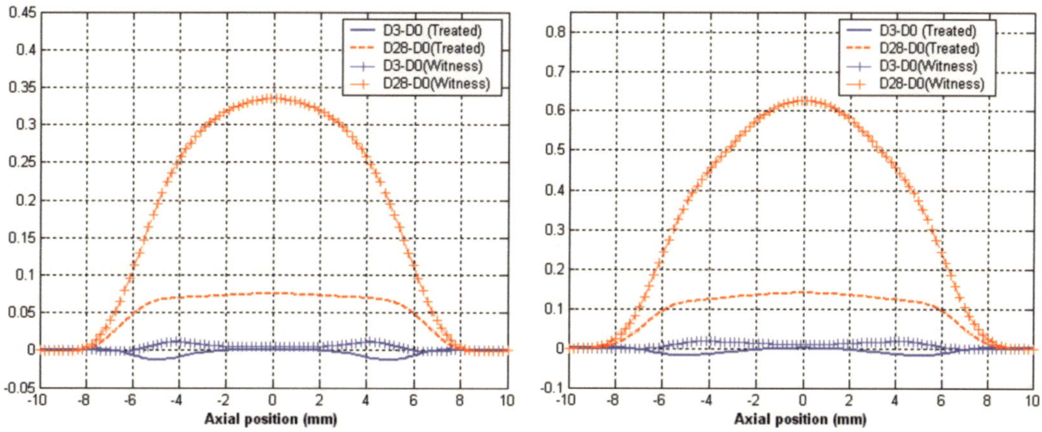

Fig. 4. Effect of gene therapy treatment on the membrane stresses (Right: σ_2, Left: σ_1).

4. Probabilistic parametric modelling of AAA uncertainties

In this section, a stochastic approach taking into account the random dispersion of the experimental measurements related to the growth of AAAs is presented. Dealing with *in-vivo* measurements of rat aortas, the experimental recorded values are often subjected to uncertainties due to the lack of accuracy. The probabilistic parametric approach is an efficient mechanical tool which allows the description of random uncertain parameters by adequate random variables. This description is performed by the attribution of suitable probability density functions (pdf) respective to the considered random variables. The construction of the pdf is not arbitrary and shall take into consideration the available information which may be, for instance, the mean of the random variable, the interval to which it belongs, the standard deviation, the higher order moment, etc.

More general, let consider a parameter x subjected to uncertainty, the random variable denoted X is the stochastic modelling associated to x. The dispersion of X is then measured by the entropy function defined by

$$S(X) = -\int_{-\infty}^{+\infty} p_X(x)\log(p_X(x))dx. \tag{7}$$

where p_X is the pdf associated to the random variable X. This function is determined according to the principle of maximum entropy (Shannon, 1948) which states that the determination of the pdf is obtained by the maximization of the uncertainty on the light of the available used information. The latter defines a set of constraints which govern the optimization problem. The mathematical resolution leads to express the pdf as

$$p_x(x) = \Pi_{[V^-,V^+]}(x)\exp\left(-\lambda_0 - \sum_{t=1}^{n} \lambda_t g_t(x)\right) \quad (8)$$

where λ_i are the Lagrange multipliers, $g_i(x)$ are the different constraints of the optimization problem and Π is the indicator function given by

$$\Pi_{[V^-,V^+]} = \begin{cases} 1 \, if \; x \in [V^-, V^+]] \\ 0 \; if \; not \end{cases} \quad (9)$$

Where $[V^-, V^+]$ represents the support of the pdf associated to the random variable X

The reader could consult (Soize, 2001; Kapur, 1992) for further information on the parametric probabilistic approach using the principle of maximum entropy.

The proposed stochastic approach is adapted to the biomechanical membrane model in order to analyze the influence of geometric parameters on the aorta stress distributions during the expansion of AAAs in the xenograft model.

In our case, the knowledge of the available information (average + support + standard deviation), the pdf of each random variable X can be expressed as

$$p_X(x) = \Pi_{[V^-,V^+]}(x)\exp(-\lambda_0(V^-,V^+,m_x,\sigma_x) - x\lambda_1(V^-,V^+,m_x,\sigma_x) - x^2\lambda_2(V^-,V^+,m_x,\sigma_x)), \quad (10)$$

where λ_0, λ_1 and λ_2 are the optimal values which minimize the convex function H

$$H(\lambda_0,\lambda_1,\lambda_2) = \lambda_0 + \lambda_1 m_x + \lambda_2 m_2 + \int_{V^-}^{V^+} \exp(-\lambda_0 - x\lambda_1 - x^2\lambda_2)dx \, . \quad (11)$$

Where m_2 denotes the second order moment linked to the average and the standard deviation of X by

$$m_2 = m_x^2 + \sigma_x^2 \, . \quad (12)$$

For instance, the values of λ_0, λ_1 and λ_2 corresponding to $\mathbf{R_a}$ (control case, at D28) are respectively equal to 134.48, -150.41 and 41.32.

Thus, for each random variable, we performed 2000 random independent realizations according to the considered pdf. Figure 5 presents the different realizations of $\mathbf{R_a}$ and $\mathbf{L_a}$ for the control case.

The numerous trials performed for the random variables $\mathbf{R_a}$ and $\mathbf{L_a}$ allow the determination of different responses/realizations corresponding to the longitudinal and circumferential normalized membrane stresses σ_1 and σ_2. Accordingly, a confidence region with a high probability of 99% can be defined in order to predict the numerous potential aorta wall stresses responses. The upper and lower bounds of this confidence interval are plotted in figure 6 and compared with the mean model result for both treated and non treated cases.

As can be noticed, the deterministic model response lies inside the confidence interval. The stochastic membrane stresses results show a similar evolution than the deterministic model. Note that the estimation error recorded for σ_1 and σ_2, in cases 1 and 2, can reach

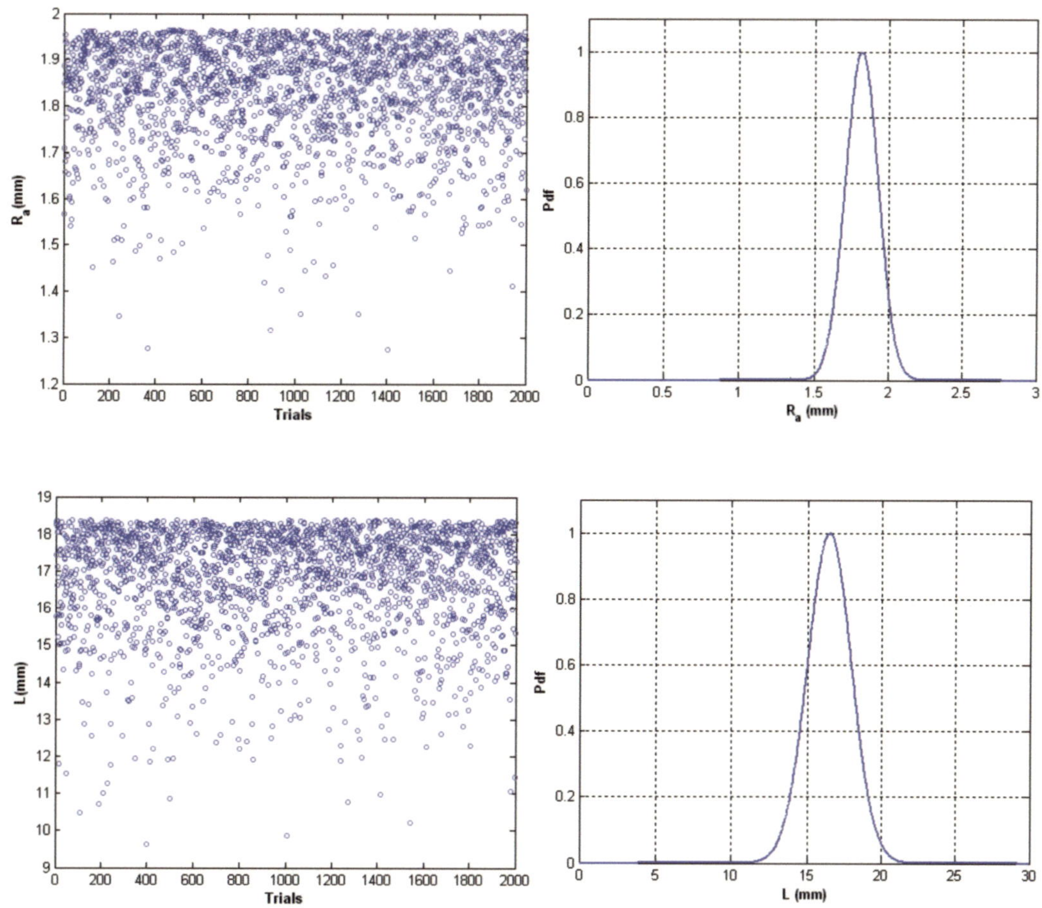

Fig. 5. Realizations and pdf of AAA radius and length

approximately 28%. The aortic mechanical stresses may be underestimated when a stochastic modelling is not considered. This last finding highlights the importance to take into account the parametric random uncertainties in order to obtain realistic estimations of the wall aorta membrane stresses.

Simulations of Monte Carlo (Kalos and Whitlock; 1992) are also carried out to show the convergence of the stochastic process by computing both the mean and the standard deviation (Std) of the Von-Mises stress for cases 1 and 2. Figure 7 illustrates this convergence reached at nearly the 1400th realization for cases 1 and 2. At convergence, the Von Mises equivalent stress is recorded. One can note that the averages of the normalized Von Mises stresses for cases 1 and 2 are respectively equal to 1.54 and 1.43.

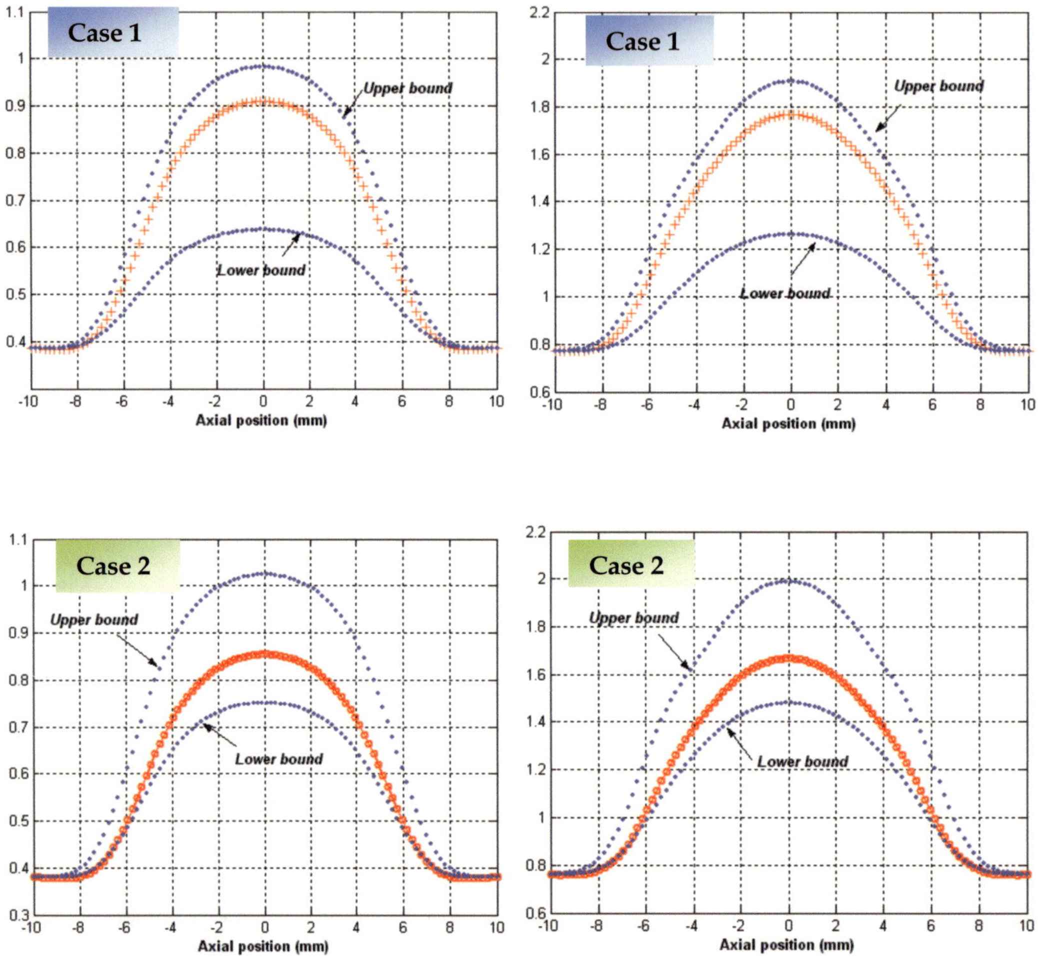

Fig. 6. Stochastic confidence intervals for the aorta membrane stresses (Right: σ_2, Left: σ_1).

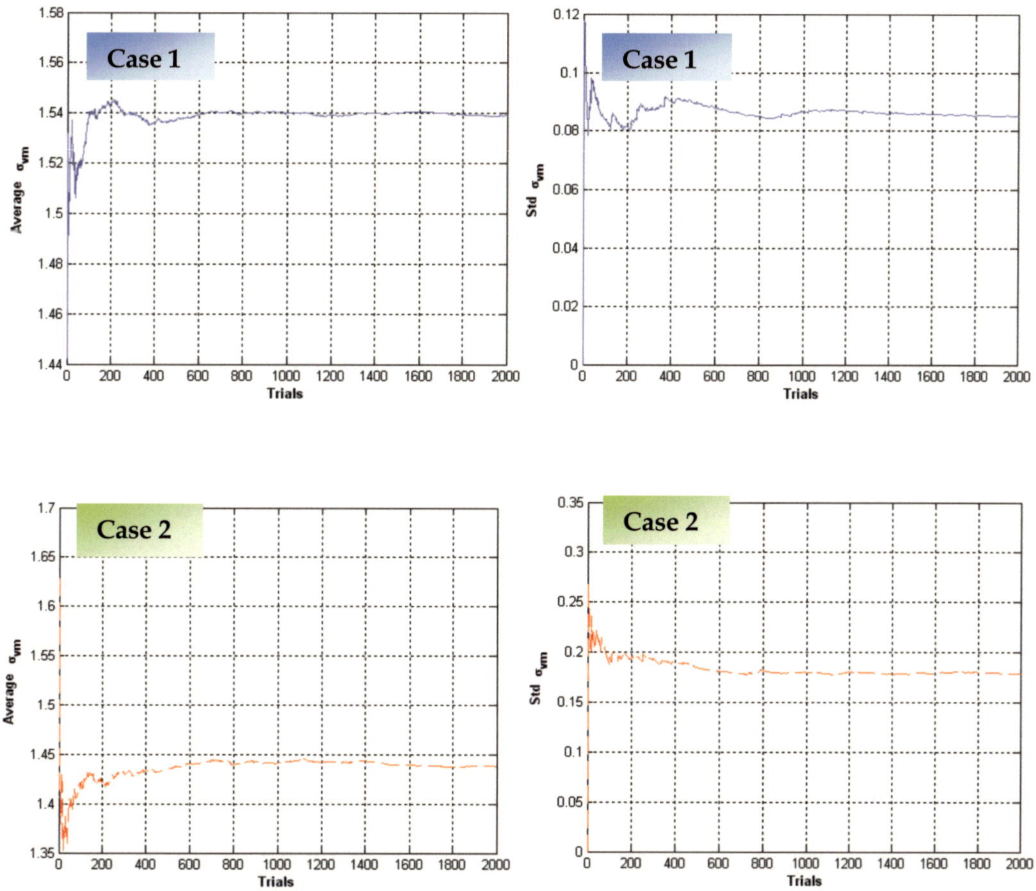

Fig. 7. Monte Carlo simulations

5. Conclusions

In this chapter, a stochastic biomechanical approach adapted to a xenograft model for AAA therapy is presented. The *in-vivo* geometric aorta characteristics (radius and length) were recorded at several days for both control and artificially damaged aortas. Thereby, experimental measurement uncertainties were considered and used for the assessment of parametric probabilistic model based on the principle of maximum entropy. It was shown that the presented endovascular gene therapy reduces significantly the stress variations while stabilizing AAA and likely prevented rupture probability of the artery. In addition, from a stochastic point of view the random experimental uncertainties were described by adequate probability density functions for a safe estimation of AAA wall stresses. Monte Carlo stochastic solver was used and it was noticed its reliability to reach convergence of the probabilistic simulations. This approach can also be generalized for other arterial diseases and can contribute to the improvement of our understanding of the arterial mechanical behavior.

6. Acknowledgment

We gratefully acknowledge Pr E. Allaire and Dr J. Dai from the Research Surgical Center of Henri Mondor Hospital for their experimental data.

7. References

Allaire E, Muscatelli-Groux, B., Guinault, A.M., Pages, C., Goussard, A., Mandet, C., Bruneval, P., Méllière, D, Becquemin, J.P., Vascular Smooth Muscle Cell Endovascular Therapy Stabilizes Already Developed Aneurysms in a Model of Aortic Injury Elicited by Inflammation and Proteolysis, Annals of Surgery 239(3), p. 417-427, 2004.

Allaire E, Schneider, F., Saucy, F., Dai, J., Cochennec, F., Michineau, S., Zidi, M., Becquemin J.P., Kirsh M, Gervais M., New Insight in Aetiopathogenesis of Aortic Diseases, European Journal of Vascular and Endovascular Surgery 37, p. 531-537, 2009.

Allaire, E., Guettier, C., Bruneval, P., Plissonnier, D., Michel, J.B., *Cell-free arterial grafts: morphologic characteristics of aortic isografts, allografts, and xenografts in rats, Journal of Vascular Surgery* 19, p. 446-56, 1994.

Anidjar, S, Salzmann, J.L., Gentric, D, Lagneau, P., Camilleri, P., Michel, J.B., *Elastase-induced experimental aneurysms in rats,* Circulation 82, p. 973–81, 1990.

Baek, S, Gleason. RL., Rajagopal, K.R., Humphrey, J.D. Theory of small on large: Potential utility in computations of fluid-solid interactions in arteries. Computer Methods in Applied Mechanics and Engineering 196, p.3070-3078, 2007.

Dai, J., Losy, F., Guinault, A.M., Pagès, C., Anegon, I., Desgranges, P., Becquemin J.P., Allaire E. Overexpression of Transforming Growth Factor-beta 1 stabilizes already-formed aortic aneurysms. A first approach to induction of functional healing by endovascular gene therapy, Circulation 112, p. 1108-1115, 2005.

Di Martino, E.S., Bohra, A., Vande Geest, J.P., Gupta, N., Makaroun, M.S., Vorp, D.A., *Biomechanical properties of ruptured versus electively repaired abdominal aortic aneurysm wall tissue,* Journal of Vascular Surgery 43(3), p. 570-576, 2006.

Dobrin, P.B., Baker, W.H., Gley, W.C., *Elastolytic and collagenolytic studies of arteries. Implications for the mechanical properties of aneurysms*, Archives of Surgery 119, p. 405-409, 1984.

Eddhahak, A., Masson, I., Allaire, E., Zidi, M., Stochastic approach to estimate the arterial pressure, European Journal of Mechanics - A/Solids 28, p. 712-719, 2009.

Elger, D.F., Blackketter, D.M., Budwig, R.S., Johansen, K.H., *The influence of shape on the stresses in model abdominal aortic aneurysms*, Journal of Biomechanical Engineering 118, p. 326–332, 1996.

Humphrey, J.D,Cardiovascular Solid Mechanics: Cells, Tissues, and Organs. Springer-Verlag, New York.

Jaynes E.T., Information theory and statistical mechanics, Physical Review 106, p. 620-630,1957.

Kalos, M.H., Whitlock, P.A., *Monte-Carlo Methods Volume 1: Basics*, John Wiley and Sons, Chistester, 1992.

Kapur, J.N., Kesavan, H.K., *Entropy Optimization Principles with Applications*, Academic Press, San Diego, 1992.

Li, Z., Kleinstreuer, C., *A new wall stress equation for aneurysm rupture prediction*, Annals of Biomedical Engineering 33, p. 209–213, 2005.

Lu, J., Zhou, X., Raghavan, M.L., *Inverse elastostatic stress analysis in pre-deformed biological structures: Demonstration using abdominal aortic aneurysms*, Journal of Biomechanics 40 p. 693–696, 2007.

Mohand-Kaci F, Eddhahak Ouni A, Dai J, Allaire, Eric and Zidi M, Stochastic modelling of wall stresses in abdominal aortic aneurysms treated by a gene therapy', Computer Methods in Biomechanics and Biomedical Engineering, First published on: 24 January 2011 (iFirst).

O'Connell , M.K., Kimura, H., Sho, E., Sho, M., Dalman, R.L., Taylor, C.A. Correlation of mechanical properties and microstructure of rat elastase-inffusion abdominal aortic aneurysms, Summer Bioengineering Conference, p. 0871-0872, 2003.

Raghavan, M.L., Webster, M.W., Vorp, D.A., *Ex-vivo biomechanical behavior of abdominal aortic aneurysm: assessment using a new mathematical model*, Annals of Biomedical Engineering 24, p. 573–582, 1996.

Rodriguez, J.F., Doblaré, M., Holzapfel, G.A., *Mechanical stresses in abdominal aneurysms: influence of diameter, asymmetry, and material anisotropy*, Journal of Biomechanical Engineering 130, 2008.

Sacks, M.S., Vorp, D.A., Raghavan, M.L., Federle, M.P., Webster, M.W., *In vivo three-dimensional surface geometry of abdominal aortic aneurysms*, Annals of Biomedical Engineering 27, p. 469-79, 1999.

Sakalihasan, N., Limet, R., Defawe O.D., *Abdominal aortic aneurysm*, Lancet 365(9470), p. 1577-1589, 2005.

Soize, C., *Maximum entropy approach for modeling random uncertainties in transient elastodynamics*, Journal of Acoustics 109, 2001.

Tang D, Yang, C, Zheng, J, Woodard, PK, Sivard, GA, Saffitz, JE, Yuan, C, 2004. 3D MRI-based multicomponent FSI models for atherosclerosis plaques. Annals of Biomedical Engineering, 32, p.947-960, 2004.

Teufelsbauer, H., Prusa, M. A., Wolff, K., Polterauer, P., Nanobashvili, J., Prager, M., Hölzenbein, T., Thurnher, S., Lammer, J., Schemper, M., Kretschmer, G., and Ihor

Huk. Endovascular Stent Grafting Versus Open Surgical Operation in Patients With Infrarenal Aortic Aneurysms : A Propensity Score -Adjusted Analysis, Circulation, 2002.
Vorp, D.A., *Biomechanics of abdominal aortic aneurysm*, Journal of Biomechanics 40, p. 1887–1902, 2007.
Watton, P.N., Hill, N.A., *Evolving mechanical properties of a model of abdominal aortic aneurysm*, Biomechanics and Modeling in Mechanobiology 8(1), p. 25-42, 2009.
Zidi M., Cheref M., Finite deformations of a hyperelastic, compressible and fibre reinforced tube. European Journal of Mechanics A/solids 21(6), p. 971-980, 2002.

12

How to Find New Ways

Simon Florian
University Hospital Düsseldorf, Germany

1. Introduction

Subject of this article is to show how research can be build up and what fields are to consider. If you want to perform modern research you have to look at different aspects of the same problem. Therefore we established three research groups to illuminate the problem of ischemia and reperfusion injury after aortic clamping. The aim of this three study groups is to find answers to questions in the field of pre- and perioperative conditioning to improve the outcome or even avoid negative effects of an ischemia reperfusion injury upcoming every day in the clinical situation of a vascular surgeon.

There is a high prevalence of hypertonia and arteriosclerosis in the industrial countries in our days. Therefore we have to expect an increase in the incidence of aortic aneurysms and the need for surgical intervention. Other reasons for aortic damage are injuries after trauma and dissections of the vascular wall. Thoracic aneurysms appear in nearly 25 % of the cases whereas abdominal aneurysms take place in round about 75 %. In most of the cases the aneurysm has to be resected operatively. During this procedure the blood flow is stopped by two clamps putted up- and downward of the aneurysm. The aneurysmatic vessel is replaced by prosthesis and blood flow is restored (Orend 1995). This means that all organs, supplied by this part of the aorta, are suffering from ischemia during the surgical procedure.

Nearly 30 % of all patients, undergoing surgical replacement of the thoracic-abdominal part of the aorta, are suffering afterwards from severe postoperative problems. These problems are caused by the inevitable ischemia of the lower body half during the clamping and the following reperfusion injury, taking place with the declamping of the aortic vessel. This is the reason why the replacement of an aortic aneurysm is a classical clinical example of an ischemia and reperfusion sequence. The most frequently upcoming complications after elective, open surgical repair of an aortic aneurysm are cardiovascular and respiratory insufficiency. Intraoperatively patients are endangered mostly by the huge change in hemodynamic situation, because clamping of the aorta causes a fulminant increase in blood pressure. Without pharmacological intervention the ejection fraction of the heart would decrease by 40 %. An ongoing overload of the heart would end in dilatation of the left ventricle with hypoperfusion of the inner heart muscle, insufficiency of the mitral valve and lung edema resulting in cardiovascular arrest (Walther 2000). Blankensteijn *et al* state in a meta-analysis of 72 studies 4.9 to 13.6 % as cardial and 3.8 to 13.5 % as pulmonal complications (Blankensteijn 1998).

Paraplegia as a consequence of spinal ischemia is the most important complication after reconstruction of the thoracic aorta. The incidence of paraplegia depends on the aneurysmatic dimension and comorbidities and ranges therefore from 0.5 %, in case of a small repair e.g. the aortic arch, to 40 % in case of a ruptured thoracic aortic aneurysm (Svensson 1993, Money 1994, Zvara 2002). Several potential reasons for postoperative paraplegia were experimentally evaluated. Main subjects were amongst others ischemia and the resulting hypoxia plus an increase of the liquor pressure during the clamping period and the reperfusion injury after declamping (Crawford 1990, Bergner 1992, Zvara 2002). Ischemia and reperfusion cause an increase of free radicals that consume the existing buffer enzymes (Gelman 1995, Willett 2001). During hypoxia mitochondrial phosphorylation slows down with a consecutive loss of ATP that causes inhibition of the membrane pumps that are responsible for cell homeostasis. Finally dysbalance of the Na^+/K^+-milieu appears accompanied by hyperkalemia, acidosis and cell edema. At the end cells undergo programmed death, called apoptosis (Abe 1995). An additional aggravating factor is that the anterior motor neurons and the spinal cord have a high metabolic rate in combination with low hypoxic tolerance (Sakurai 1998), that make the neurons extremely sensitive to fluctuations in oxygen supply. Another important thing is the time factor, because clamping shorter than 30 minutes shows only little impact on the neurological tissue while longer ischemia periods coincide with a high risk for neurological damage like e.g. paraplegia (Hatori 2000, Wahlberg 2002, Roques 2003). Adequate blood supply for the spinal tissue can be measured electro physiologically by using somatosensoric (SEP) or motor evoked potentials (MEP). SEP´s show mainly the signal transduction of the dorsal part of the spinal cord while the MEP´s allow the monitoring of the neurons of the anterior horn and of the tractus corticospinalis. Experiments comparing these two methods showed that SEP´s react with a delay on spinal cord ischemia and have a high wrong positive rate. In contrast 18 out of 38 patients that underwent thoracic-abdominal reconstruction of the aorta showed pathological MEP-results. This changing's in MEP measurement were attenuated by protective procedures e.g. reinsertion of segmental arteries. A loss of more than 75 % of the baseline MEP amplitude was taken as a sign for an ischemic spinal cord dysfunction. Paraplegia rate in this study, using MEP monitoring, was 0 % (de *Haan 1999, Meylaerts 1999, 2000*).

The risk for renal complications is about 15 to 20 % and depends on location of aneurysm, mainly of the lower thoracoabdominal or infrarenal aorta (Back 2005) and on potentially existing preoperative damages of the renal tissue of the patients. Creatinine levels over 230 mmol/L and - or renal ischemia time over 60 minutes increase the risk of postoperative necessary dialysis, that occurs in 5 to 10 % of the cases (Kazautchian 1994). In patient with acute kidney failure that results in postoperative dialysis prognosis worsen dramatically with an increase of mortality up to 75 %. The higher the preoperative creatinine level the poorer the postoperative outcome of the patients (Svensson 1993). These facts show the need for new strategies to attenuate the harmful impact of ischemia and reperfusion on the spinal cord and the renal tissue. Before patients can benefit from new e.g. drugs and therapies that avoid tissue damage, experiments must be done, that ensure safety to humans. Therefore a valid experimental model to investigate new strategies in the field of ischemia and reperfusion is warranted. The next chapters show how our group is working on different aspects of the same problem, namely ischemia and reperfusion, to show up new strategies and hopefully give answers to questions of clinical problems in a vascular department.

2. Large animal model

For the realisation of a valid large animal model pigs are the appropriate species. Anatomically (position and configuration of the thoracic and abdominal organs, spinal cord and blood supply) metabolically as well as physio- and pathophysiologically pigs show the biggest homology with humans (Dodds 1982). We used pigs of both gender with a body weight of 40 to 50 kg in average and about 3 to 4 month of age. Furthermore other animal models were described before by other experimental groups (de Haan 1999, Hellberg 2000, Meylaerts 1999, 2000). Therefore we adapted the experimental setup to fit our special needs to examine ischemia and reperfusion in a standardised model (Schelzig 2003, Kick 2007). Another advantage of a large animal model is the easy surgical preparation, the possibility for neurological examinations and the acquisition of enough blood samples for further analytics. Via femoral cut down, catheter sheaths were introduced into the *Aa. femorales sinistra* and *dextra* for distal blood pressure recording and placement of inflatable balloon catheters. One catheter was placed directly above the porcine aortic bifurcation, the other one directly downstream of the *A. subclavia sinistra* as shown in Figure 1.

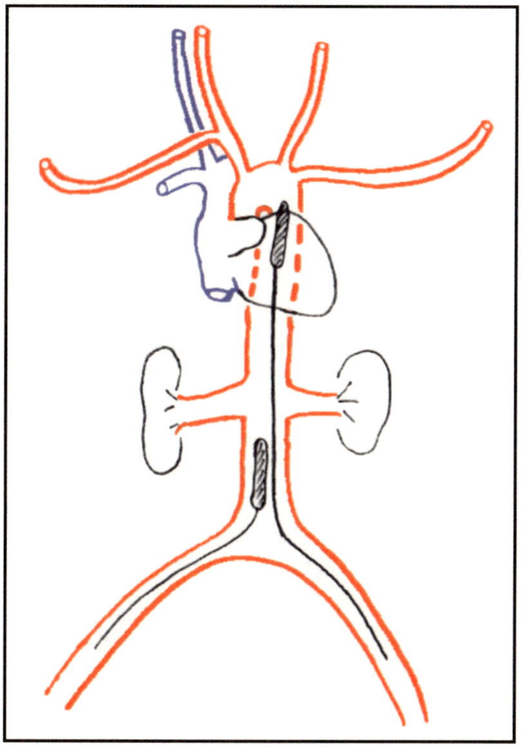

Fig. 1. Position of the two inflatable balloon catheters.

This approach was chosen in order to prevent any perfusion of the spinal cord via collateral flow distal to the proximal balloon, which could result from variable origin of the *A. radicularis magna anterior*. The intra-aortic balloon occlusion was used in order to avoid the mechanical injury, related to a clamp placement and release *per se*. A mini-laparotomy was performed to place a catheter into the bladder for save and controlled urine sampling. To examine the neurological function of the spinal cord we established motor evoked potentials (MEP) that were already described above. Three electrodes were placed in the pig's calvarium and one in the soft palate for electric stimulation of the motor cortex. Answers of the peripheral nerves were assessed in the lower limbs. After this model was well established over several years we tested different substances to see if there is any benefit compared to control groups. The next chapters give a short overview of some of the studies performed with this animal model.

2.1 Erythropoietin (EPO)

One of the first drugs we tested was erythropoietin (EPO). The reasons for choosing a substance that is known for so many years were the experimental results of other groups that discovered new aspects of EPO. Experiments dealing with apoptosis and neurological disability after ischemic impact on the spinal cord showed that EPO had not only some positive effects but seemed to attenuate the damage to the motor neurons at a notable range (Celik 2002). There were also reports of improved renal tissue function after ischemia and reperfusion in animal models (Ates 2005, Forman 2007). Interestingly EPO was already in focus of human studies dealing with stroke and also reporting beneficial effects in the patients outcome, even though this results were only preliminary (Ehrenreich 2002). After we were sure that EPO would be an interesting candidate to take a closer look at, we had the problem of which doses to take, because most of the experiments in literature used high EPO doses. Only some experimental groups examined doses comparable to those used in hospital dealing with anemia (Silver 2006) also showing positive effects on spinal cord and kidney damage after trauma and ischemia and reperfusion (Kaptanoglu 2004, Abdelrahman 2004). Therefore we started our large animal experiments dealing with "low dose" EPO and its effects on spinal cord and kidney function after an ischemia and reperfusion sequence.

14 anesthetized, ventilated and instrumented pigs twice received EPO (n=8; 300IU/kg both over 30 minutes before as well as over 4 hours during reperfusion) or vehicle (n=6). During the early reperfusion period i.v. noradrenaline was titrated continuously as required to maintain MAP > 80 % of the baseline level. Kidney function was assessed by PAH- and creatinine-clearance, spinal cord function by motor evoked potentials and lower extremity reflexes, respectively. DNA damage in whole blood samples was evaluated with the alkaline version of the comet assay. Oxidative stress was determined by isoprostane, catalase and superoxiddismutase in blood and renal tissue. After 8 hours of reperfusion post mortem tissue samples were taken for histological evaluation. Kidney and spinal specimen were analysed for apoptosis (TUNEL-assay). Spinal cord damage was quantified using the Nissl staining. Results show that conditions were stable throughout the whole experiments, meaning that as well hemodynamics as parameters of gas exchange were comparable between both groups without significant differences. This is a strongly recommended requirement to gain results that allow comparison of the experimental groups. Interestingly the amount of given noradrenaline, needed to keep blood pressure in the targeted range, was significantly lower in the EPO treated group. The fact of stable hemodynamics in combination with lower need for catecholamine may indicate an improved peripheral vascular resistance. It is also possible that vasoconstrictor vessel response is improved by EPO. Because of the shortness noradrenaline must be given, it is very likely that with EPO treated animals also have an improved cardiac function. These findings fit well with

findings in other experiments demonstrating positive effects of EPO on the heart of rats after myocardial infarction (Moon 2005). Although there were no clinical differences related to the spinal cord function, assessed by lower limbs reflexes and MEP-Amplitudes, we saw a significant higher number of intact neurons in the thoracic histological Nissl-stainings. This benefit unfortunately was lost in the lumbar histological staining, while HE-staining in both, the thoracic and the lumbar slices, showed cytoplasmatic swelling and vacuolisation as an indicator for spinal cord injury.

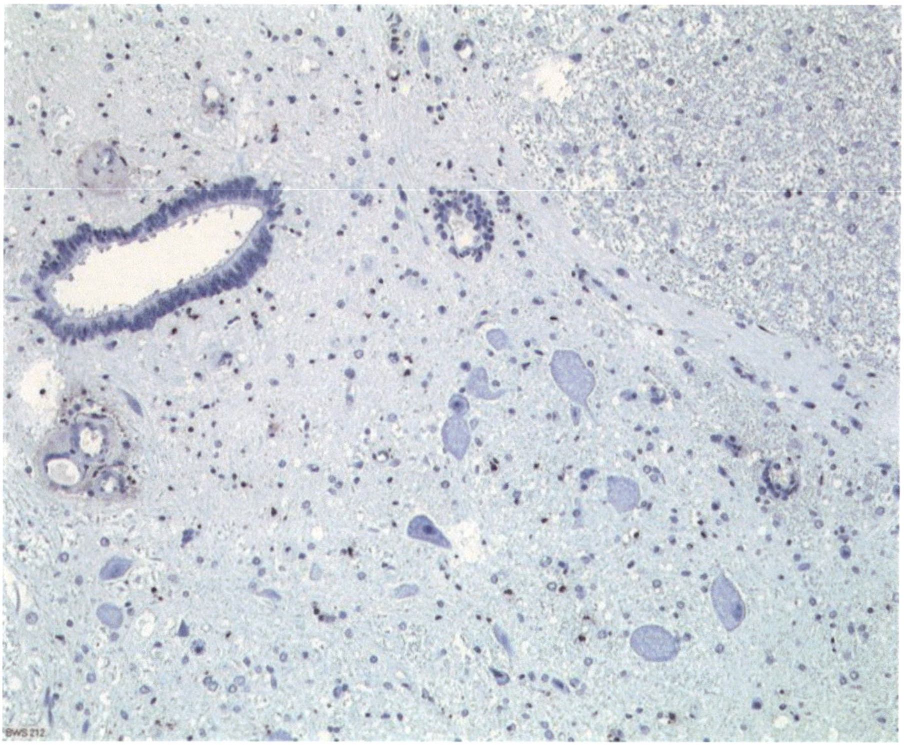

Fig. 2. Nissl-staining of a spinal cord slice showing swollen neurons as a sign of hypoxic injury.

Finally TUNEL-staining of microglia and astrocytes also imposed with less damage in the thoracic slices, but not at the lumbar level. These results show a positive effect of EPO on the neurological tissue, but this does not mean necessarily also an intact clinical outcome. One forth of the neurons was damaged by hypoxia, what might be too less for a proper function. The results of the kidney function showed an improvement as well of the creatinine clearance as of the fractional Na-excretion. Important in this context is that renal hemodynamics, namely renal blood flow, were comparable between the two groups meaning that differences between the groups are no artefacts caused by different postischemic perfusion. Urine production however was comparable between the groups. Interestingly these renal differences had no equivalent in the histological HE- or the TUNEL-staining. At least even systemic parameters of oxidative stress and antioxidant enzyme activity showed no intergroup differences. We can only have a guess why we have clinical relevant effects of EPO on the glomerular and tubular kidney function but see no histological or oxidative stress parameters. One point of view might be that 45 minutes of ischemia is a relatively low challenge on renal tissue so that temporarily improved global renal function must not result in histological changing's demonstrating a severe damage to the kidney tissue. This aspect is underlined by the gentle increase in plasma creatinine that indicates a possible recovering of the kidneys without any therapeutic intervention. The other point is that a reperfusion period of 8 hours might be too short to see already histological damages in renal tissue when the ischemic stress was not very excessive. In conclusion we can say that EPO has beneficial effects on cardiac and vascular hemodynamics, it improves the surviving of neuronal tissue and it protects kidney from acute failure. The lesson we learned out of that, was, that we can not examine two different organs in one single experimental setup and therefore have to split experiments in future. On the one hand we will have the spinal cord group with shorter clamping period and on the other hand we will have the kidney branch with prolonged ischemia time (Simon 2008).

2.2 H_2S – proof of principle

The second substance we focused on was the hydrogen sulfide (H_2S), because there was a remarkable study in mice. In this experiment mice were exposed to an atmosphere with 80 ppm H_2S. Just by inhaling this gas atmosphere the animals fell in a "suspended animation-like" metabolic status. This is characterised by reduced metabolism, hypothermia and reduced O_2 demand. The interesting fact in this context was that exposition of the animals to normal atmosphere reversed all of the mentioned effects without resulting in neurological damage (Blackstone 2005). This is of specific interest while H_2S was known as a toxic agent harmful to humans (Couch 2005, Truong 2006), but recently came to mind as a third gaseous mediator (Lowicka 2007). One explanation might be the cytochrome oxidase c inhibition and the resulting reduction of the mitochondrial respiratory chain work und thus protecting animals from getting harmed by lethal hypoxia (Khan 1990, Blackstone 2007). To get further information if a "suspended animation-like" status is clinically relevant we wanted to know if we can translate the mice experiments in our large animal model, because small animals drop their body temperature much easier than large animals or humans and this might be a very important difference. Two major hypotheses were investigated: Is it possible to induce a reduced metabolic status in our large animal model as described in mice by using H_2S as an i.v. formulation, to avoid airway irritation of the sulfide gas. Second aim was to see if H_2S has any effect on the cardiovascular system, because sulfide was reported to be protective to the post-ischemic heart function (Johansen 2006, Zhu 2007). After an initial bolus H_2S was given continuously with doses of 2 mg/kg per h until the end of the experiment. Control group received instead of sulfide only vehicle. After 2 hours of drug infusion the aortic blood flow was arrested for 30 minutes by using balloon catheters as described above. This occlusion time was chosen to investigate hemodynamics and metabolic changings and cardiovascular reaction without the adulteration of a huge inflammation reaction caused by the ischemia and reperfusion sequence. Reperfusion monitoring was 8 hours long with the followed killing of the animals in deep anaesthesia. The results showed that sulfide caused indeed a fall of heart rate and of cardiac output as well and came hand in hand with a reduction of noradrenaline in time and total amount, but did not affect stroke volume. Important in this context is that neither mean arterial nor venous pressure differed between the groups so that it is plausible that changing's of cardiac output was caused solely by the fall of heart frequency and that the vasoconstrictor response to the noradrenaline infusion was improved although in literature H_2S is described as an endogenous vasodilator (Bhatia 2005, Fiorucci 2006). Core temperature decreased in the H_2S stronger than in the control group and reached significance at the end of experiment. This loss of temperature came together with a lowered O_2 uptake and CO_2 production after 2 hours of reperfusion and remained until the end of experiment after 8 hours of reperfusion.

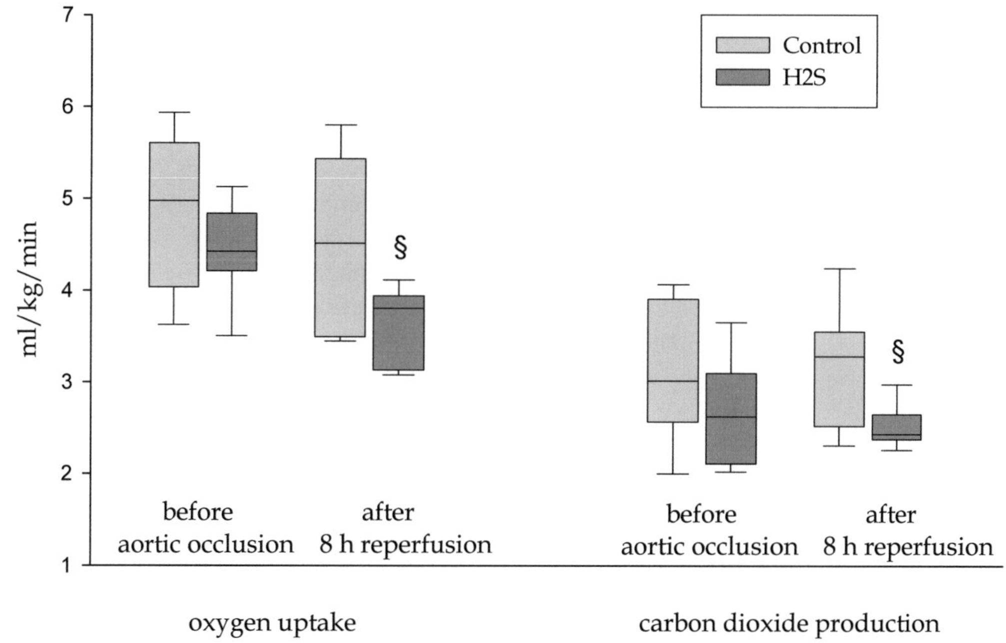

§ depicts $p < 0.05$ control vs. sulfide.

Fig. 3. O_2 uptake and CO_2 production in the vehicle (light whiskers) and sulfide-treated (dark whiskers) animals. All data are median (quartiles, range), n = 8 in each group.

This reduction of metabolism also caused consequently less need for anaerobic generation of ATP and therefore also less glucose turnover. As we planed there was no intergroup difference between the parameters of inflammation and oxidative stress, namely isoprostan levels, nitrate plus nitrite and TNF-α. The reason for that mild inflammation and oxidative stress response is the relatively short ischemia, giving us the opportunity to study just the effects of sulfide per se. What we found unfortunately was a significant lower pO_2 level in the sulfide group at the end of the experiments while pCO_2 and acid-base status didn't change. The reason for this loss of lung function was seen when the lung was taken out at the end of the last experiment. There was a diffuse lung haemorrhage suggesting that longterm infusion of sulphide in high doses can cause pulmonary toxicity. In conclusion we demonstrated in our large animal model that i.v. H_2S reduces significantly metabolism and energy expenditure. It also reduced noradrenaline requirements during the early reperfusion period and might have positive effects on the cardiovascular system, but may cause pulmonary irritations up to acute lung failure. (Simon 2008)

2.3 H_2S – 90 minutes of kidney ischemia

With the knowledge of the previous H_2S experiment, we wanted to develop further the idea of a "suspended animation-like" status and its benefits to kidneys suffering from an ischemia and reperfusion sequence, especially since sulfide showed beneficially effects in renal I/R injury (Tripatara 2009, Xu 2009). These effects were also seen in porcine models dealing with myocardial I/R injury and in isolated kidney preparations, mainly by the reduction of inflammatory response and oxidative stress (Sodha 2009, Hosgood 2010). Therefore we were interested if H_2S could reduce the renal tissue damage in our large animal model, described above with a special interest in the global kidney function, the animal metabolism, body temperature and parameters of inflammation and oxidative stress. After the initial bolus was given, the infusion rate was again 2 mg/kg per h for the first two hours but then was halved to 1 mg/kg per h. During the 90 minutes of aortic clamping the infusion rate was only 0.5 mg/kg per h, to avoid toxic accumulation. For the rest of the procedure please see above. As already described, it is important to keep animals in comparable conditions to avoid artefacts. Hemodynamics, gas exchange, acid-base and electrolyte parameters did not differ between the two groups prior to aortic occlusion, except for a little difference in blood pressure level in the sulfide group that was a little bit lower compared to the control group. Again H_2S caused a fall of body temperature and heart rate and reduced again the need for noradrenaline. Postischemic acidosis and hyperkalemia were attenuated by sulfide. While there were comparable renal perfusion conditions the kidney function differed in favour for the H_2S animals. Plasma creatinine and creatinine clearance showed an improved function of the renal tissue while there was no difference in the fractional Na^+-excretion. At the first glance it looks as if sulfide would not benefit renal tubular cells, but there is evidence, that it influences Na^+-exchange directly, because H_2S caused a 5 fold increase in fractional excretion while there was only a rise of 50 to 80 % in glomerular filtration (Xia 2009). Control animals showed "renal failure" and a "stage 2 kidney injury" in the RIFLE and AKIN classification (Cruz 2009). Sulfide caused only a mild increase of IL-6, IL-1β and nitrite + nitrate what came hand in hand with lower oxidative DNA base damage, measured with the comet assay, and iNOS expression, underlining the anti-inflammatory and NO-release attenuating effect of H_2S (Sodha 2009, Tripatara 2008, Hosgood 2010). The drop in body temperature is unlikely to be the reason as there is a deeper hypothermia recommended to affect inflammation in a relevant manner (Chen 2005). Heme oxygenase-1 (HO-1) and cleaved caspase-3 were similar in both groups while sulfide reduced expression of the anti-apoptotic protein Bcl-xL and increased nuclear transcription factor NF-κB. Interestingly NF-κB not only has inflammatory properties, but also quite the opposite, especially in renal tissue and may contribute to the anti-inflammatory effect seen in our experiment (Lawrence 2005, Panzer 2009). Contrary to the missing anti-inflammatory effect of the lower body temperature, there might be a beneficial effect of mild hypothermia on the protective properties of NF-κB during I/R injury (Kuboki 2007). The most important change in histopathology was the reduction of the "glomerular tubularization", while the rest of the histological staining only showed mild glomerular swelling, flattening of tubulus epithelium and intra-tubular deposits. Even TUNEL-staining showed comparable results between the two groups. This seems to be in contrast with other authors, evaluating more severe histological damages to the renal tissue after I/R injury (Forman 2007, Sanchez-Conde 2008).

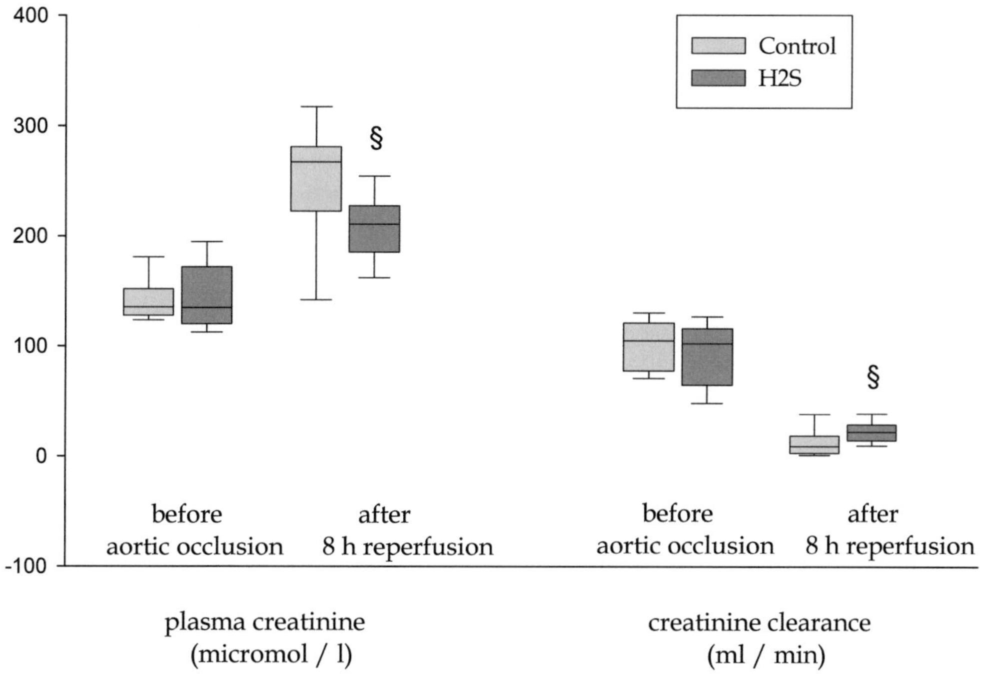

§ $p<0.05$ versus control group.

Fig. 4. Blood creatinine levels and creatinine clearance in the control (light whiskers) and sulfide-treated animals (dark whiskers). All data are median (quartiles, range), control n=10, sulfide n=9,

The crucial point seems to be again the relatively short reperfusion period, because other experiments show comparable results after short post ischemic monitoring (Behrends 2000). This time factor seems also to be involved in the missing differences of HO-1 with a potential latency up to 24 hours (Calvert 2009). In conclusion we demonstrated in a clinically relevant porcine I/R injury model, that i.v. sulfide administration improved kidney function coming together with an anti-inflammatory effect and reduced DNA damage and NO release. The higher NF-κB activation was probably due to the drop in temperature (Simon 2011).

3. Small animal model

We established a small animal model to give answers to questions of the longer outcome of potential therapies, because in our pig model, with sacrifice of the animal at the end of the experiment the neurological outcome cannot be determined. The killing of the pigs at the end of the experiments is necessary, because of the positioning of the proximal balloon catheter, as described above, and the resultant hemodynamic imbalance as well as the ischemia of the abdominal organs. Much more compelling would be to monitor for several days the postoperative neurological outcome of awake animals after such an I/R injury. In New Zealand White Rabbit's spinal ischemia can be induced by cross-clamping of the infrarenal aorta due to strictly segmental blood supply of the spinal cord and can be therefore taken as a model for thoracic aortic clamping in pigs and humans respectively (Zivin 1980). In this way it is possible to keep the surgical impact relatively small, to avoid ischemia of the visceral organs and to keep hemodynamics stable without pharmacological intervention. Inspired by the experiments and experiences of our large animal model and the EPO drug (Simon 2008) we were interested now to examine the effects of a carbamylated derivative of EPO, the so called cEPO. Compared to EPO, whose neuroprotective abilities have been discussed above, the cEPO is lacking of the erythropoietic component (Doggrell 2004), but with all of the tissue protective characteristics of the native EPO. Cytoprotective effects are transmitted by a two-piece receptor, that has on the one hand an EPO receptor and on the other hand a special β-subunit. Experiments with mice lacking this subunit, showed no tissue protective effects (Brines 2004). This is of special interest, because erythropoiesis might be undesired in ill patients with hypertonia. 20 New Zealand White Rabbits were randomly distributed to either the control or the cEPO therapy group and were anesthetized by a mixture of ketamine (50mg/kg body weight) and xylazine (5mg/kg). Blood pressure, heart rate, oxygen saturation and temperature were monitored intraoperatively. In preliminary trials a clamping time of 15 min was defined as being optimal. After this clamping time all animals imposed initially with complete paraplegia and a recovering during the first 24 hours with a following incomplete re-paraplegia as a sign of the reperfusion injury. Animals received vehicle or cEPO over a period of 30 minutes prior to ischemia and with the same doses during the first 30 minutes of reperfusion. Neurological tests took place at 6h, 24h, 36h, 48h, 60h, 72h, 84h and 96h of reperfusion using a modified form of the Tarlov-score, describing the motoric-neurological function of the lower limbs, with a point score. After 96 h the spinal cord was taken out for histopathological examination.

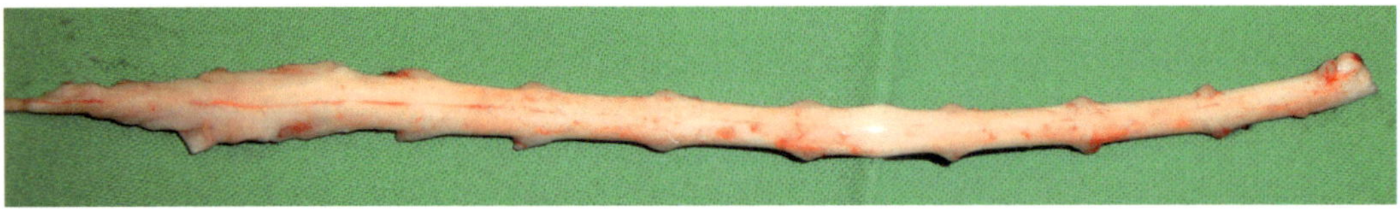

Fig. 5. Spinal cord explanted "in toto" after 96 hours of reperfusion (Th3-L5).

In the results the control and the therapy animals showed postoperatively complete paraplegia as supposed (Tarlov = 0). After 6 h of reperfusion control animals recovered a little in the neurological examination (Tarlov = 4.25). This improvement remained until 36 h of reperfusion with a subsequent deterioration until 96 h at the end of the experiment (Tarlov = 3.625). Aetiopathology in the cEPO group was similar to the control group with a primary recovering up to 24 h after surgery (Tarlov = 4.25) and a tableau until 36 h (Tarlov = 4) and a subsequent worsening until 96 h (Tarlov = 3.5). There was unfortunately no significant difference between the two groups. Histopathological examination did not reveal any injury in thoracic sections of the spinal cord whereas damage in lumbal sections correlated significantly with neurological symptoms (p=0.007). The treatment group (cEPO) and the placebo group showed no differences in neurological or histopathological outcome. Again we learned a lot out of this animal model especially that the time factor varies between different animal models. Even literature can not answer questions to the correct ischemia duration in a rabbit model, because some groups had good results after 15 minutes (Lee 2005) others needed 25 minutes (Jacobs 1992) or 30 minutes (Oz 2007) or even 40 minutes (Lafci 2008). We have to state that in our small animal model with rabbits a clamping time of 15 minutes may be questioned, because, as described above, we saw a fast recovering from paraplegia meanwhile the first 24 hours with no animal imposing with a complete paraplegia to the end after 96 hours.

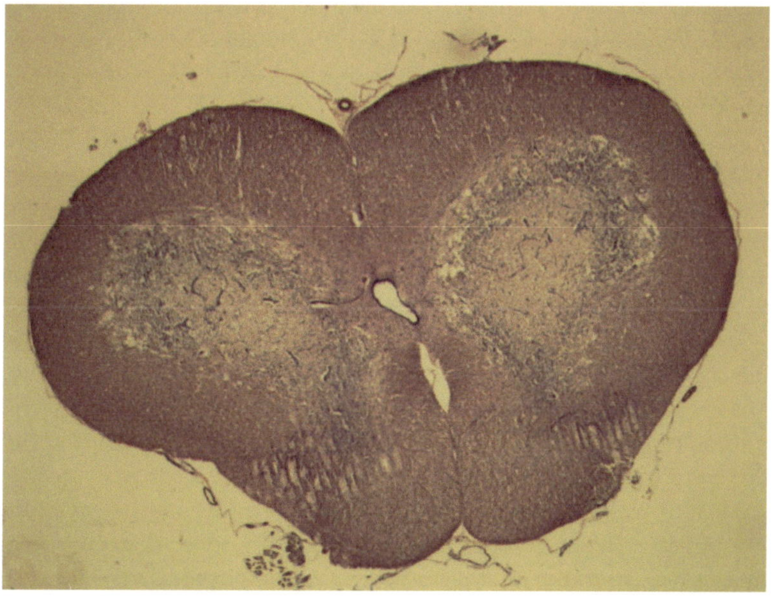

Fig. 6. Slice of the necrotic lumbar spinal cord (L2) with cellular inflammation reaction.

Our decision to work with a clamping time of 15 minutes is based on our aim to keep clamping time and surgery as short as possible to spare the animals. Looking now at the results we have to say that there is no difference between the groups and that we can not exclude the possibility that clamping time was too short. The neuronal damage was not big enough to see potential benefits of the treatment group, because the control group came out well, too. Therefore we can only speculate if the results are due to the short clamping time or just to the ineffectiveness of the cEPO drug. Statistically we found a huge range of variance in our results, what might be not unusual (Zivin 1980), but may disturb our database to see relevant intergroup differences. Therefore further investigations are warranted. In conclusion this is a highly reproducible model which allows clinical neurological assessment after aortic cross-clamping. Using this model promising pharmaceutics, influencing ischemia tolerance, can be tested clinically and histopathologically. In the initial experimental series with a cross-clamping time of 15 min no significant improvement of the clinical or histological damage could be achieved by administration of cEPO, what might be due to a too short clamping time (Simon 2010).

4. Cell culture

Cell culture is a possibility to illuminate processes on the level of genes and proteins as well as changings during hypoxia and reoxigenation. Additional substances and / or therapies can be tested before realising cost and time intensive large animal models. Subjects of interest are tubular and neuronal cells as representative tissue samples of the organs examined in our animal models described above. To realise this aim we used permanent human (HEK293) and porcine (LLC-PK1 and PK15) renal cells. Evaluation of the system was performed by determination of the hypoxia inducing factor 1 alpha (HIF1α) which plays an important role of the O_2 regulation in every cell (Ivan 2001, Jaakkola 2001, Bardos 2004). We also determined expression of Proteinkinase beta 1 (AMPKβ1), which is activated by an elevated AMP/ATP ratio due to cellular and environmental stress, such as heat shock, hypoxia and ischemia (Hardie 2004). In both, human (HEK293) und porcine (LLC-PK1) kidney cells we saw that cells are quite tolerant to short (1-2 h) and middle (4-8 h) hypoxic periods, but a distinct upregulation of protein expression occurs after 18 to 24 hours of cultivation under hypoxic conditions. After 24 h of hypoxia the cells where reoxygenised. For characterisation of the system examinations of the cell morphology, distribution of intact, apoptotic and necrotic cells as well as expression of multiple apoptotic relevant genes on protein level were done. Induction of hypoxia is performed by manipulation of the O_2 content of the cultivating medium, induced by a devolatilization of the cultivation medium and by using a standardised hypoxic chamber which is flushed with nitrogen. In this way we were able to combine different hypoxic timepoints with diverse reoxygenation durations. After putting the hypoxia medium on the cells they were cultivated in a hypoxic chamber. We compared normoxic cells with hypoxic ones. Expressions of the normoxic cells were taken as baseline and compared to hypoxic and reoxygenised cells, each with or without treatment. Target genes were caspase 3 and cleaved caspase 3 as a marker for apoptosis, HIF-1α (Hypoxia induced factor) to evaluate hypoxia, Bcl-2 and Bcl2xL as antiapoptotic markers as well as Bax, as a proapoptotic marker of mitochondrial apoptosis. By using these methods it is possible to see differences in the gene expression in cells cultivated during hypoxic and normoxic conditions and how these things change under the treatment with potentially protective substances. After 24 hours of hypoxia we basically found expression of pro-apoptotic stimuli like Bax or rather severely deranged ratio of Bax and Bcl-2. We have Cytochrome c release, which can lead to activation of caspase 9 that processes caspase 3 and initiates to the formation of the apoptosome. And we have distinct release of other apoptotic factors, e.g. "Second-mitochondria-derived activator of caspase" in short Smac/Diablo, which counteracts the effect of inhibitors of apoptosis. These data are a second validation for our hypoxia model, because the intrinsic pathway of apoptosis begins when injury occurs within the cell, such as e.g. DNA damage, hypoxia and depravation of survival factors. Western blot was used to detect gene expression on protein level. Therefore proteins are isolated out of the target cells and then were separated by size using the "sodium dodecylsulfate polyacrylamide" gel electrophoresis (SDS-Page) and blotted on a nitrocellulose membrane. After treatment with a specific antibody, amplifying the primary antibody by a second one, it can be detected if a protein is expressed or not, compared to a standard protein in defined volume. To identify morphologic changings in mitochondria, cells were stained with the MitoTrackerRed, a mitochondria specific fluorescent dye. MitoTrackerRed Dyes stain mitochondria in living cells and its accumulation in the cell depends on the membrane potential. This means that a loss of fluorescence is caused by a decreased mitochondrial activity.

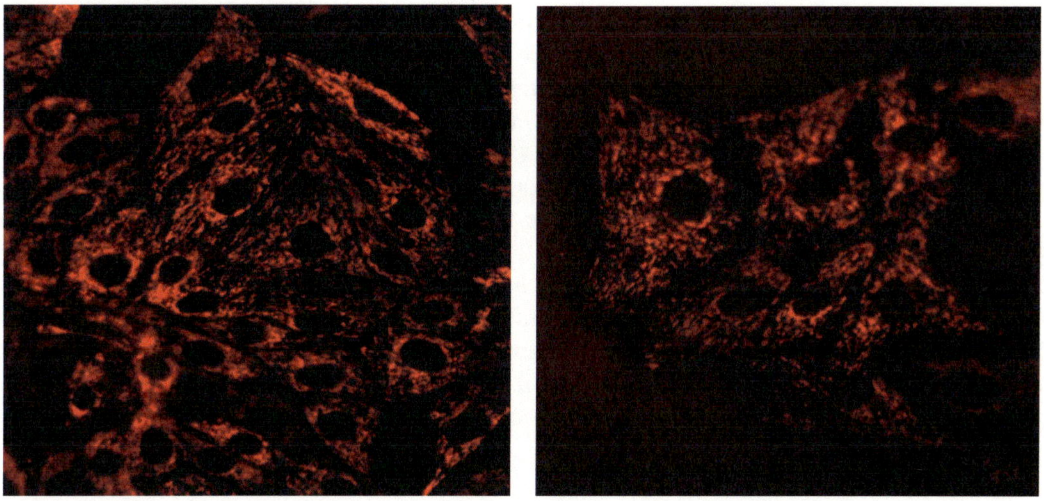

Fig. 7. MitoTrackerRed-staining in normoxic cells (left) and in cells after 24 hours of hypoxia (right).

We saw microscopic mitochondrial structures such as shape, localisation inside the cell and number of active mitochondria. Mitochondria seemed to be much more compact and after long terms of hypoxia, they partly seem to be more diffuse and also a loss of active mitochondria could be detected. Oxidative stress occurring during ischemia and reperfusion injury affects mitochondrial function and therefore respiratory chain. Thus, in addition, to follow changes in respiratory chain during hypoxic period and reoxygenation oxygraphical studies (Oxygraph, Oroboros; Austria) were performed. With that method by titration of inhibitors and substrates it is possible to follow changes in several complexes of the respiratory chain. Therefore it is possible to distinguish activities and dysfunction of the respiratory chain in particular. A classic titration protocol starts with state 1 respiration, which means endogenous substrates, no adenylates, with inorganic phosphates in the mitochondrial respiration medium. As expected we monitored a lowered state 1 respiration in hypoxic cells and a recovery after 24 h of reoxygenation. Another interesting point is the maximum respiration capacity of the cells and again, we found distinct lowered values in hypoxic cells and a slowly recovery after reoxygenation. We always compared normoxic cells with hypoxic ones. After these experiments we looked at the effects of EPO and cEPO on hypoxic cells. We tested two approaches. At first we admitted substances before the 24 hour hypoxic period and as second attempt during this period. What we saw is a downregulation of HIF-1α expression to nearly normoxic control level under high EPO / cEPO doses (100 - 1000 IU/ 5 ml medium) given during hypoxia in human and pig kidney cells. Concerning activities on mitochondrial bases, we analysed Bcl-2 as an anti-apoptotic mitochondrial marker and its antagonist Bax. We found a loss of Bcl-2 after 24 h hypoxic stress and a rise of Bax. So the Bcl-2/Bax ratio is severely deranged, which contributes to cellular apoptosis. But we also found these expressions re-adjusted with the help of EPO or cEPO. In addition we examined cellular proliferation, based on a luminescent assay. The assay, determining the number of viable cells in culture based on quantification of the ATP, is an indicator of metabolically active cells. The amount of ATP is directly proportional to the number of cells present in culture. What we saw, was no influence of cEPO in the control cells. As expected there was a reduced proliferation rate after 24 h of hypoxia, but also improved proliferation with cEPO treated cells. After 24h of hypoxia and 24h of reoxygenation nearly control level was reached again. In the long run we will work with primary renal and spinal cord cells, because I/R injury not only affect kidney but also spinal cord. Therefore we are interested in working with neuronal cells. Yet we did first steps with hippocampal primary neurons extracted from rat embryos, but in the near future it is planned not only to deprive oxygen but also to test a combination of oxygen and glucose deprivation. Also of particular importance is the examination of DNA damage during hypoxia, reoxygenation and drug treatment. Further projects will also deal with the effects of hypothermia on the cell system. The cell culture project is still developing and we learn a lot day by day so that these experiments, described above, are only the very beginning of our studies with cell culture and serves until now more or less only as a standardisation model with further projects and publications coming in the near future.

5. Conclusion

Aim of our studies is to examine systematically the phenomenon of the ischemia and reperfusion injury in common and in the aortic surgery in special. These experiments are important to develop pre- and perioperative concepts to improve clinical outcome of patients in the future. The models described above started their evolution 10 years ago and developed and expanded over the years. It is possible to study not only acute but also elective surgery situations and therefore might give answers to problems in the everyday life of a vascular surgeon to reduce morbidity and mortality in the aortic surgery.

6. Acknowledgment

The research of our group "Ischemia and reperfusion during aortic surgery" is kindly supported by the "Deutsche Gesellschaft für Gefäßchirurgie und Gefäßmedizin" and the "Deutsche Forschungsgemeinschaft".

7. References

Abdelrahman, M; Sharples, EJ; McDonald, MC et al (2004). *Erythropoietin attenuates the tissue injury associated with hemorrhagic shock and myocardial ischemia. Shock* 2004;22:63-69

Abe, A; Aoki, M (1995). *Itoyama. Ischemic delayed neuronal death: a mitochondrial hypothesis.* Stroke 26:1478–1489

Ates, E; Yalcin, AU; Yilmaz, S; Koken, T; Tokyol, C (2005). *Protective effect of erythropoietin on renal ischemia and reperfusion injury. ANZ J Surg* 2005;75:1100-1105

Back, MR; Bandyk, M; Bradner, M; Cuthbertson, D; Johnson, BL; Shames, ML; Bandyk, DF (2005). *Critical analysis of outcome determinants affecting repair of intact aneurysms involving the visceral aorta.* Ann Vasc Surg. 2005;19:648-56

Bárdos, JI; Chau, NM; Ashcroft, M (2004). *Growth factor-mediated induction of HDM2 positively regulates hypoxia-inducible factor 1alpha expression.* Mol Cell Biol. 2004;24(7):2905-14

Bhatia, M (2005). *Hydrogen sulfide as a vasodilator.* IUBMB Life 2005;57:603-606

Behrends, M; Walz, MK; Kribben, A; Neumann, T; Helmchen, U; Philipp, T; Schulz, R; Heusch, G (2000). *No protection of the porcine kidney by ischaemic preconditioning.* Exp Physiol 2000;85:819-827

Bergner, R.; Porto, J.; Fedoronko, B. (1992). *Selective deep hypothermia of the spinal cord prevents paraplegia after aortic crossclamping in the dog model.* J Vasc Surg, 1992; 15: 62 - 72

Blackstone, E; Morrison, M; Roth, MB (2005). *H_2S induces a suspended animation-like state in mice.* Science 2005; 308:518

Blackstone, E; Roth, MB(2007). *Suspended animation-like state protects mice from lethal hypoxia.* Shock 2007;27:370–372

Blankensteijn, JD.; Lindenburg, FP.; Van der Graaf, Y.; Eikelboom, BC. (1998). *Influence of study design on reported mortality and morbidity rates after abdominal aortic aneurysm repair.* Br J Surg 1998; 85: 1624–30

Brines, M; Grasso, G; Fiordaliso, F et al (2004). *Erythropoietin mediates tissue protection through an erythropoietin and common beta-subunit heteroceptor.* Proc Natl Acad Sci USA 2004;101:14907–14912

Calvert, JW; Jha, S; Gundewar, S; Elrod, JW; Ramachandran, A; Pattillo, CB; Kevil, CG; Lefer, DJ (2009). *Hydrogen sulfide mediates cardoprotection through Nrf2 signaling.* Circ Res 2009; 105:365-374

Celik, M; Gokmen, N; Erbayraktar, S; et al (2002). *Erythropoietin prevents motor neuron apoptosis and neurologic disability in experimental spinal cord ischemic injury.* Proc Natl Acad Sci U S A 2002;99:2258-2263

Chen, Z; Chen, H; Rhee, P; Koustova, E; Ayuste, EC; Homma, K; Nadel, A; Alam, HB (2005). *Induction of profound hypothermia modulates the immune/inflammatory response in a swine model of lethal hemorrhage.* Resuscitation 2005;66:209-216

Couch, L; Martin, L; Rankin, N (2005). *Near death episode after exposure to toxic gases from liquid manure.* NZ Med J 2005;118:1-4

Crawford, E.; Svensson, L.; Hess, K.R. (1990). *A prospective randomized study of cerebrospinal fluid drainage to prevent paraplegia after high-risk surgery on the thoraco-abdominal aorta.* J Vasc Surg. 1990 13: 36 - 46

Cruz, DN; Ricci, Z; Ronoc, C (2009). *Clinical review: RIFLE and AKIN – time for reappraisal.* Crit Care 2009;13:211

Dodds, WJ (1982). *The pig model for biomedical research.* Fed Proc 1982; 41: 247-56

Doggrell, SA (2004). *A neuroprotective derivative of erythropoietin that is not erythropoietic.* Expert Opin Investig Drugs 2004;13:1517–1519

Ehrenreich, H; Hasselblatt, M; Dembowski, C et al (2002). *Erythropoietin therapy for acute stroke is both safe and beneficial.* Mol Med 2002;8:495-505

Fiorucci, S; Distrutti, E; Cirino, G; Wallace, JL (2006). *The emerging roles of hydrogen sulphide in the gastrointestinal tract and liver.* Gastroenterology 2006;131:250-271

Forman, CJ; Johnson, DW; Nicol, DL (2007). *Erythropoietin administration protects against functional impairment and cell death after ischaemic renal injury in pigs.* BJU Int 2007;99:162–65

Gelman, S (1995). *The pathophysiology of aortic cross-clamping and unclamping.* Anesthesiology 82(4):1026–1060

de Haan, P; Kalkman, CJ; Meylarts, SAG; Lips, J; Jacobs, MJHM (1999). *Development of spinal cord ischemia after clamping of noncritical segmental arteries in the pig.* Ann Thorac Surg 1999; 68: 1278-84

Hardie DG (2004). *The AMP-activated protein kinase pathway - new players upstream and downstream.* J Cell Sci 2004;117: 5479-5487

Hatori, N; Yoshizu, H; Shimizu, M; Hinokiyama, K; Takeshima, S; Kimura, T; Iizuka, Y; Tanaka, S (2000). *Prognostic factors in the surgical treatment of ruptured abdominal aortic aneurysms*. Surg-Today.2000; 30(9): 785-90

Hellberg, A; Koga, I; Christiansson, L; Stiernstrom, H; Wiklund, L; Bergquist, D; Karacagil, S (2000). Influence *of segmental spinal cord perfusion on intrathecal oxygen tension during experimental thoracic aortic crossclamping*. J Vasc Surg 2000; 31: 164-170

Hosgood, SA; Nicholson, ML (2010). *Hydrogen sulphide ameliorates ischaemia-reperfusion injury in an experimental model of non-heart-beating donor kidney transplantation*. Br J Surg 2009;97:202-209

Ivan, M; Kondo, K; Yang, H; Kim, W; Valiando, J; Ohh, M; Salic, A; Asara, JM; Lane, WS; Kaelin, WG Jr. (2001). *HIFa targeted for VHL-mediated destruction by proline hydroxylation: implications for O2 sensing*. Science 2001;292: 464-468

Jaakkola, P; Mole, DR; Tian, YM; Wilson, MI; Gielbert, J; Gaskell, SJ; Kriegsheim, Av; Hebestreit, HF; Mukherji, M; Schofield, CJ; Maxwell, PH; Pugh, CW; Ratcliffe, PJ (2001). *Targeting of HIF-1a to the von Hippel-Lindau ubiquitylation complex by O2-regulated prolyl hydroxylation*. Science 2001;292: 468-472

Jacobs, TP; Kempski, O; Mc Kinley, D et al (1992). *Blood flow and vascular permeability during motor dysfunction in a rabbit model of spinal cord ischemia*. Stroke 1992;23:267–373

Johansen, D; Ytrehus, K; Baxter, GF (2006). *Exogenous hydrogen sulfide (H_2S) protects against regional myocardial ischemia/reperfusion injury. Evidence for a role of K_{ATP} channels*. Basic Res Cardiol 2006;10:53–60

Khan, AA; Schuler, MM; Prior, MG; Yong, S; Coppock, RW; Florence, LZ; Lillie, LE (1990). *Hydrogen sulfide exposure on lung mitochondrial respiratory chain enzymes in the rat*. Toxicol Appl Pharmacol 1990;103:482-490

Kaptanoglu, E; Solaroglu, I; Okutan, O; Surucu, HS; Akbiyik, F; Beskonakli, E (2004). *Erythropoietin exerts neuroprotection after acute spinal cord injury in rats: effect on lipid peroxidation and early ultrastructural findings*. Neurosurg Rev 2004;27:113-120

Kazautchian, PO. *Protection of Kidney's from ischemic injuries through surgeries of aneurysms of thoracoabdominal and abdominal location*. In: Thoracic and Thoracoabdominal Aortic Aneurysms: 177 - 187 Hrsg.: Weimann S. Monduzzi Edition, Bologna (1994)

Kick, J; Hauser, B; Bracht, H; Albicini, M; Öter, S; Simon, F; Ehrmann, U; Garrel, C; Sträter, J; Brückner, UB; Leverve, XM; Schelzig, H; Speit, G; Radermacher, P; Muth, CM (2007). *Effects of a Cantaloupe melon extract/wheat gliadin biopolymer during aortic cross-clamping*.Intensive Care Med. 2007 Apr;33(4):694-702

Kuboki, S; Okaya, T; Schuster, R; Blanchard, J; Denenberg, A; Wong, HR; Lentsch, AB (2007). *Hepatocyte NF-κB activation is hepatoprotective during ischemia-reperfusion injury asn is augmented by ischemic hypothermia*. Am J Physiol Gastrointest Liver Physiol 2007;292:G201-G207

Lafci, B; Yasa, H; Ilhan, G et al (2008). *Protection of the spinal cord from ischemia: comparative effects of levosimendan and iloprost*. Eur Surg Res 2008;41(1):1–7

Lawrence, T; Bebien, M; Liu, GY; Nizet, V; Karin, M (2005). *IKKα limits macrophage NF-κB activation and contributes to the resolution of inflammation*. Nature 2005;434:1138-1142

Lee, J-C; Hwang, IK et al (2005). *Histochemical and electron microscopic study of motoneuron degeneration following transient spinal cord ischaemia at normothermic conditions in rabbits*. Anat Histol Embryol 2005; 34:252–257

Łowicka, E; Bełtowski, J (2007). *Hydrogen sulfide (H_2S) – the third gas of interest for pharmacologists. Pharmacol Res* 2007;59:4-24

Meylaerts, SA; De-Haan, P; Kalkman, CJ; Lips, J (1999). *The influence of regional spinal cord hypothermia on transcranial myogenic motor-evoked potential monitoring and the efficacy of spinal cord ischemia detection.* J-Thorac-Cardiovasc-Surg.1999 Dec; 118(6): 1038-45

Meylaerts, SA; De-Haan, P; Kalkman, CJ; Jaspers, J; Vanicky, I; Jacobs, MJ (2000). *Prevention of paraplegia in pigs by selective segmental artery perfusion during aortic cross-clamping.* J-Vasc-Surg. 2000 Jul; 32(1): 160-70

Money, SR; Hollier, LH (1994). *The management of thoracoabdominal aneurysms.* Adv-Surg. 1994; 27: 285-94

Moon, C; Krawczyk, M; Paik, D; Lakatta, EG; Talan, MI (2005). *Cardioprotection by recombinant human erythropoietin following acute experimental myocardial infarction: dose response and therapeutic window. Cardiovasc* Drugs Ther 2005;19:243-250

Orend, KH.; Liewald, F.; Kirchdorfer, B.; Sunder-Plassmann, L. (1995). *Management of descending aortic dissection.* Ann Ital Chir. 1995; 66: 821-4

Oz Oyar, E; Korkmaz, A (2008). *Aortic cross-clamping-induced spinal cord oxidative stress in rabbits: the role of a novel antioxidant adrenomedullin.* J Surg Res 2007;147(1):143- 147

Panzer, U; Steinmetz, OM; Turner, JE; Meyer-Schwesinger, C; von Ruffer, C; Meyer, TN; Zahner, G; Gómez-Guerrero, C; Schmid, RM; Helmchen, U; Moeckel, GW; Wolf, G; Stahl, RA; Thaiss, F (2009). *Resolution of renal inflammation: a new role for NF-κB1 (p50) in inflammatory kidney diseases.* Am J Physiol Renal Physiol 2009;297:F429-F439

Roques, X; Remes, J; Laborde, M-N; Guibaud, J-P; Rosato, F; MacBride, T; Baudet, E (2003). *Surgery of chronic traumatic aneurysm of the aortic isthmus: benefit of direct suture.* Eur-J-Cardiothorac-Surg.2003 Jan; 23(1): 46-9

Sakurai, M; Hayashi, T; Abe, K; Tabayashi, K (1998). *DElayed selective motor neuron death and Fas antigen induction after spinal cord ischemia in rabbits.* Brain Res 1998, 797(1):23-28

Sánchez-Conde, P; Rodríguez-López, JM; Nicolás, JL; Lozano, FS; García-Criado, FJ; Cascajo, C; Gonzáleeez-Sarmiento, R; Muriel, C (2008). *The comparative abilities of propofol and sevoflurane to modulate inflammation and oxidative stress in the kidney after aortic cross-clamping.* Anesth Analg 2008;106:371-378

Schelzig, H; Sunder-Plassmann, L; Träger, K; Georgieff, M; Radermacher, P; Fröba, G (2003). *Ischämie and Reperfusion des intestinalen und hepatischen Stromgebiets bei thorakalem crossclamping.* Gefäßchirurgie 2003; 8: 92-99

Silver, M; Corvin, MJ; Bazan, A; Gettinger, A; Enny, C; Corwin, HL (2006). *Efficacy of recombinant human erythropoietin in critically ill patients admitted to a long-term acute care facility: a randomized, double-blind, placebo-controlled trial.* Crit Care Med 2006;34:2310-2316

Simon, F; Scheuerle, A; Calzia, E; Bassi, G; Oter, S; Duy, CN; Kick, J; Brückner, UB; Radermacher, P; Schelzig, H (2008). *Erythropoietin during porcine aortic balloon occlusion-induced ischemia/reperfusion injury.* Crit Care Med. 2008 Jul;36(7):2143-50

Simon, F; Giudici, R; Duy, CN; Schelzig, H; Öter, S; Gröger, M; Wachter, U; Vogt, J; Speit, G; Szabó, C; Radermacher, P; Calzia, E (2008). *Hemodynamic and metabolic effects of hydrogen sulfide during porcine ischemia/reperfusion injury.* Shock. 2008;30(4):359-64

Simon, F; Thiere, M; Erhart, P; Orend, KH; Schelzig, H; Oberhuber, A (2010). *Präklinisches Kleintiermodell zur Erforschung von Ischämie- und Reperfusionsschäden des Rückenmarks nach Crossclamping der Aorta.* Gefässchirurgie 2010;15(6): 463-7

Simon, F; Scheuerle, A; Gröger, M; McCook, O; Stahl, B; Wachter, U; Vogt, J; Speit, G; Hauser, B; Möller, P; Calzia, E; Szabó, C; Schelzig, H; Georgieff, M; Radermacher, P; Wagner, F (2011). *Effects of intravenous sulphide during porcine aortic occlusion-induced kidney ischemia/reperfusion injury*. Shock 2011;35(2): 156-163

Sodha, NR; Clements, RT; Feng, J; Liu, Y; Bianchi, C; Horvath, EM; Szabó, C; Stahl, GL; Sellke, FW(2009). *Hydrogen sulfide therapy attenuates the inflammatory response in a porcine model of myocardial ischemia/reperfusion injury.* J Thorac Cardiovasc Surg 2009;138:977-984

Svensson, L.G.; Crawford, E.S.; Hess, K.R.; Coselli, J.S.; Safi, H.J. (1993). *Experience with 1509 patients undergoing thoracoabdominal aortic operations.* J Vasc Surg 1993; 17: 357 – 370

Tripatara, P; Patel, NS; Brancaleone, V; Renshaw, D; Rocha, J; Sepodes, B; Mota-Filipe, H; Perretti, M; Thiemermann, C (2009). *Characterisation of cystathionine gamma-lyase/hydrogen sulphide pathway in ischaemia/reperfusion injury of the mouse kidney: an in vivo study.* Eur J Pharmacol 2009;606:205-209

Truong, DH; Eghbal, MA; Hindmarsh, W; Roth, SH; O'Brien, PJ (2006). *Molecular mechanisms of hydrogen sulfide toxicity. Drug Metabol Rev 2006;* 38:733-744

Walther, A.; Bardenheuer, H-J. (2000). *The abdominal aortic aneurysm. Anesthesiologic considerations and perioperative management in conservative surgical treatment.* Anaesthesist. 2000 Jul; 49(7): 690-703

Wahlberg, E; Dimuzio, P-J; Stoney, R-J (2002). *Aortic clamping during elective operations for infrarenal disease: The influence of clamping time on renal function.* J-Vasc-Surg.2002 Jul; 36(1): 13-8

Willett, WC; Stampfer, MJ (2001). *Clinical practice. What vitamins should I be taking, doctor*? N Engl J Med 345(25):1819–1824

Xia, M; Chen, L; Muh, RW; Li, PL; Li, N (2009). *Production and actions of hydrogen sulfide, a novel gaseous bioactive substance, in the kidneys.* J Pharmacol Exp Ther 2009;329:1056-1062

Xu, Z; Prathapasinghe, G; Wu, N; Hwang, SY; Siow, YL; O, (2009). *Ischemia-reperfusion reduces cystathionine-beta-synthase-mediated hydrogen sulfide generation in the kidney.* Am J Physiol Renal Physiol 2009;297:F27-F35

Zhu, YZ; Wang, ZJ; Ho, P; Loke, YY; Zhu, YC; Hunag, SH; Tan, CS; Whiteman, M; Lu, J; Moore, PK (2007). *Hydrogen sulfide and its cardioprotective effects in myocardial ischemia in experimental rats.* J Appl Physiol 2007;102:261-268

Zivin, JA; DeGirolami, U (1980). *Spinal cord infarction: a highly reproducible stroke model.* Stroke 11(2):200–202

Zvara, D (2002). *Thoracoabdominal aneurysm surgery and thr risk of paraplegia.* J Extra Corpor Technol. 2002 Mar; 34(1):11-7

13

Ischaemic Postconditioning Reduces Reperfusion Injury After Aortic Revascularization Surgery

Gabor Jancso, Endre Arató and Lászlo Sinay
University of Pécs, Faculty of Medicine,
Department of Vascular Surgery,
Hungary

1. Introduction

In vascular surgery during the manipulation on the vessels the periferial tissues always suffer from a more or less severe ischaemia. In acute ischaemia the time of ischaemia could be also serious, thus after reconstruction we always have to face with reperfusion injury. The aim to reduce these extent of these reperfusion injury associated pathways has real clinical importance in vascular surgery.

Reperfusion injury is an inherent response to the restoration of blood flow after ischaemia, and is initiated at the very early moments of reperfusion, lasting potentially for days. The extent of the oxidative stress and the consecutive generalized inflammatory response depends on the ischaemic-time, the ischaemic tissue volume, and the general state of the endothelium-leukocyte-tissue functional complex (diabetes, chronic ischaemia, drugs). The pathogenesis of reperfusion injury is a complex process involving numerous mechanisms exerted in the intracellular and extracellular environment.

2. Pathophysiology of reperfusion injury

Reperfusion injury is not a mere worsening of the ischaemia-induced damage, but it is secondary to events that are specifically induced by reperfusion. In fact, reperfusion injury is due to complex mechanisms involving mechanical, extra-cellular and intracellular processes. The modern hypothesis of the pathogenesis of reperfusion injury has been reviewed by Piper and al.[1] In patients with acute periferial ischaemia, it is now widely accepted that periodically reopening the occluded artery is accompanied by a reduction of the extent of necrosis and a major reduction of short- and long-term mortality. However, together with a definite protective effect on ischaemic tissues, post-ischaemic reperfusion may bring with it unwanted consequences that may partly counteract its beneficial effects. This phenomenon has thus been named reperfusion injury.

2.1 Causes of reperfusion injury

It seems that in the tissue ischaemia/reperfusion (I/R) can induce various forms of cell death, such as programmed cell death, apoptosis, oncosis and necrosis[2]. Apoptosis can be caused by both prolonged ischaemia/hypoxia and by reperfusion[3]. In contrast to programmed cell death, apoptosis and oncosis, which are pre-mortal processes, necrosis is a post-mortal event. According to this viewpoint necrosis is not a form of cell death but the end stage of cell death processes.

The mechanisms of reperfusion-induced cell death are not completely understood, but it seems that the occurrence of **oxidative stress** related to the generation of ROS may play an important role[4]. ROS have downstream effects, which results in the initiation of a highly orchestrated acute inflammatory response through the release of cytokines, activation of vascular endothelial cells and leukocytes with expression of cell surface adhesion molecules, and up-regulation of a program of pro-inflammatory genes, which contribute to the onset and maintenance of post-ischaemic inflammation[5]. When the occlusion of the artery branch that perfuse the ischaemic tissue is removed, the superoxide anion (O^{2-}) production increases as a result of the activation of various enzymatic complexes. The superoxide anion and other ROS strongly oxidize the myocardial fibres already damaged by the ischaemia, thus favouring the apoptosis[6]. It reacts with the nitric oxide, forming peroxynitrite ($ONOO^-$). Therefore, $ONOO^-$, represents a sign of a reduced availability of nitric oxide[7] and it participates with O^{2-} in the lesion of tissues[8]. Superoxide anion dependent damages are reduced if O^{2-} is transformed to hydrogen peroxide (H_2O_2) by the superoxide-dismutase. However, since in the presence of Fe^{2+} or Cu^{2+}, the H_2O_2 can be transformed in hydroxyl anion (HO^-), which is more toxic than O^{2-} and H_2O_2, an increase in toxicity can occur. Reperfusion injury is also due to cellular Ca^{2+} overload. The Ca^{2+}-overload, which starts during ischaemia, is further increased during reperfusion.

The overload of Ca^{2+} increases the cellular osmolarity favouring swelling (explosive swelling) of skeletal muscle cells; it can also favour the expression of proapoptotic elements from mitochondria[9]. It is noteworthy that altered cytosolic Ca^{2+}-handling during ischaemia may induce structural fragility and excessive contractile activation upon reperfusion, as also indicated from a progressive increase of ventricular diastolic pressure and contraction band necrosis[10].

Ca^{2+}-overload is also considered to be responsible for the opening of mPTP. Although, mPTP opening is strongly inhibited by acidosis during ischaemia, it is favoured by ATP depletion, oxidative stress and high intramitochondrial Ca^{2+} concentrations, conditions all occurring during myocardial reperfusion[11].

Intriguingly, the nuclear factor kappa B (NFkB) plays a double-edge sword role in tissue-protection. Activation of NFkB is essential for late preconditioning, in which NFkB is involved in the up-regulation of iNOS and COX-2 genes. However, in the longer time the role NFkB is also important in reperfusion injury. It contributes to the exacerbation of the tissues lesions sustaining inflammatory reactions. The activation of NFkB is induced from several agents included hydrogen peroxide[12]. NFkB determine an up-regulation of the genes responsible of the production of molecules of cellular adhesion. These molecules favour the adhesion of leukocytes to the endothelium and possibly the migration within the cells[13]. Moreover, the reduced nitric oxide availability determined by I/R participates to the activation of transcription codifying for molecules of cellular adhesion[14]. Therefore, tissue damages during reperfusion among others can be due to the cellular/mitochondrial overload of Ca^{2+}, to the liberation of ROS, to the activation of mPTP, to the reduced availability of nitric oxide and to the activation of the NFkB. The nitric oxide deficiency can also cause vasoconstriction and formation of micro-thrombi into the lumen of the small vessels[15]. These mechanisms, combined with the adhesion of the leucocytes to the endothelium, can lead to the so-called 'no-reflow phenomenon`[16]. In summary, reperfusion injury is due to several mechanisms that include Ca^{2+} overload, ROS generation, reduced availability of nitric oxide, mPTP opening and to the activation of the NFkB, which lead to the augmented expression of molecules of cellular adhesion, leukocyte infiltration and no-reflow phenomenon.

3. Effects of reperfusion injury

Among the outcomes of reperfusion injury are included: (1) endothelial and vascular dysfunction and the sequels of impaired arterial flow, which may concur with the 'no-reflow phenomenon'; (2) metabolic and contractile dysfunction; (3) arrhythmias in case of myocardial I/R; (4) cellular death by cellular swelling, and apoptosis. One may anticipate that effective treatment during reperfusion may reduce tissue injury. However, the complexity of mechanisms suggests that one single intervention aimed to contrast just one or two of these mechanisms may not be sufficient. (*Figure 1*)

4. Definition of postconditioning

The concept of 'Ischaemic PostC' was first described by Vinten-Johansen's group[17]. This study was performed in a canine model of 1 hr coronary occlusion and 3 hrs reperfusion. In this study the PostC algorithm was 30 sec. of reperfusion followed by 30 sec. of coronary occlusion, which were repeated for three cycles at the onset of reperfusion. Although this seminal study used the term 'Ischaemic PostC', subsequent studies of these and other authors omit the term 'Ischaemic' because it is not clear whether the brief periods of ischaemia, the preceding and/or the subsequent periods of reperfusion, or their combination, provide the key stimulus for cardioprotection. In general, PostC can be defined as intermittent interruption of coronary flow in the very early phase of a reperfusion, which leads to protection against reperfusion injury. The duration and number of these stuttering periods of reperfusion and ischaemia has been one of the aims of early studies on this topic.

5. Protective effects of postconditioning

Ischaemic PostC was already examined mostly in myocardium, thus the protective effects are known in the myocardium. Our study was the first to examine the effect of PostC in peripheral tissues.

Depending on species, models and other factors, PostC reduces the infarct size by ~20–70% versus matched controls with matched risk areas. There is an emerging agreement across multiple models and species that PostC may reduce endothelial dysfunction and endothelial activation, thus leading to a reduced endothelial/leukocyte interaction and to a reduced ROS formation. Reduced incidence of apoptosis and arrhythmias has also been observed. Whether PostC reduces post-ischaemic stunning it has not yet been clarified.

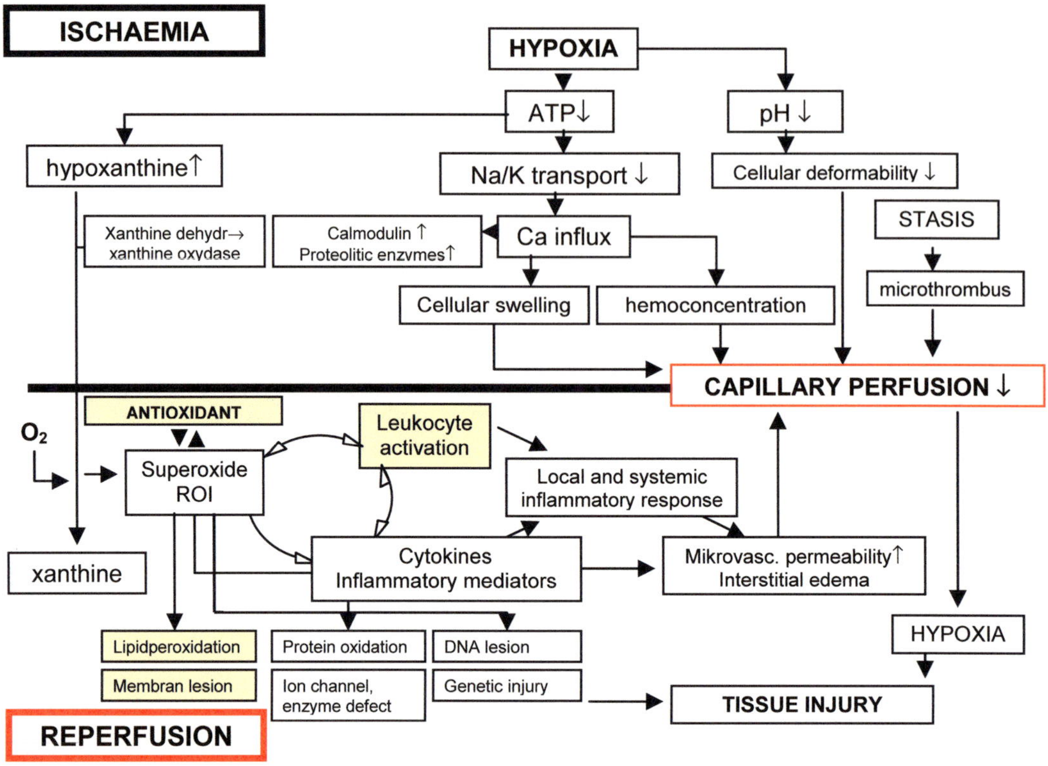

Fig. 1. Simplified presentation of the mechanism of ischaemic-reperfusion injury. Emphasizing, that the engine of reperfusion injury is the ROI - cytokine - leukocyte positive feedback circle.

Hypoxia leads to intracellular ATP depletion with a consecutive hypoxanthine elevation. In the early seconds of reperfusion, when the molecular oxygen appears in the cell, the - xanthine oxidase catalised - hypoxanthine-xanthine conversion will produce a mass of superoxide radicals. Superoxide radical and the other reactive oxygen intermediates will damage the membrane-lipids (through lipidperoxidation), the proteins (causing enzyme defects and ion channel injury) and the DNA. These are the main pathways of the cellular oxidant injury. The endogenous antioxidant system defends against these radical injuries. [18] Reactive oxygen species (ROS) will also induce local and systemic inflammatory responses through the inducing of cytokine expression and leukocyte activation. Inflammatory process leads to increased microvascular permeability, interstitial edema, and capillary perfusion depletion. The oxidative and inflammatory pathways will lead to a complex reperfusion injury. [19] (ROI - reactive oxygen intermediers; ATP - adenosine triphosphate; DNA - deoxyribonucleic acid)

6. Reduction of necrosis

In their seminal study Vinten-Johansen and coworkers [20] reported that PostC causes massive salvage of the myocardium. The infarct size was reduced by ~45% when the initial minutes of reperfusion were 'stuttered' compared to an abrupt and complete reperfusion. These findings have been confirmed by several laboratories as well[21]. As mentioned, in multiple species and models, PostC reduces infarct size by ~20–70% versus matched controls with matched risk areas[22]. Studies from Przyklenk's laboratory and other laboratories confirmed the infarct size reduction in rat isolated heart model[23]. It has been showed that in hearts perfused with constant flow the infarct size reduction by PostC is greater than that observed in the same model perfused at constant pressure [24].

7. Reduction of apoptosis

Apoptosis is a genetically programmed cell death that occurs in reperfusion injury[25]. The reduction in apoptosis may involve the inhibition of caspase-3 and caspase-9 and preservation of Bcl- 2/Bax ratio. So far the only study that reported a reduction of apoptosis by PostC is of Zhao et al. [26] in which a reduced apoptosis was detected with TUNEL assay and the presence of DNA ladders in a model of isolated neonatal cardiomyocytes that underwent hypoxic PostC. We also examined anti- and proapoptotic factors in our periferial PostC model.

8. Reduction of endothelial dysfunction

The endothelial cell dysfunction is a common characteristic of various heart pathologies[27]. In their seminal study Zhao et al.[28] reported that postischaemic endothelial dysfunction was attenuated by PostC. In this study, incremental doses of acetylcholine were used to evaluate the endothelium dependent vasodilatation of coronary vessels isolated from the post-ischaemic region. The authors demonstrated that vasodilatation of postconditioned vessels was improved with respect to that observed in post-ischaemic control vessels. The vasodilator response was similar to that observed in preconditioned vessels and to that observed in vessels from non-ischaemic region.

9. Reduction of endothelial activation and neutrophil adherence

PostC decreases the expression of P-selectin, an adhesion molecule on the surface of endothelial cells. Moreover, it has been observed both a reduction in neutrophils adhesion on the post-conditioned coronary artery endothelium and accumulation of neutrophils in the area at risk[29]. A reduction in superoxide anion generation in the perivascular area has also been observed in the proximity of risk area of postconditioned hearts[30]. Whether the reduced neutrophil accumulation, the subsequent ROS production and the pro-inflammatory response is a cause or consequence of necrosis, apoptosis and vascular injury is not clear. In fact, PostC exerts marked cardioprotection in leukocyte-free models (isolated buffer perfused hearts and isolated cardiomyocytes)[31].

10. Possibilities of postconditioning

It has been reported that PostC-induced necrosis reduction persists up to 72 hrs[32]. These are important studies because they demonstrate that the protection by PostC represents a long-term protective effect and not a mere attenuation of event involved in early reperfusion injury.

In some studies the protocol of classical preconditioning and PostC were combined in order to see whether or not the protection by these two protocols was additive, relative to the protection of each protocol alone. The results are inconsistent. In a canine model, Halkos et al. [33] showed that the combination of protocols is neither additive for infarct size reduction, ROS production nor for post-ischaemic endothelial dysfunction. Similar results were obtained by Tsang et al. [34] and by us [35] in isolated perfused rat hearts. However, Yang et al. [36] demonstrated in an in vivo rabbit model that the combination of the two protocols reduced infarct size significantly more than either manoeuvre alone. The different results may be due to species difference and/or different I/R and PostC protocols. Recently, Bolli's group reported that cardioprotection induced by late preconditioning is enhanced by PostC via a COX-2-mediated mechanism in conscious rats[37]. It remains to de ascertained whether such additive effect between late preconditioning and PostC can be observed in other species and/or models.

Very few studies tested the differences between male and female hearts with regard to PostC effectiveness. In a specifically designed study it has been reported that while the PostC protective effect against stunning was observed in isolated male rat hearts after both 20 min. and 25 min. ischaemia, the protective effect was present in female rat hearts exposed to 20 min of ischaemia, but absent in those exposed to 25 min. ischaemia[38]. In a preliminary study, it has been observed that after 30 min. ischaemia the PostC protective effect against infarction is less effective in female than in male rat hearts. The importance of PostC warrants further studies to elucidate the signal pathways and differences in males and female hearts. It has been reported that cardioprotection by PostC is dependent on the PostC algorithm in aged and STAT3 (signal transducer and activator of transcription 3)-deficient hearts. Moreover it seems that the reduced levels of STAT3 with increasing age may contribute to the age-related loss of PostC protection[39].

In clinical practice ischaemic postconditioning seems even as effective as ischaemic preconditioning. Furthermore, PostC could be used after ischaemia, thus it coud be used in acute ischaemia as well. Threre are many more details in the pathogenesis and clinical applicability of PostC, it seems to be an effective tool in cardiology and vascular surgery to reduce reperfusion injury.

11. Effects of ischaemic postconditioning in human vascular surgery

11.1 Aims

Ischaemic postconditioning was found effective to reduce reperfusion injury not only in experimental animal models, but in humans as well in cardiac interventions. In our investigations we focused on the effect of ischaemic PostC in human revascularization operations. After aorto-bifemoral bypass surgery we applied ischaemic PostC and observed the protective effect.

To describe the oxidative stress we measured the serum malondialdehyde level - to quantify the rate of lipidperoxidation, and the antioxidant enzymes (SOD, GSH, SH). To see the inflammatory changes we measured serum MPO levels, free radical production of leukocytes, and the expression of leukocyte CD11a and 18 adhesion molecules.

11.2 Patients and methods

Patient selection for this prospective randomized study performed according to the Helsinki Declaration (1996), considering the statute of Hungarian Ministry of Health

(35/2005.(VIII:26.)) with the permission of local ethical board of the Pécs University Medical School (No of permission: 2498). Blood samples were collected in three Vacutainer tube containing trisodium citrate (3.8%) and one containing K3-EDTA (7.5%; Becton Dickinson, UK; blue or purple, respectively), before, and two and 24 hours, then one week after the surgery. All human subjects provided formal informed consent.

12. Aorto-bifemoral bypass surgery

In general anaesthesia median laparatomy was performed. After physical examination of the abdominal organs we prepared the distal abdominal aorta. Intravenous 7500 IU unfractionated heparine was given. After occlusion of the aorta a 3 cm longitudinal aortotomy was made. High pressure inflow could be detected from the central aorta. Dacron Y-graft (size depending on the diameter of the vessels) proximal end-to-side anastomosis was sutured with 4/0 Premilene (polypropilene monophylament, B-Braun Aesculap, Tuttlingen, Germany).

We isolated the common femoral artery and its sidebranches (deep and superficial femoral artery). 3 cm longitudinal arteriotomy was made on the common femoral artery. Exploration of distal flow was checked Fogarty catheter. The distal branches of Y-graft are tunneled under the inguinal ligament, and on both sides an end-to-side anastomosis was performed to the common femoral artery with 5/0 Premilene running suture. Followed by haemostasis, drain was placed, and the wound was closed.

All patients completing the study suffered from general atherosclerosis with distal aortic or aorto-biiliac occlusion. All patients received antiplatelet therapy (at least 75 mg Aspirin) before the recruitment. Low molecular weight heparin was administered in the perioperative period. Ten healthy blood donors served as controls for the measurements (Control group). The patients with other chronic inflammatory disease, or gangrene were excluded from the study. After intragroup analysis the patients with significantly deviating results (caused by polytransfusion, extreme intraoperative blood loss, or any postoperative complication) we excluded from the study.

13. Human ischaemic postconditioning protocol

In the postconditioned group (10 patients) after the completion of the distal anastomosis, before starting the reperfusion we made two cycles of 30 sec reperfusion-reocclusion on the graft. After this two cycles of reperfusion-reocclusion we let the continuous reperfusion to the distal artery.

In the ischaemia-reperfusion group (10 patients) after the distal anastomosis we started the continuous perfusion.

14. The measurement of oxidative stress parameters

Measurement of malondialdehyde (MDA):

Malondialdehyde was determined in anticoagulated whole blood, by photometric method[40].

Measurement of reduced glutathione (GSH) and plasma thiol (SH) groups:

GSH and plasma SH levels were determined from anticoagulated whole blood (ethylene diamine tetraacetic acid (EDTA)) by Ellman's reagent according to the method of Sedlak and Lindsay[41].

Measurement of Superoxide dismutase (SOD) activity in washed red blood cell (RBC):

The main principle of this measurement was that adrenaline is able to spontaneously transform to adrenochrome (a detectable colorful complex). This transformation can be blocked by SOD, and SOD containing cells or tissues. The difference in the rate of rise of control and sample curves obtained at 415 nm, are proportional to SOD activity[42].

15. Measurement of inflammatory response, leukocyte activation

Determination of free radical production from whole blood:

Free radical production was induced by 30 μl phorbol-12 myristate 13-acetate (PMA; 0,2μg/ml) (Sigma Aldrich Budapest); in the mixture of whole blood (20 μl), phosphate buffered saline (1400 μ) and 50 μl luminol (3.33 μg/ml; Boehringer Mannheim Gmbh Germany), and was detected by Chrono-Log Lumino-aggregometer.

16. Serum myeloperoxidase assay

Anticoagulated blood was centrifuged with 2000g, and 200 μl plasma was mixed with 1 ml working solution (0,1 M sodium-citrate 10,9 ml, 0,05% Triton-X 100 5 μl, 1mM H_2O_2 1 ml, 0,1% o-dianisidine 100 μl). The mixture was incubated at 37 °C for 5 minutes, then 1 ml 35% perchloric acid was added. Photometry were done at 560 nm. Plasma myeloperoxidase was expressed as nM/l. Hematologic measurement: Red blood cell count, white blood cell count, platelet numbers, haemoglobin concentration, haematocrit level were measured by Minitron automatic analysator (Diatron Ltd, Budapest, Hungary).

17. Leukocyte adhesion molecule measurement

The leukocytes were marked with fluorescein isotiocianide (FITC) labeled antibodies for adhesion molecules (CD11, CD11b, CD18, CD49d, és CD97) (Becton Dickinson Biosciences, Pharmingen, USA), and measurements were performed on BD FacsCalibur (Becton Dickinson Biosciences, Pharmingen, USA) flowcytometer.[43 44]

18. Hematology test

Red blood cell count, white blood cell count, platelet numbers, haemoglobin concentration and haematocrit level were measured by Minitron automatic analysator (Diatron Ltd, Budapest, Hungary).

19. Statistical analysis

Data are expressed as mean ± SE, or percentage. For analysis of data, paired and unpaired Student's t-test, and one-way analysis of variance (ANOVA) were used. Statistical significance was established at $p<0.05$.

20. Results

Plasma malondialdehyde concentration before surgery was similar to the control group. A significant increase was detected in both group right after the reconstruction, but this elevation was significantly higher in the non-conditioned group. Same results were measured 24 hours later and the MDA plasma concentration decreased to the initial values after 7 days. (*Figure 2*)

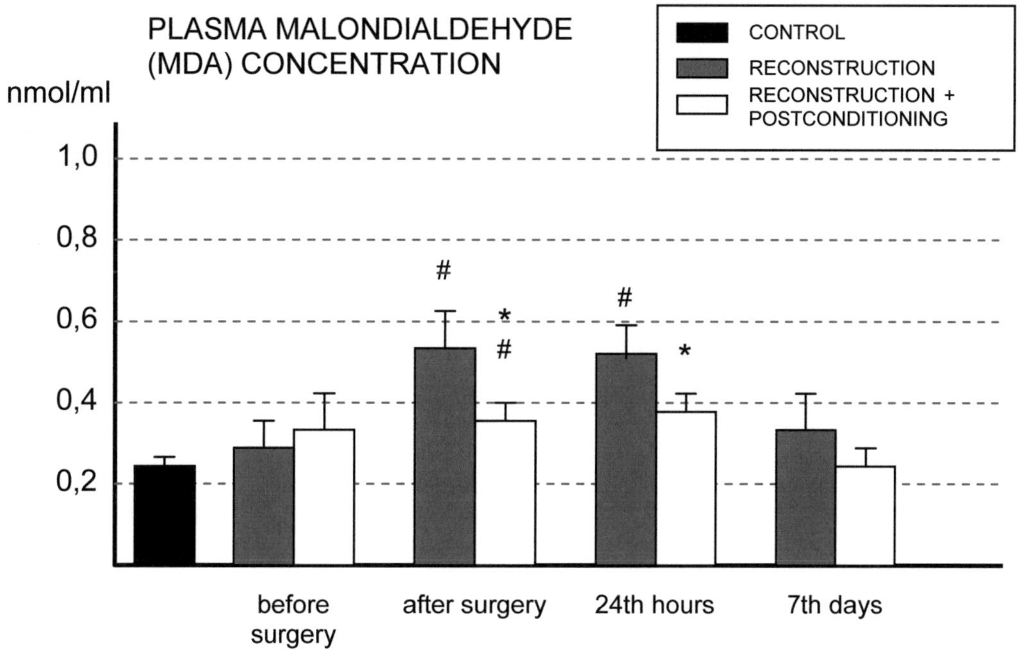

Fig. 2. Changes in plasma malondialdehyde concentration in the patients following the operations. (# $p<0.05$ vs before surgery; * $p<0.05$ vs non-conditioned group)

Measuring the antioxidant enzyme plasma levels we observed that the thiol group concentration in non-conditioned group significantly decreased in the early reperfusion period. The 24 hours values did not show significant changes compared to control and initial values, but after a week in the non-conditioned group a slight decrease was detectable (the second waves of reperfusion injury: mediated by not the ischaemia-reperfusion, but the inflammatory response activated leukocytes[45]).

In the plasma level of reduced glutathion, a significant decrease was detectable in the early reperfusion in both groups. From the first day a continuous elevation was observed until the 7th day and the plasma level in both groups returned to the values before surgery. (*Figure 3*)

The activity of superoxide dismutase before surgery was lower in both groups compared to the control group, and did not show any changes right after the operation. 24 hours later in the non-conditioned group we detected a significant decrease, which disappeared at the end of the week. (*Figure 4*)

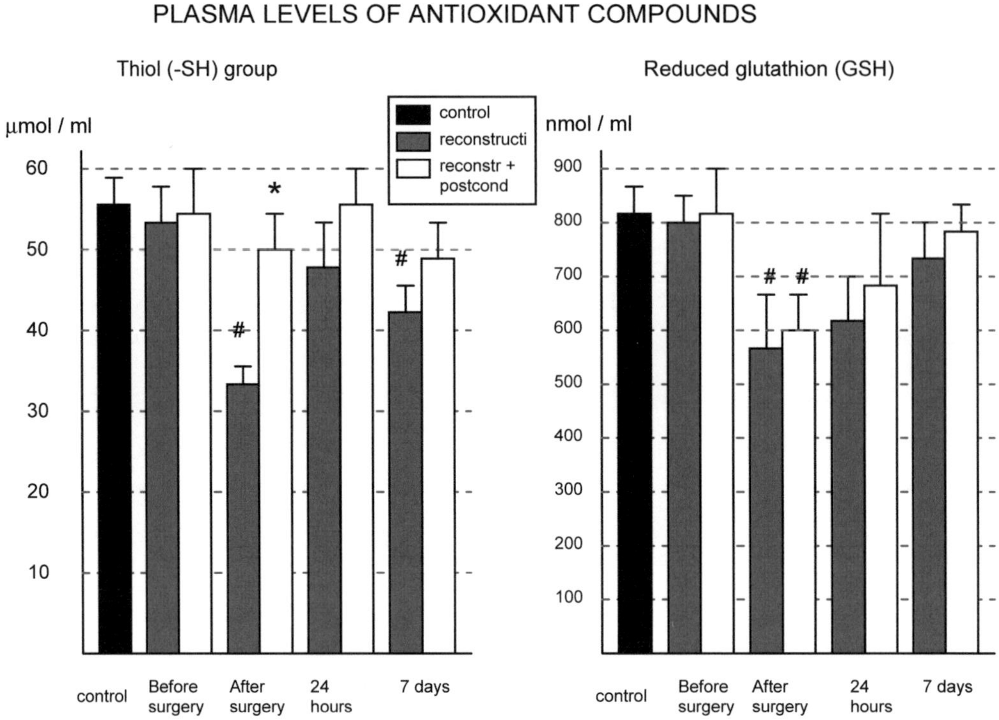

Fig. 3. Changes in antioxidant compounds (thiol group, reduced glutahtion) plasma levels during the examined perioperative period. (# p<0.05 vs before surgery; * p<0.05 vs non-conditioned group)

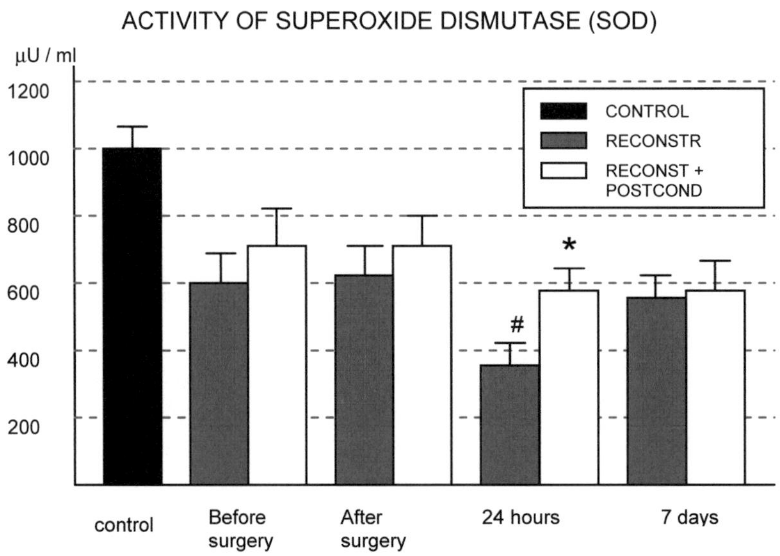

Fig. 4. Changes in blood superoxide dismutase activity during the examined perioperative period. (# p<0.05 vs before surgery; * p<0.05 vs non-conditioned group)

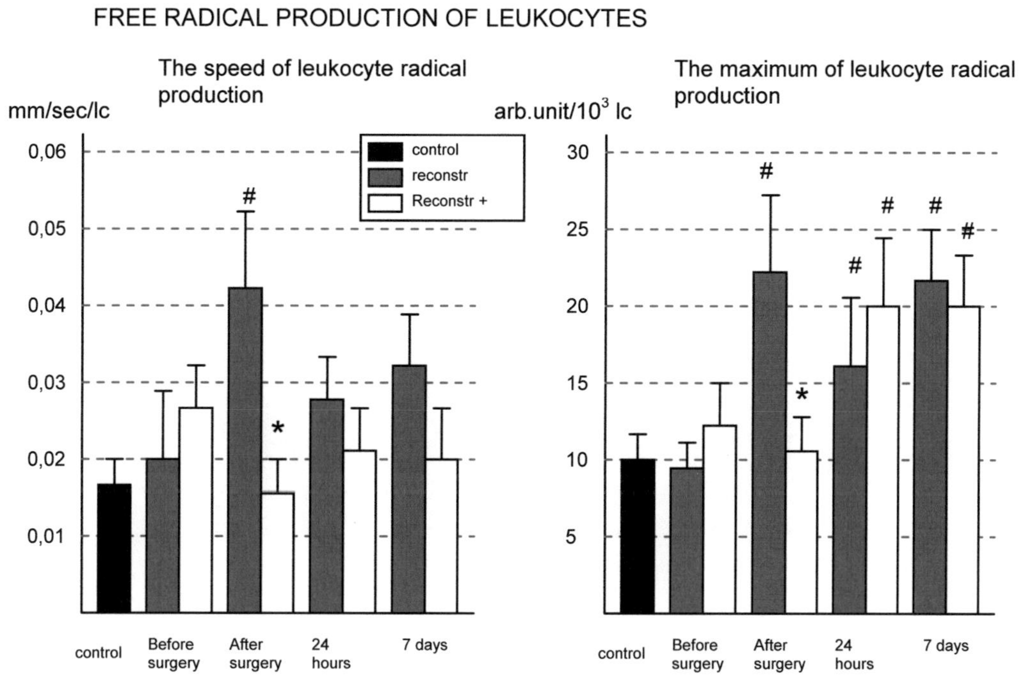

Fig. 5. Changes in the PMA induced free radical production of leukocytes during the perioperative period. We demonstrated the result of the speed and the maximum of radical production. (# $p<0.05$ vs before surgery; * $p<0.05$ vs non-conditioned group)

Leukocyte activation increased significantly immediately after revascularisation surgery in the non-conditioned group, and this elevation could not be observed in the postconditioned group. In the late reperfusion period the maximum of leukocyte-derived free radical production were elevated in both group withouth significant difference between the two groups. (*Figure 5*)

The plasma myeloperoxidase (MPO) concentration was higher in both investigated groups than in healthy control group. We did not observed any significant changes until the 7th day. On the last day of the protocol the plasma MPO concentration elevated significantly in the non-conditioned group, and this elevation was not detectable in the postconditioned group. (*Figure 6*)

Granulocyte surface adhesion molecules were detected by flowcytometer. The detectable expression of CD11a adhesion molecules were significantly lower in the postoperative first samples than before surgery. There was no significant difference at this time between the two groups. After 24 hours in the non-conditioned group a significant expression was observed, which was not detected in the postconditioned group. At the end of the one week period the values reached the starting values.

CD18 showed a significant decrease in the immediate reperfusion period in both groups, and after these changes were the same as the control values. (*Figure 7*)

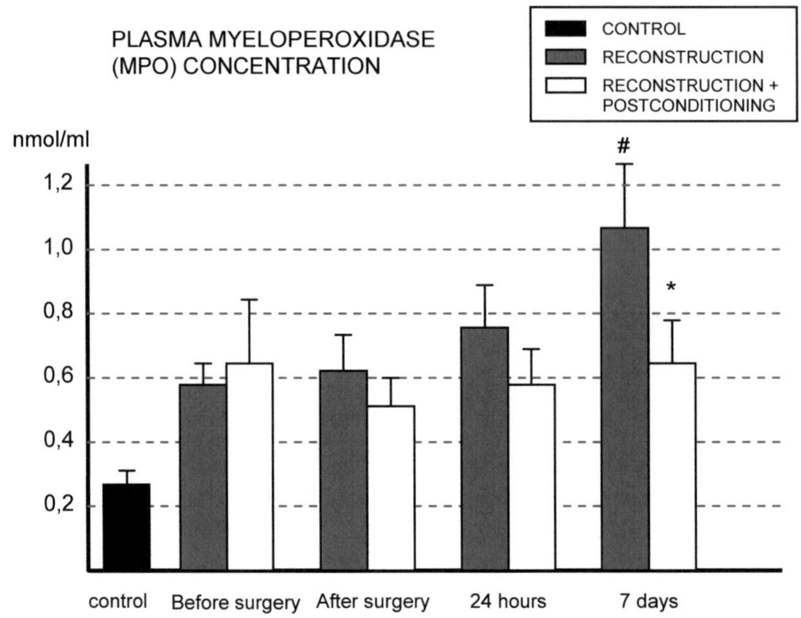

Fig. 6. Changes in plasma myeloperoxidase following operation (# p<0.05 vs before surgery; * p<0.05 vs non-conditioned group)

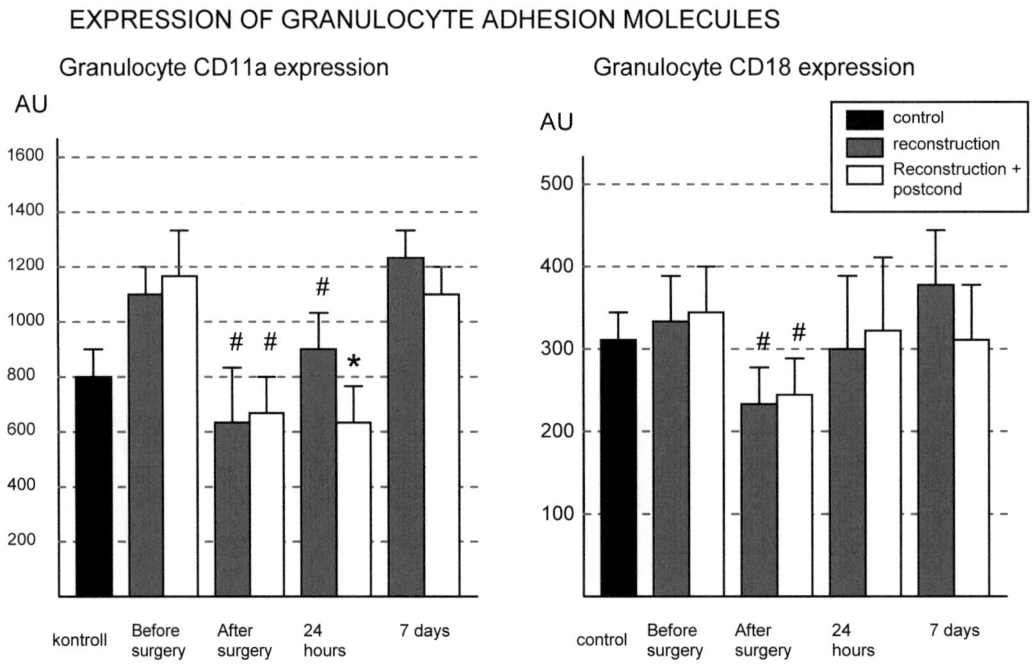

Fig. 7. The graphs show the changes in expression of granulocyte adhesion during the examined perioperative period. (AU= arbitary unit) (# p<0.05 vs before surgery; * p<0.05 vs non-conditioned group)

In the results of the red blood cell count, white blood cell count, platelet numbers, haemoglobin concentration and haematocrit level we did not detected any difference between the two groups of patient.

21. Discussion

In the last 3 years the literature of ischaemic postconditioning exponentially increased in the experimental cardiology. The beneficial effects of the manoeuver has been confirmed in various models, including human results as well, and the cellular and biochemical background is intensively examined. Until now this is the first study to evaluate the effect of ischaemic postconditioning on peripheral tissues in abdominal aortic surgery.

Our results demonstrated that after a prolonged ischaemia, postconditioning can reduce free radical production, TNF-alpha expression and leukocyte activation in the early phase of reperfusion in an animal model of abdominal aortic surgery. In this model we also confirmed that PostC could induce antiapoptotic signaling pathways in the skeletal muscle and in far organs as well.

In our human model we could confirm that ischaemic PostC could decrease in some points the revascularization surgery evoked oxidative stress and inflammatory response.

We have demonstrated that the protective effect of postconditioning is a complex process, involving many cell types, the generation of oxidants, cytokines, and inflammatory pathways, has not only one target, but acts on a diverse site. This complexity, the powerful protective effect and the simplicity in the surgery (lasts for a few minutes) can make the manoeuver really a powerful tool of surgeons.

22. Mechanisms involved in postconditioning

The mechanisms of protection by PostC were initially attributed mainly to improved endothelial function and to the events reducing the detrimental effects of lethal reperfusion injury, such as reduced edema, reduced oxidative stress, reduced mitochondrial calcium accumulation, reduced endothelium damage and reduced inflammation. However, subsequent studies suggest that protection is mediated through the recruitment of signal transduction pathways as in the case of ischaemic preconditioning. Therefore, a distinction in passive and active mechanisms can be proposed. Of course an intricate cross-talk among these events/mechanisms exists, thus this distinction can be useful for a better understanding of the phenomenon, but we must not forget that a single event/mechanism may not be effective if it occurs alone. (*Figure 8*)

23. Passive mechanisms

Among passive mechanisms we can consider those strictly related with hydrostatic force – hereafter named as 'Mechanical mechanisms' – and those related with reduced endothelial adhesion of leucocytes and subsequent reduction of inflammatory process that we call 'Cellular mechanisms'.

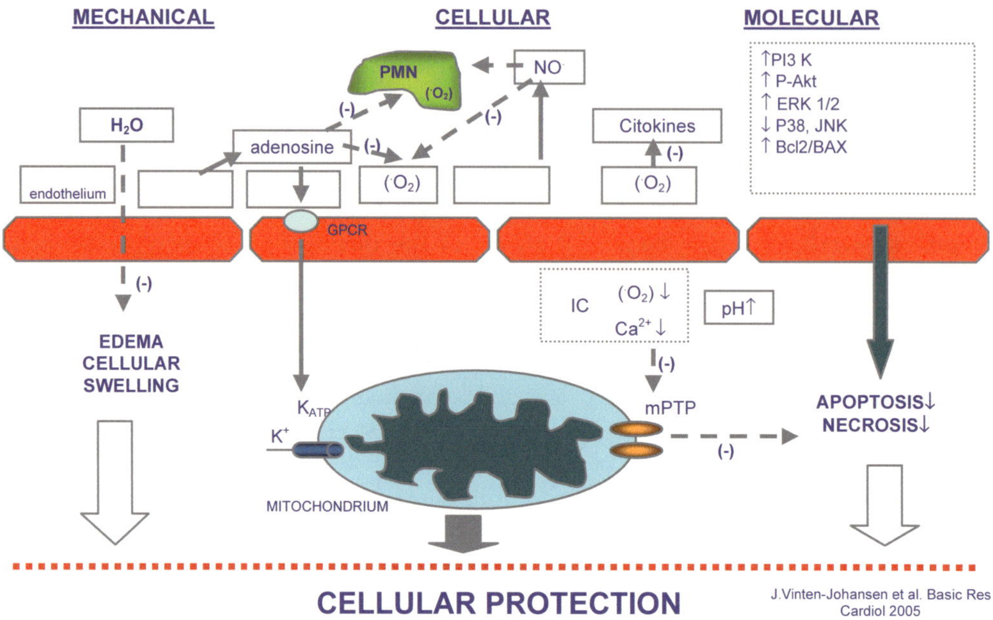

Fig. 8. A schematic figure on the mechanisms of ischaemic postconditioning.

24. Mechanical mechanisms

With regard to mechanical or haemodynamic mechanisms, it has been suggested that the stuttering of reperfusion and pressure during PostC manoeuvres may limit the hydrostatic forces in a very important moment, thus limiting early edema and consequent damages. In experiments performed in isolated heart models, the effect of the PostC on the infarct area has been studied perfusing the hearts either with constant pressure or with constant flow. It has been compared the role of these two types in perfusion in affecting the infarct area during PostC. In the constant pressure model the infarct area was less reduced by PostC than it was with the model of the constant flow reperfusion after PostC[46]. Considering that during the short period of restoration of flow in the PostC manoeuvres the capillary pressure increases less in the constant flow model, than in the constant pressure model (i.e. at the beginning of reperfusion in the constant flow model there is smaller hydrostatic pressure and so smaller transcapillary pressure), it was argued that in the constant-flow model a reduced edema and consequent reduced damages may explain the increased effectiveness of PostC. In other words, in the constant flow model the effectiveness of PostC is greater than in the constant pressure model supports the idea that the reduction of hydrostatic forces during PostC manoeuvres may play an important role in determining the protective effects.

25. Cellular mechanisms

Among the cellular mechanisms we consider acute inflammatory response. It occurs through the release of cytokines, activation of vascular endothelial cells and leukocytes with expression of cell surface adhesion molecules, and up-regulation of a program of proinflammatory genes. PostC delays the onset and reduces the maintenance of post-ischaemic inflammation[47]. As stated before, whether this is a cause or an effect of PostC protection remains to be elucidated.

26. Active mechanisms (intracellular mechanisms)

Studies have identified a signalling pathway that is recruited at the time of reperfusion and which is similar in ischaemic preconditioning and PostC. This pathway includes the survival kinases phosphatidylinositol 3-kinase (PI3K)-Akt and Erk1/2, the major components of the reperfusion-injury salvage kinase pathway, termed the RISK- pathway, which may influence the mPTP, a non-specific pore of the mitochondrial membrane whose opening in the first few minutes of myocardial reperfusion promotes cell death[48]. Delayed washout of endogenously produced adenosine and activation of the adenosine receptor also seems to be required for PostC protection[49], by activating the survival pathway.

Thus delayed washout of adenosine in the setting of PostC might recruit RISK at the time of reperfusion through the activation of adenosine responsive G-protein-coupled receptors. It seems that adenosine receptors are repopulated during PostC manoeuvres. While in murine hearts adenosine A2a and A3 subtypes [50] have been seen to be involved, in rabbit hearts PostC seems to depend on A2b subtype [51]. An important role of the redox environment has also been observed[52].

Therefore, similar to preconditioning, PostC has been proposed to be triggered by receptor stimulation, mediated by one or more complex and interrelated signal transduction pathways, and, ultimately, achieved via phosphorylation of one or more end-effectors of cardioprotection[53].

27. Triggers of postconditioning

Ligands, such as adenosine [54] and bradykinine [55] what accumulate during PostC manoeuvres may initiate the cascade that lead to PostC protection. It has been recently reported that inhibition of opioid receptors with opioid antagonists administered 5 min. before reperfusion in the absence or presence of PostC, reversed the infarct sparing effect of PostC in an in vivo rat model[56]. The activation of protein kinase C and G (PKC and PKG) and opening of mitochondrial K_{ATP} channels after PostC (see below) would be consistent with the involvement of BK and endogenous opioids. Nitric oxide and ROS may be included among the triggers. Nitric oxide is demonstrated to act both as a trigger and as a mediator of the preconditioning response in a variety of species. The role of endogenous NO in classic ischaemic preconditioning was controversial. Cohen and Downey's group suggested that exogenously administered NO could trigger the preconditioned state through a free radical-mediated process not shared by endogenous NO. Very recently these authors questioned whether their observation was due to a bias in the experimental model. These authors are now on the opinion that endogenous NO participates in triggering in vivo preconditioning[57]. Among the autocaids released by the ischaemic heart there is BK that may induce nitric oxide release (*Figure 3*). It has been suggested that the mechanism whereby NO protects myocardium includes the activation of guanylate-cyclase[58]. As an inducer of the protection, nitric oxide may also directly open the mitochondrial K_{ATP}

channels[59]. Therefore, nitric oxide acting on mitochondria may play a relevant role in protection both through activation of these channels and via modulation of respiratory chain; both mechanisms favor ROS signalling, which can trigger protection[60]. A relevant role of nitric oxide may also be attributed to the endothelial protection brought by this molecule [61] or to its role as antioxidant under certain conditions [62].

The one-electron-reduction product of nitric oxide, HNO/NO– (nitrosyl hydride/nitroxyl anion), has been scarcely studied in an I/R scenario. In our laboratory low doses of Angeli's salt, a donor of HNO/NO–, have been seen to induce early/classical preconditioning against myocardial damages[63]. Intriguingly, the protective effects of HNO/NO– generated by Angeli's salt were more potent than the protective effects induced by equimolar concentration of the pure nitric oxide donor diethylamine/nitric oxide (DEA/NO). While the HNO/NO– donor seems deleterious in reperfusion[64], there is evidence that NO may also be involved in the cardioprotection by ischaemic PostC. When the nitric oxide synthase (NOS) inhibitor N-omega-nitro-L-arginine methyl esther (LNAME) was given 5 min. before start of reperfusion of *in vivo* rabbit hearts, the infarct limiting effect was abolished[65]. We have shown that nitric oxide participates in PostC, but NOS inhibitors given for the entire reperfusion period only blunted the protective effect of PostC[66] . Paradoxically, the same inhibitor, given only during PostC manoeuvres completely blocked the protective effects[67]. At the moment, we do not have an explanation for this apparent paradox. In a previous study, we argued that nitric oxide may be produced in post-conditioned heart both by NOS and by non-enzymatic mechanisms. Nitric oxide can then activate the guanyl cyclase to produce cyclic guanosine monophosphate (cGMP), which mediates protection [68] (see also below). The infusion of a NOS inhibitor only during PostC manoeuvres may alter the equilibrium between ROS and nitric oxide thus leading to the production of the wrong kind of radical which does not trigger the protective pathway. It can be argued that in the absence of this protection the stronger limitation of nitric oxide production by NOS may be protective during reperfusion. In fact, data have demonstrated that NOS inhibitors can attenuate I/R damage[69]. Also, the different doses of nitric oxide inhibitors applied and the different basal levels of nitric oxide endogenously produced may explain these disparities.

The beneficial and deleterious effects of nitric oxide and nitrite in pathophysiological conditions and contradictory results about the effects of nitric oxide during reperfusion have been reviewed by Bolli in 2001[70], Wink et al. in 2003[71], Pagliaro in 2003[72] and Schulz et al. in 2004 [73]. ROS could also be included among the triggers of PostC. In fact, ROS scavengers such as N-acetylcysteine and 2-mercapto-propionylglycine given during PostC manoeuvres prevent the protective effects[74]. It is possible that the low pH during the PostC cycles prevents mPTP opening, while the intermittent oxygen bursts allow mitochondria to make enough ROS in a moment in which other enzymes, able to produce massive quantity of ROS, are not yet re-activated. Then mitochondrial ROS may activate PKC and put the heart into a protected state. The importance of the role of acidosis in the triggering of PostC protection has been recently confirmed by two independent laboratories[75]. Acidosis may also prevent mPTP opening in the early reperfusion (see below). Recently, it has been reported that redox signaling and a low pH at the time of myocardial reperfusion are also required to mediate the cardioprotection triggered by ischaemic preconditioning[76].

28. Mediators of postconditioning

We considered ROS among triggers as they are necessary during PostC manoeuvres. Nevertheless, PostC activated the RISK pathway, with increased expression of the phosphorylated form of endothelial nitric oxide synthase (eNOS) as one of the results[77]. Thus it is likely that after NOS activation the cGMP is produced and PKG is activated; then mitochondrial ATP-dependent potassium (mK_{ATP}) channels are opened and ROS produced. Therefore cGMP, PKG, mKATP and ROS may be considered as mediators of PostC protection, which are likely to be upstream to PKC activation. We demonstrated that cGMP production is increased during reperfusion of postconditioned hearts[78]. Moreover we showed that in these hearts mKATP and PKC must also be active (i.e. they should not be blocked) during late reperfusion[79]. Regarding the role of mK_{ATP} channels a couple of papers indicate that the mKATP channel is important for PostC[80]. In these studies two different mK_{ATP} channel blockers (glibenclamide and 5-hydroxidecanoate) abolished the protective effect of PostC [81].

It is interesting that many of the RISK elements (e.g. PI3K/Akt and MEK1/2-ERK) involved in the signaling pathway in preconditioning and protection against reperfusion injury have recently been documented also in PostC[82]. Some differences, however, may exist between pre- and PostC (see also Table 1 and Table 2). Darling et al. [83] showed an increase of phospho-ERK, but not of PI3K/Akt in PostC, while Yang et al.[84] showed that ERK is involved in PostC, but not in preconditioning. These findings may explain a certain degree of additive protection between ischaemic preconditioning and PostC, as observed by Yang et al.[85]. Yet in contrast with Yang et al.[86], Cao et al.[87] reported that ERK is present in preconditioning trigger pathway. The reasons for the differences are not clear. Different species and/or protocols may play a role[88]. Different methods of tissue sampling also be may play a role[89]. Besides protein kinase C, the possible roles for tyrosine kinase, and members of the MAPK family other than ERK1/2 in PostC has been suggested[90]. (*Figure 9*)

Focal disorganization of gap junction distribution and down-regulation of connexin 43 (Cx43) are typical features of myocardial remodelling [91] and Cx43 - especially Cx43 localized in mitochondria - has been indicated as one key element of the signal transduction cascade of the protection by preconditioning. However, Cx43 does not seem to be important for infarct size reduction by PostC [92]. These results, together with the above reported differences on kinase activation by pre- and PostC, suggest a certain degree of differences between the protective pathways activated by these two procedures.

29. End-effectors of postconditioning

Mitochondrial PTPs opening represents a fundamental step of reperfusion injury. Among the potential mechanisms responsible for mPTP opening during reperfusion, Ca^{2+}-overload has received particular attention. In particular, mitochondrial Ca^{2+}-overload occurring during ischaemia must bring mitochondria closer to the threshold at which mPTP opening takes place, favouring the occurrence of mPTP opening during reperfusion, a phenomenon described as mitochondrial priming[93]. Additionally, reduced mitochondrial Ca^{2+} overload during ischaemia has been pointed out as a potentially important mechanism of ischaemic and pharmacological preconditioning[94].

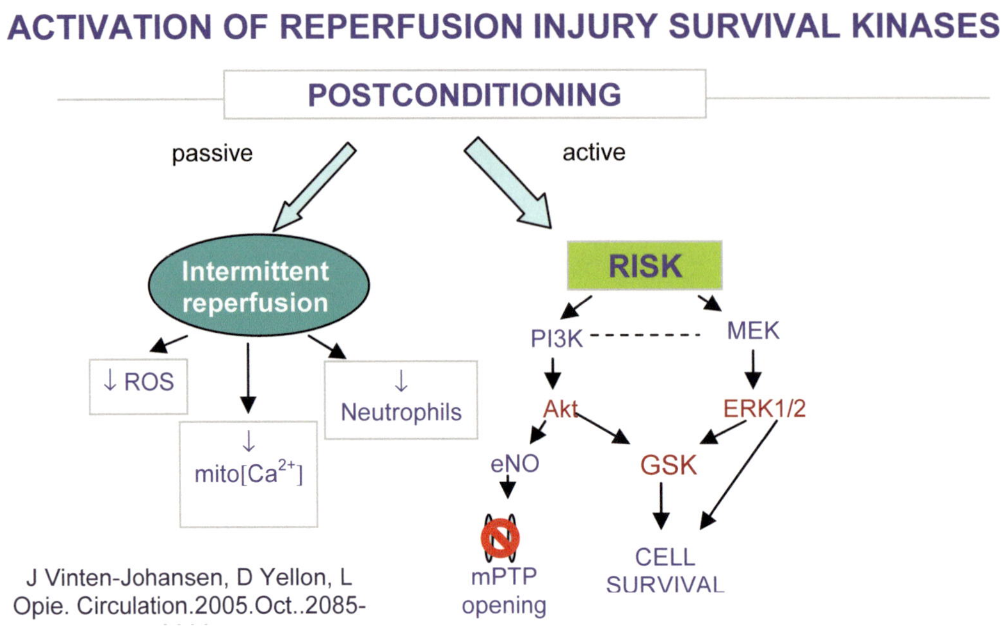

Fig. 9. Possible contexts in the activation of reperfusion injury survival kinases in ischaemic postconditioning

Neonatal rat cardiomyocytes subjected to 3 hrs of hypoxia and 6 hrs of re-oxygenation, "hypoxic PostC" with alternating exposure to three cycles of 5 min. hypoxic and normoxic conditions preceding re-oxygenation reduced intracellular and mitochondrial Ca^{2+} loading compared to non-postconditioned cardiomyocytes. This was associated with a reduction in cardiomyocyte death assessed by propidium iodide and lactate dehydrogenase release[95]. However, the signalling pathways and physiological consequences of this lower intracellular Ca^{2+} by PostC are not known at present, especially in vivo. For instance, it cannot be excluded that reduced mitochondrial Ca^{2+} overload could actually be a consequence of a more preserved Ca^{2+} handling by the sarcoplasmic reticulum in postconditioned cardiomyocytes rather than a cause of protection. It has been reported that PostC reduces calcium-induced opening of the mPTP in mitochondria isolated from the myocardial area at risk[96]. PostC was also associated with a reduction in infarct size after both acute and long-term (72 hrs) reperfusion. Bopassa et al.[97] demonstrated in isolated perfused rat hearts that maintenance of mPTP closure was associated with PI3K activation, which is consistent with the activation of survival kinase pathways described above, but the functional involvement of these pathways and regulation of the mPTP in vivo is not yet clear. It seems that in the PostC scenario the inhibition of GSK3 contributes to the prevention of mPTP opening[98]. Taken together it would appear that the trigger pathway for PostC involves the following sequence of events: occupation of surface receptors (adenosine and NOS and non-enzymatic processes to make nitric oxide, activation of cGMP-dependent kinase (PKG), opening of mK_{ATP}, production of ROS and finally activation of PKC and MAPKs as well as inhibition of GSK3 which put the heart into a protected state. The protect state may include a central role of the prevention of mPTP opening by acidosis in the early phase and by the aforementioned mechanisms in the late reperfusion (*Figures 2 and 3*).

30. Cytoprotection by pre- and postconditioning is redox-sensitive

It has been already established that preconditioning triggering, that is the period that precedes the index ischaemia, is redox sensitive. This was demonstrated by both avoiding preconditioning with ROS scavengers and inducing preconditioning with ROS generators given before the index ischaemia [99]. Also, several metabolites, including acetylcholine, BK, opioids and phenylephrine, trigger preconditioning-like protection via a mK_{ATP}-ROS dependent mechanism[100]. As stated in the case of reperfusion injury, ROS are also implicated in the sequel of myocardial reperfusion injury[101]. These studies supported the paradigm that ROS may be protective in pre-ischaemic phase, but are deleterious in the post-ischaemic phase. Thus the main idea was that ROS play an essential, though double-edged, role in cardioprotection: they may participate reperfusion injury or may play a role as signaling elements of protection in pre-ischaemic phase[102]. The importance of ROS signalling (as opposed to excess ROS in the development of injury) has been examined closely in great detail in recent years[103]. Intriguingly, and in contrast to the above-described theory of ROS as an obligatory part of reperfusion induced damage, some studies suggest the possibility that some ROS species at low concentrations could protect ischaemic hearts[104]. Yet, from the above reported mechanisms of PostC, it appears that also ischaemic PostC is a cardioprotective phenomenon that requires the intervention of redox signaling to be protective[105]. Moreover, as mentioned, very recently it has been shown that redox signalling is also required at the time of myocardial reperfusion to mediate the cardioprotection elicited by ischaemic preconditioning[106]. Therefore, the role of ROS in reperfusion may be reconsidered as they are not only deleterious. This fact may help to understand the variability in the results of studies aimed at proving a role of ROS in reperfusion injury. For instance, negative results came from trials in which free radical scavengers such as recombinant human superoxide dismutase or vitamin E were administered to patients with coronary artery disease or risk factors for cardiovascular events[107]. In addition to the dual role of ROS (beneficial versus deleterious), among the reasons why these scavengers did not show any consistent benefit in these human studies may be: (1) the type of ROS generated (e.g. superoxide dismutase only removes the superoxide and not the hydroxyl radical); (2) the site of ROS generation (e.g. most scavengers scarcely enter into the cells) and (3) the rate of reaction between two ROS and/or scavengers. The importance of the rate of reaction can be understood if we consider that, despite a five times lower concentration of nitric oxide with respect to superoxide dismutase, 50% or more of the available superoxide will react with nitric oxide to form ONOO– instead of reacting with superoxide dismutase[108]. Notwithstanding the evidence of a protective role of ROS signalling in reperfusion, we were unable to reproduce cardioprotection with ROS generation by purine/xanthine oxidase given at reperfusion[109].

Since ROS scavengers (N-acetyl-L-cysteine or 2-mercapto-propionylglycine), given at the beginning of reperfusion, abolished both IP- and PostC-induced protection[110] it is likely that the type, the concentration and/or the compartmentalization of ROS may play a pivotal role in triggering protection at reperfusion time. We are performing studies in the attempt to clarify this issue.

31. Conclusion

Postconditioning has the advantage of being a way to influence and modify reperfusion injury after it has occurred. This may open a therapeutic alternative in situations of unexpected and uncontrolled ischaemic-reperfusion injury, for instance in the situation where technical complications occur during surgery, making a simple procedure into a complicated one, and making aortic cross-clamping longer than anticipated.

We think, that many more examinations are needed to describe and understand in details the mechanism of ischaemic PostC. We are sure, that this manoeuver is easy to perform, quick, and does not any expensive instruments, so it may have a place in the therapeutic arsenal of vascular surgeons.

32. References

[1] Piper HM, Meuter K, Schafer C. Cellular mechanisms of ischaemia-reperfusion injury. Ann Thorac Surg. 2003; 75: S644–8.
[2] Takemura G, Fujiwara H. Morphological aspects of apoptosis in heart diseases. J Cell Mol Med. 2006; 10: 56–75.
[3] Van Cruchten S, Van Den Broeck W. Morphological and biochemical aspects of apoptosis, oncosis and necrosis. Anat Histol Embryol. 2002; 31: 214–23.
[4] Tritto I, Ambrosio G. Role of oxidants in the signaling pathway of preconditioning. Antioxid Redox Signal. 2001; 3: 3–10.
[5] Zhao ZQ, Vinten-Johansen J. Myocardial apoptosis and ischemic preconditioning. Cardiovasc Res. 2002;55: 438–55.
[6] Ambrosio G, Flaherty JT, Duilio C,Tritto I, Santoro G, Elia PP, Condorelli M, Chiariello M. Oxygen radicals generated at reflow induce peroxidation of membrane lipids in reperfused hearts. J Clin Invest. 1991; 87: 2056–66.
[7] Kaeffer N, Richard V, Thuillez C. Delayed coronary endothelial protection 24 hours after preconditioning: role of free radicals. Circulation. 1997; 96: 2311–6
[8] Lefer AM, Lefer DJ. Endothelial dysfunction in myocardial ischaemia and reperfusion: role of oxygenderived free radicals. Basic Res Cardiol. 1991; 86: 109–16.
[9] Zhao ZQ. Oxidative stress-elicited myocardial apoptosis during reperfusion. Curr Opin Pharmacol. 2004; 4: 159–65.
[10] Hoffman JW Jr, Gilbert TB, Poston RS, Silldorff EP. Myocardial reperfusion injury: etiology, mechanisms, and therapies. J Extra Corpor Technol. 2004; 36: 391–411.
[11] Gateau-Roesch O, Argaud L, Ovize M. Mitochondrial permeability transition pore and postconditioning. Cardiovasc Res. 2006; 70: 264–73.
[12] Schreck R, Albermann K, Baeuerle PA. Nuclear factor kappa B: an oxidative stress-responsive transcription factor of eukariotic cells. Free Radical Res Commun. 1992; 17: 221–37.
[13] Baldwin AS. The transcription factor NFkB and human disease. J Clin Invest. 2001; 107: 3–6.
[14] Lefer AM, Lefer DJ. The role of nitric oxide and cell adhesion molecules on the microcirculation in ischaemia-reperfusion. Cardiovasc Res. 1996; 32: 743–51.
[15] Radomski MW, Palmer RM, Moncada S. Comparative pharmacology of endothelium-derived relaxing factor, nitric oxide and prostacyclin in platelets. Br J Pharmacol. 1987; 92: 181–7.
[16] Reffelmann T, Kloner RA. The "no-reflow" phenomenon: basic science and clinical correlates. Heart. 2002; 87: 162–8.
[17] Zhao ZQ, Corvera J, Halkos ME, Kerendi F,Wang NP, Guyton RA, Vinten-Johansen J. Inhibition of myocardial injury by ischemic postconditioning during reperfusion:

comparison with ischemic preconditioning. Am J Physiol Heart Circ Physiol. 2003; 285: H579–88.
[18] LB Becker , New concepts in reactive oxygen species and cardiovascular reperfusion physiology, Cardiovasc Res, 15 (2004), 461-70.
[19] KA Kaminski, Bonda TA, Korecki J, Musial WJ, Oxidative stress and neutrophil activation-the two keystones of ischaemia/reperfusion injury, Int J Cardiol, 86 (2002), 41-59. Review.
[20] Zhao ZQ, Corvera J, Halkos ME, Kerendi F,Wang NP, Guyton RA, Vinten-Johansen J. Inhibition of myocardial injury by ischemic postconditioning during reperfusion: comparison with ischemic preconditioning. Am J Physiol Heart Circ Physiol. 2003; 285: H579–88.
[21] Darling CE, Jiang R, Maynard M, Whittaker P, Vinten-Johansen J, Przyklenk K. 'Postconditioning' via stuttering reperfusion limits myocardial infarct size in rabbit hearts: role of ERK 1/2. Am J Physiol Heart Circ Physiol. 2005; 289: H1618–26.
[22] Yang XM, Philipp S, Downey JM, Cohen MV. Postconditioning's protection is not dependent on circulating blood factors or cells but involves adenosine receptors and requires PI3-kinase and guanylyl cyclase activation. Basic Res Cardiol. 2005; 100: 57–63.
[23] Kerendi F, Kin H, Halkos ME, Jiang R, Zatta AJ, Zhao ZQ, Guyton RA, Vinten-Johansen J. Remote postconditioning. Brief renal ischaemia and reperfusion applied before coronary artery reperfusion reduces myocardial infarct size via endogenous activation of adenosine receptors. Basic Res Cardiol. 2005; 100: 404–12.
[24] Penna C, Cappello S, Mancardi D, Raimondo S, Rastaldo R, Gattullo D, Losano G, Pagliaro P. Post-conditioning reduces infarct size in the isolated rat heart: role of coronary flow and pressure and the nitric oxide/cGMP pathway. Basic Res Cardiol. 2006; 101: 168–79.
[25] Gottlieb RA, Burleson KO, Kloner RA, Babior BM, Engler RL. Reperfusion injury induces apoptosis in rabbit cardiomyocytes. J Clin Invest. 1994; 94: 1621–8.
[26] Sun HY, Wang NP, Halkos M, Kerendi F, Kin H, Guyton RA, Vinten-Johansen J, Zhao ZQ. Postconditioning attenuates cardiomyocyte apoptosis via inhibition of JNK and p38 mitogen-activated protein kinase signaling pathways. Apoptosis. 2006; 11: 1583–93.
[27] Heltianu C, Costache G, Gafencu A, Diaconu M, Bodeanu M, Cristea C, Azibi K, Poenaru L, Simionescu M. Relationship of eNOS gene variants to diseases that have in common an endothelial cell dysfunction. J Cell Mol Med. 2005; 9: 135–42.
[28] Zhao ZQ, Corvera J, Halkos ME, Kerendi F,Wang NP, Guyton RA, Vinten-Johansen J. Inhibition of myocardial injury by ischemic postconditioning during reperfusion: comparison with ischemic preconditioning. Am J Physiol Heart Circ Physiol. 2003; 285: H579–88.
[29] Zhao ZQ, Corvera J, Halkos ME, Kerendi F,Wang NP, Guyton RA, Vinten-Johansen J. Inhibition of myocardial injury by ischemic postconditioning during reperfusion: comparison with ischemic preconditioning. Am J Physiol Heart Circ Physiol. 2003; 285: H579–88.
[30] Schwartz LM, Lagranha CJ. Ischemic postconditioning during reperfusion activates Akt and ERK without protecting against lethal myocardial ischaemia-reperfusion injury in pigs. Am J Physiol Heart Circ Physiol. 2006; 290: H1011–8.

[31] Sun HY, Wang NP, Kerendi F, Halkos M, Kin H, Guyton RA, Vinten-Johansen J, Zhao ZQ. Hypoxic postconditioning reduces cardiomyocyte loss by inhibiting ROS generation and intracellular Ca2+ overload. Am J Physiol Heart Circ Physiol. 2005; 288: H1900–8.
[32] Mykytenko J, Kerendi F, Reeves JG, Kin H, Zatta AJ, Jiang R, Guyton RA, Vinten-Johansen J, Zhao ZQ. Long-term inhibition of myocardial infarction by postconditioning during reperfusion. Basic Res Cardiol. 2007; 102: 90–100.
[33] Halkos ME, Kerendi F, Corvera JS,Wang NP, Kin H, Payne CS, Sun HY, Guyton RA,Vinten-Johansen J, Zhao ZQ. Myocardial protection with postconditioning is not enhanced by ischemic preconditioning.Ann Thorac Surg. 2004; 78: 961–9.
[34] Tsang A, Hausenloy DJ, Mocanu MM, Yellon DM. Postconditioning: a form of "modified reperfusion" protects the myocardium by activating the phosphatidylinositol 3-kinase-Akt pathway. Circ Res. 2004; 95: 230–2.
[35]Penna C, Cappello S, Mancardi D, Raimondo S, Rastaldo R, Gattullo D, Losano G, Pagliaro P. Post-conditioning reduces infarct size in the isolated rat heart: role of coronary flow and pressure and the nitric oxide/cGMP pathway. Basic Res Cardiol. 2006; 101: 168–79.
[36] Yang XM, Proctor JB, Cui L, Krieg T, Downey JM, Cohen MV. Multiple, brief coronary occlusions during early reperfusion protect rabbit hearts by targeting cell signaling pathways. J Am Coll Cardiol. 2004; 44: 1103–10.
[37] Sato H, Bolli R, Rokosh GD, Bi Q, Dai S, Shirk G, Tang XL. The cardioprotection of the late phase of ischemic preconditioning is enhanced by postconditioning via a COX-2-mediated mechanism in conscious rats. Am J Physiol Heart Circ Physiol. 2007; 293: H2557–64.
[38] Crisostomo PR,Wang M,Wairiuko GM,Terrell AM, Meldrum DR. Postconditioning in females depends on injury severity. J Surg Res. 2006; 134: 342–7.
[39] Boengler K, Buechert A, Heinen Y, Roeskes C, Hilfiker-Kleiner D, Heusch G, Schulz R. Cardioprotection by ischemic postconditioning is lost in aged and STAT3-deficient mice. Circ Res. 2008; 102: 131–5.
[40] Ohakawa HN, Okishi N, Yagi K: Assay for lipid peroxides in animal tissues by thiobarbituric acid reaction. Anal Biochem, 1979; 95: 351-8
[41] Sedlak J, Lindsay RH: Estimation of total protein-bound and non-protein sulphydryl groups in tissue with Ellman'sreagent, Anal Biochem, 1968; 25: 192-205
[42] Misra HP, Fridovich I. The role of superoxide anion in the autooxidation of epinephrine and a simple assay for superoxide dismutase. J Biol Chem 1972. 247: 3170-3175.
[43] Albelda SM, Smith CW, Ward PA. Adhesion molecules and inflammatory injury. FASEB J. 1994, 8: 504-512.
[44] Menger MD, Vollmar B. Adhesion molecules as determinations disease: from molecular biology to surgical research. BR. J. Surg. 1996, 83: 588-601.
[45] Arató E. PhD Thesis 2006 Univ of Pécs
[46] Penna C, Cappello S, Mancardi D, Raimondo S, Rastaldo R, Gattullo D, Losano G, Pagliaro P. Post-conditioning reduces infarct size in the isolated rat heart: role of coronary flow and pressure and the nitric oxide/cGMP pathway. Basic Res Cardiol. 2006; 101: 168–79.
[47] Zhao ZQ, Corvera J, Halkos ME, Kerendi F,Wang NP, Guyton RA, Vinten-Johansen J. Inhibition of myocardial injury by ischemic postconditioning during reperfusion:

comparison with ischemic preconditioning. Am J Physiol Heart Circ Physiol. 2003; 285: H579–88.
[48] Hausenloy DJ, Yellon DM. The mitochondrial permeability transition pore: its fundamental role in mediating cell death during ischaemia and reperfusion. J Mol Cell Cardiol. 2003; 35: 339–41.
[49] Y Itoh, Takaoka R, Ohira M, Abe T, Tanahashi N, Suzuki N. Reactive oxygen species generated by mitochondrial injury in human brain microvessel endothelial cells. Clin Hemorheol Microcirc. 2006;34(1-2):163-8.
[50] Kin H, Zatta AJ, Lofye MT, Amerson BS, Halkos ME, Kerendi F, Zhao ZQ, Guyton RA, Headrick JP, Vinten-Johansen J. Postconditioning reduces infarct size via adenosine receptor activation by endogenous adenosine. Cardiovasc Res. 2005; 67: 124–33.
[51] Philipp S,Yang XM, Cui L, Davis AM, Downey JM, Cohen MV. Postconditioning protects rabbit hearts through a protein kinase C-adenosine A2b receptor cascade. Cardiovasc Res. 2006; 70: 308–14.
[52] Penna C, Rastaldo R, Mancardi D, Raimondo S, Cappello S, Gattullo D, Losano G, Pagliaro P. Postconditioning induced cardioprotection requires signalling through a redox-sensitive mechanism, mitochondrial ATP-sensitive K+ channel and protein kinase C activation. Basic Res Cardiol. 2006; 101: 180–9.
[53] Hausenloy DJ, Tsang A, Yellon, DM. The reperfusion injury salvage kinase pathway: a common target for both ischemic preconditioning and postconditioning. Trends Cardiovasc Med. 2005; 15: 69–75.
[54] Philipp S,Yang XM, Cui L, Davis AM, Downey JM, Cohen MV. Postconditioning protects rabbit hearts through a protein kinase C-adenosine A2b receptor cascade. Cardiovasc Res. 2006; 70: 308–14.
[55] Penna C, Mancardi D, Rastaldo R, Losano G, Pagliaro P. Intermittent activation of bradykinin B2 receptors and mitochondrial KATP channels trigger cardiac postconditioning through redox signaling. Cardiovasc Res. 2007; 75: 168–77.
[56] Kin H, Zatta AJ, Jiang R, Reeves JG. Activation of opioid mediates the infarct size reduction by postconditioning. J Mol Cell Cardiol. 2005; 38: 827.
[57] Cohen MV, Yang XM, Downey JM. Nitric oxide is a preconditioning mimetic and cardioprotectant and is the basis of many available infarct-sparing strategies. Cardiovasc Res. 2006; 70: 231–9.
[58] Dawn B, Bolli R. Role of nitric oxide in myocardial preconditioning. Ann N Y Acad Sci. 2002; 962: 18–41.
[59] Sasaki N, Sato T, Ohler A, O'Rourke B, Marban E. Activation of mitochondrial ATP-dependent potassium channels by nitric oxide. Circulation. 2000; 101: 439–45.
[60] Moncada S, Erusalimsky JD. Does nitric oxide modulate mitochondrial energy generation and apoptosis? Nat Rev Mol Cell Biol. 2002; 3: 214–20.
[61] Gattullo D, Linden RJ, Losano G, Pagliaro P, Westerhof N. Ischaemic preconditioning changes the pattern of coronary reactive hyperaemia in the goat: role of adenosine and nitric oxide. Cardiovasc Res. 1999; 42: 57–64.
[62] Ridnour LA, Thomas DD, Mancardi D, Espey MG, Miranda KM, Paolocci N, Feelisch M, Fukuto J, Wink DA. The chemistry of nitrosative stress induced by nitric oxide and reactive nitrogen oxide species. Putting perspective on stressful biological situations. Biol Chem. 2004; 385: 1–10.

[63] Pagliaro P, Mancardi D, Rastaldo R, Penna C, Gattullo D, Miranda KM, Feelisch M, Wink DA, Kass DA, Paolocci N. Nitroxyl affords thiol-sensitive myocardial protective effects akin to early preconditioning. Free Radic Biol Med. 2003; 34: 33–43.
[64] Ma XL, Gao F, Liu GL, Lopez BL, Christopher TA, Fukuto JM, Wink DA, Feelisch M. Opposite effects of nitric oxide and nitroxyl on postischemic myocardial injury. Proc Natl Acad Sci USA. 1999; 96: 14617–22.
[65] Yang XM, Proctor JB, Cui L, Krieg T, Downey JM, Cohen MV. Multiple, brief coronary occlusions during early reperfusion protect rabbit hearts by targeting cell signaling pathways. J Am Coll Cardiol. 2004; 44: 1103–10.
[66] Penna C, Cappello S, Mancardi D, Raimondo S, Rastaldo R, Gattullo D, Losano G, Pagliaro P. Post-conditioning reduces infarct size in the isolated rat heart: role of coronary flow and pressure and the nitric oxide/cGMP pathway. Basic Res Cardiol. 2006; 101: 168–79.
[67] Penna C, Mancardi D, Rastaldo R, Losano G, Pagliaro P. Intermittent activation of bradykinin B2 receptors and mitochondrial KATP channels trigger cardiac postconditioning through redox signaling. Cardiovasc Res. 2007; 75: 168–77.
[68] Pagliaro P, Rastaldo R, Penna C, Mancardi D, Cappello S, Losano G. Nitric oxide (NO)-cyclic guanosine monophosphate (cGMP) pathway is involved in ischemic postconditioning in the isolated rat heart. Circulation. 2004; 110: III 136.
[69] Patel VC,Yellon DM, Singh KJ, Neild GH,Woolfson RG. Inhibition of nitric oxide limits infarct size in the in situ rabbit heart. Biochem Biophys Res Commun. 1993; 194: 234–8.
[70] Bolli R. Cardioprotective function of inducible nitric oxide synthase and role of nitric oxide in myocardial ischaemia and preconditioning: an overview of a decade of research. J Mol Cell Cardiol. 2001; 33: 1897–918.
[71] Wink DA, Miranda KM, Katori T, Mancardi D, Thomas DD, Ridnour L, Espey MG, Feelisch M, Colton CA, Fukuto JM, Pagliaro P, Kass DA, Paolocci N. Orthogonal properties of the redox siblings nitroxyl and nitric oxide in the cardiovascular system: a novel redox paradigm. Am J Physiol Heart Circ Physiol. 2003; 285: H2264–76.
[72] Pagliaro P. Differential biological effects of products of nitric oxide (NO) synthase: it is not enough to say NO. Life Sci. 2003; 73: 2137–49.
[73] Schulz R, Kelm M, Heusch G. Nitric oxide in myocardial ischaemia/reperfusion injury. Cardiovasc Res. 2004; 61: 402–13.
[74] Downey JM, Cohen MV. A really radical observation–a comment on Penna et al. in Basic Res Cardiol (2006) 101:180–189. Basic Res Cardiol. 2006; 101: 190–1.
[75] Cohen MV,Yang XM, Downey JM. The pH hypothesis of postconditioning: staccato reperfusion reintroduces oxygen and perpetuates myocardial acidosis. Circulation. 2007; 115: 1895–903.
[76] Hausenloy DJ, Wynne AM, Yellon DM. Ischemic preconditioning targets the reperfusion phase. Basic Res Cardiol. 2007; 102: 445–52.
[77] Tsang A, Hausenloy DJ, Mocanu MM, Yellon DM. Postconditioning: a form of "modified reperfusion" protects the myocardium by activating the phosphatidylinositol 3-kinase-Akt pathway. Circ Res. 2004; 95: 230–2.
[78] Pagliaro P, Rastaldo R, Penna C, Mancardi D, Cappello S, Losano G. Nitric oxide (NO)-cyclic guanosine monophosphate (cGMP) pathway is involved in ischemic postconditioning in the isolated rat heart. Circulation. 2004; 110: III 136.

[79] Penna C, Rastaldo R, Mancardi D, Raimondo S, Cappello S, Gattullo D, Losano G, Pagliaro P. Postconditioning induced cardioprotection requires signalling through a redox-sensitive mechanism, mitochondrial ATP-sensitive K+ channel and protein kinase C activation. Basic Res Cardiol. 2006; 101: 180–9.

[80]Yang XM, Philipp S, Downey JM, Cohen MV. Postconditioning's protection is not dependent on circulating blood factors or cells but involves adenosine receptors and requires PI3-kinase and guanylyl cyclase activation. Basic Res Cardiol. 2005; 100: 57–63.

[81] Penna C, Rastaldo R, Mancardi D, Raimondo S, Cappello S, Gattullo D, Losano G, Pagliaro P. Postconditioning induced cardioprotection requires signalling through a redox-sensitive mechanism, mitochondrial ATP-sensitive K+ channel and protein kinase C activation. Basic Res Cardiol. 2006; 101: 180–9.

[82] Hausenloy DJ, Tsang A, Yellon, DM. The reperfusion injury salvage kinase pathway: a common target for both ischemic preconditioning and postconditioning. Trends Cardiovasc Med. 2005; 15: 69–75.

[83] Darling CE, Jiang R, Maynard M, Whittaker P, Vinten-Johansen J, Przyklenk K. 'Postconditioning' via stuttering reperfusion limits myocardial infarct size in rabbit hearts: role of ERK 1/2. Am J Physiol Heart Circ Physiol. 2005; 289: H1618–26.

[84] Yang XM, Philipp S, Downey JM, Cohen MV. Postconditioning's protection is not dependent on circulating blood factors or cells but involves adenosine receptors and requires PI3-kinase and guanylyl cyclase activation. Basic Res Cardiol. 2005; 100: 57–63.

[85] Yang XM, Philipp S, Downey JM, Cohen MV. Postconditioning's protection is not dependent on circulating blood factors or cells but involves adenosine receptors and requires PI3-kinase and guanylyl cyclase activation. Basic Res Cardiol. 2005; 100: 57–63.

[86] Yang XM, Philipp S, Downey JM, Cohen MV. Postconditioning's protection is not dependent on circulating blood factors or cells but involves adenosine receptors and requires PI3-kinase and guanylyl cyclase activation. Basic Res Cardiol. 2005; 100: 57–63.

[87] Cao Z, Liu L, Van Winkle DM. Met5-enkephalininduced cardioprotection occurs via transactivation of EGFR and activation of PI3K. Am J Physiol Heart Circ Physiol. 2005; 288: 1955–64.

[88] Vinten-Johansen J, Zhao ZQ, Zatta AJ, Kin H, Halkos ME, Kerendi F. Postconditioning A new link in nature's armor against myocardial ischaemiareperfusion injury. Basic Res Cardiol. 2005; 100: 295–310.

[89] Darling CE, Jiang R, Maynard M, Whittaker P, Vinten-Johansen J, Przyklenk K. 'Postconditioning' via stuttering reperfusion limits myocardial infarct size in rabbit hearts: role of ERK 1/2. Am J Physiol Heart Circ Physiol. 2005; 289: H1618–26.

[90] Zhao ZQ, Vinten-Johansen J. Postconditioning: reduction of reperfusion-induced injury. Cardiovasc Res. 2006; 70: 200–11.

[91] Kostin S. Zonula occludens-1 and connexin 43 expression in the failing human heart. J Cell Mol Med. 2007; 11: 892–5.

[92] Heusch G, Büchert A, Feldhaus S, Schulz R. No loss of cardioprotection by postconditioning in connexin 43-deficient mice. Basic Res Cardiol. 2006; 101: 354–6.

[93] Weiss JN, Korge P, Honda HM, Ping P. Role of the mitochondrial permeability transition in myocardial disease. Circ Res. 2003; 93: 292–301.

[94] Murata M, Akao M, O'Rourke B, Marban E. Mitochondrial ATP-sensitive potassium channels attenuate matrix Ca(2+) overload during simulated ischaemia and reperfusion: possible mechanism of cardioprotection. Circ Res. 2001; 89: 891–8.
[95] Sun HY, Wang NP, Kerendi F, Halkos M, Kin H, Guyton RA, Vinten-Johansen J, Zhao ZQ. Hypoxic postconditioning reduces cardiomyocyte loss by inhibiting ROS generation and intracellular Ca2+ overload. Am J Physiol Heart Circ Physiol. 2005; 288: H1900–8.
[96] Argaud L, Gateau-Roesch O, Raisky O, Loufouat J, Robert D, Ovize M. Postconditioning inhibits mitochondrial permeability transition. Circulation. 2005; 111: 194–7.
[97] Bopassa JC, Ferrera R, Gateau-Roesch O, Couture-Lepetit E, Ovize M. PI 3-kinase regulates the mitochondrial transition pore in controlled reperfusion and postconditioning. Cardiovas Res. 2006; 69: 178–85.
[98] Gateau-Roesch O, Argaud L, Ovize M. Mitochondrial permeability transition pore and postconditioning. Cardiovasc Res. 2006; 70: 264–73.
[99] Tritto I, Ambrosio G. Role of oxidants in the signaling pathway of preconditioning. Antioxid Redox Signal. 2001; 3: 3–10.
[100] Zhao ZQ. Oxidative stress-elicited myocardial apoptosis during reperfusion. Curr Opin Pharmacol. 2004; 4: 159–65.
[101] Pagliaro P. Differential biological effects of products NO. Life Sci. 2003; 73: 2137–49.
[102] Zhao ZQ. Oxidative stress-elicited myocardial apoptosis during reperfusion. Curr Opin Pharmacol. 2004; 4: 159–65.
[103] Yao Z, Tong J, Tan X, Li C, Shao Z, Kim WC, vanden Hoek TL, Becker LB, Head CA, Schumacker PT. Role of reactive oxygen species in acetylcholineinduced preconditioning in cardiomyocytes. Am J Physiol Heart Circ Physiol. 1999; 277: H2504–9.
[104] Urschel WC. Cardiovascular effects of hydrogen peroxide: current status. Dis Chest. 1967; 51: 180–92.
[105] Tsutsumi YM, Yokoyama T, Horikawa Y, Roth DM, Patel HH. Reactive oxygen species trigger ischemic and pharmacological postconditioning: In vivo and in vitro characterization. Life Sci. 2007; 81: 1223–7.
[106] Hausenloy DJ, Wynne AM, Yellon DM. Ischemic preconditioning targets the reperfusion phase. Basic Res Cardiol. 2007; 102: 445–52.
[107] Flaherty JT, Pitt B, Gruber JW, Heuser RR, Rothbaum DA, Burwell LR, George BS, Kereiakes DJ, Deitchman D, Gustafson N. Recombinant human superoxide dismutase (h-SOD) fails to improve recovery of ventricular function in patients undergoing coronary angioplasty for acute myocardial infarction. Circulation. 1999; 89: 1982–91.
[108] Kloner RA, Jennings RB. Consequences of brief ischaemia: stunning, preconditioning and their clinical implications. Circulation. 2001; 104: 2981–9.
[109] Penna C, Mancardi D, Rastaldo R, Losano G, Pagliaro P. Intermittent activation of bradykinin B2 receptors and mitochondrial KATP channels trigger cardiac postconditioning through redox signaling. Cardiovasc Res. 2007; 75: 168–77.
[110] Hausenloy DJ, Wynne AM, Yellon DM. Ischemic preconditioning targets the reperfusion phase. Basic Res Cardiol. 2007; 102: 445–52.